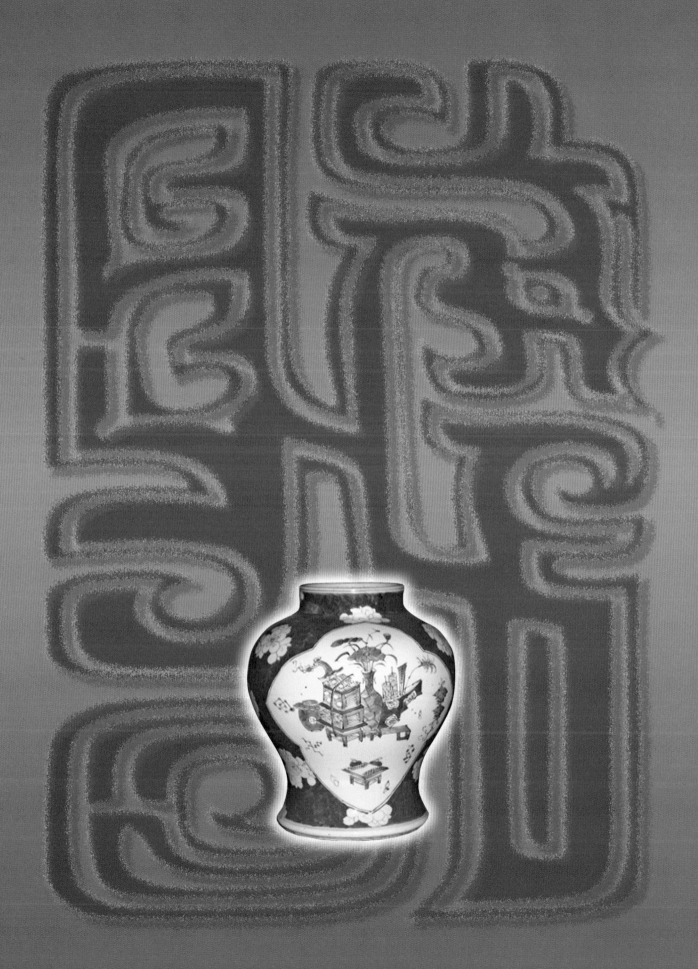

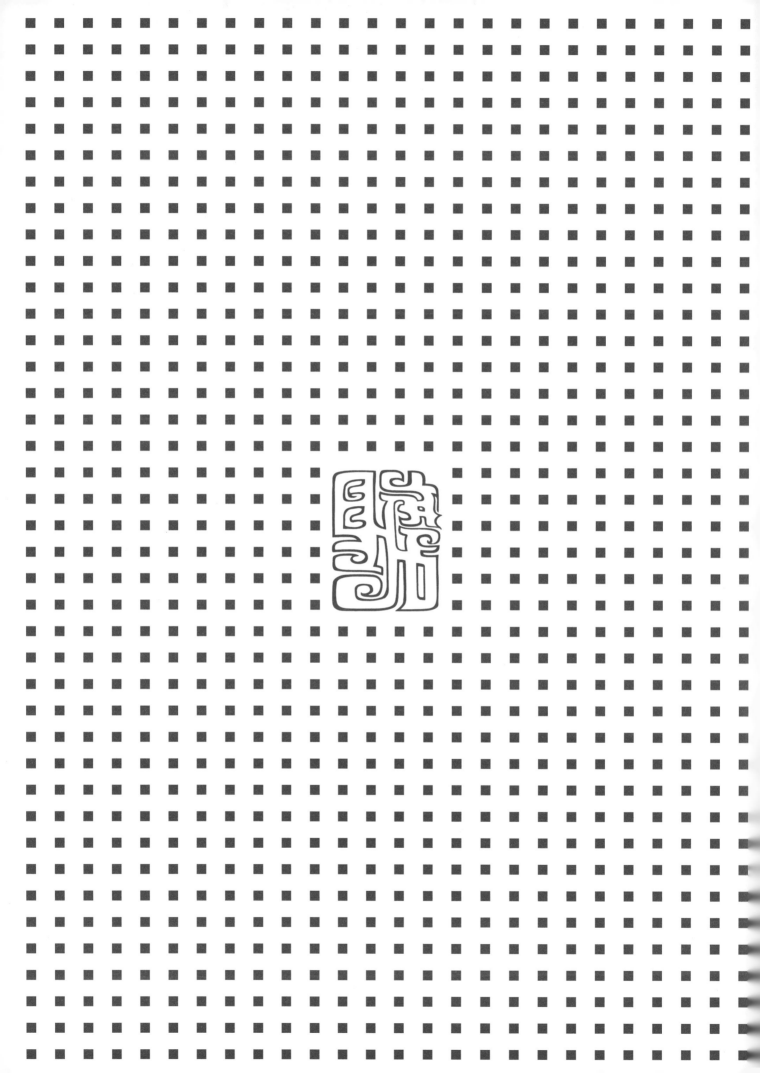

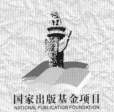

国家出版基金项目
NATIONAL PUBLICATION FOUNDATION

中华医药卫生

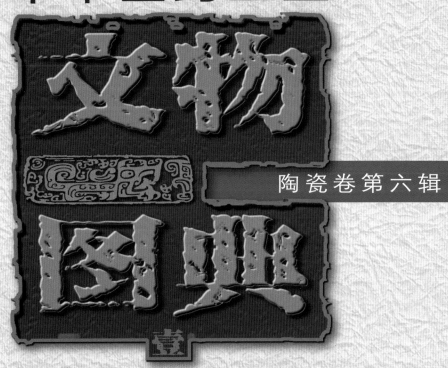

陶瓷卷第六辑

主　编　李经纬　梁　峻　刘学春
总主译　白永权
主　译　陈向京

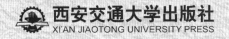

西安交通大学出版社
XI'AN JIAOTONG UNIVERSITY PRESS

图书在版编目 (CIP) 数据

中华医药卫生文物图典 . 1. 陶瓷卷 . 第 6 辑 . / 李经纬,

梁峻，刘学春主编 .— 西安：西安交通大学出版社，2016.12

ISBN 978-7-5605-7033-4

Ⅰ . ①中… Ⅱ . ①李… ②梁… ③刘… Ⅲ . ①中国医药学—

古代陶瓷—中国—图录 Ⅳ . ① R-092 ② K870.2

中国版本图书馆 CIP 数据核字（2015）第 013596 号

书　　名　中华医药卫生文物图典（一）陶瓷卷第六辑

主　　编　李经纬　梁　峻　刘学春

责任编辑　秦金霞

出版发行　西安交通大学出版社

　　　　　（西安市兴庆南路 10 号　邮政编码 710049）

网　　址　http://www.xjtupress.com

电　　话　（029）82668805 82668502（医学分社）

　　　　　（029）82668315（总编办）

传　　真　（029）82668280

印　　刷　中煤地西安地图制印有限公司

开　　本　889mm×1194mm　1/16　印张 40.75　字数 663 千字

版次印次　2017 年 12 月第 1 版　2017 年 12 月第 1 次印刷

书　　号　ISBN 978-7-5605-7033-4

定　　价　1200.00 元

读者购书、书店添货、如发现印装质量问题，请通过以下方式联系、调换。

订购热线：（029）82665248　（029）82665249

投稿热线：（029）82668805　（029）82668502

读者信箱：medpress@126.com

铭记感受历史

自信自重自强

书贺

中华医药卫生文物图典问世

陈可冀 谨题
二〇一七年六月

陈可冀　中国科学院院士、国医大师

精修醫藥衛生文物

圖典功著當代

深究岐黃學術思想

淵源惠澤千秋

中華醫藥衛生文物圖典出版誌慶

丁酉孟秋 孫光榮 敬題於北京

孫光荣　国医大师

中華醫藥衛生文物圖典出版

彰顯中醫藥
文化精神

體現中醫藥
歷史價值

歲次丁酉夏　王琦

王琦　国医大师

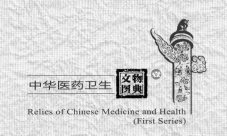

中华医药卫生
Relics of Chinese Medicine and Health
(First Series)

中华医药卫生文物图典（一）
丛书编撰委员会

主　编　李经纬　梁　峻　刘学春

副主编　廖　果　吴鸿洲　康兴军　和中浚　刘小斌　杨金生

　　　　郑怀林　徐江雁　白建疆　黄　煌

编　委　李洪晓　梁永宣　王强虎　董树平　马　健　王　霞

　　　　张雅宗　朱德明　包哈申　张建青　郑　蓉　庄乾竹

　　　　李宏红　刘哲峰　王宏才　陈润东

总主译　白永权

主　译　陈向京　聂文信　范晓晖　温　睿　赵永生　杜彦龙

　　　　吉　乐　李小棉　郭　梦　陈　曦

副主译（按姓氏音序排列）

　　　　董艳云　姜雨孜　李建西　刘　慧　马　健　任宝磊

　　　　任　萌　任　莹　王　颇　习通源　谢皖吉　徐素云

　　　　许崇钰　许　梅　詹菊红　赵　菲　邹郝晶

译　者（按姓氏音序排列）

迟征宇　邓　甜　付一豪　高　琛　高　媛　郭　宁

韩　蕾　何宗昌　胡勇强　黄　鋆　蒋新蕾　康晓薇

李静波　刘雅恬　刘妍萌　鲁显生　马　月　牛笑语

唐云鹏　唐臻娜　田　多　铁红玲　佟健一　王　晨

王　丹　王　栋　王　丽　王　媛　王慧敏　王梦杰

王仙先　吴耀均　席　慧　肖国强　许子洋　闫红贤

杨姣姣　姚　晔　张　阳　张　鋆　张继飞　张梦原

张晓谦　赵　欣　赵亚力　郑　青　郑艳华　朱江嵩

朱瑛培

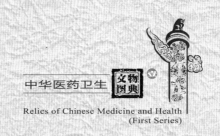

中华医药卫生 文物图典

Relics of Chinese Medicine and Health
(First Series)

本册编撰委员会

主　编　李经纬　梁　峻　刘学春

副主编　廖　果　吴鸿洲　康兴军　和中浚　刘小斌　杨金生
　　　　郑怀林　徐江雁　白建疆　黄　煌

编　委　李洪晓　梁永宣　王强虎　董树平　马　健　王　霞
　　　　张雅宗　朱德明　包哈申　张建青　郑　蓉　庄乾竹
　　　　李宏红　刘哲峰　王宏才　陈润东

总主译　白永权

主　译　陈向京

副主译　董艳云

译　者　邹郝晶　许　梅　王　丽　王　晨　高　媛　郑艳华
　　　　王梦杰　张晓谦　刘妍萌　许子洋

丛书策划委员会

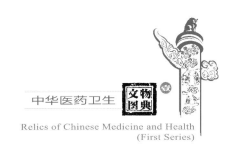

中华医药卫生 文物图典

Relics of Chinese Medicine and Health
(First Series)

序 言

　　探索天、地、人运动变化规律以及"气化物生"过程的相互关系，是人类永恒的课题。宇宙不可逆，地球不可逆，人生不可逆业已成为共识。天地造化形成自然，人类活动构成文化。文物既是文化的载体，又是物化的历史，还是文明的见证。

　　追求健康长寿是人类共同的夙愿。中华民族之所以繁衍昌盛，健康文化起了巨大的推动作用。由于古人谋求生存发展、应对环境变化产生的智慧，大多反映在以医药卫生为核心的健康文化之中，所以，习总书记说："中医药学是中国古代科学的瑰宝，也是打开中华文明宝库的钥匙"。

　　秉持文化大发展、大繁荣理念，中国中医科学院李经纬、梁峻等为负责人的科研团队在完成科技部"国家重点医药卫生文物收集调研和保护"课题获2005年度中华中医药学会科技二等奖基础上，又资鉴"夏商周断代工程""中华文明探源工程"等相关考古成果，用有重要价值的新出土文物置换原拍摄质量较差的文物，适当补充民族医药文物，共精选收载5000余件。经西安交通大学出版社申报，《中华医药卫生文物图典（一）》（以下简称《图典》）于2013年获得了国家出版基金的资助，并经专业翻译团队翻译，使《图典》得以面世。

　　文物承载的信息多元丰富，发掘解读其中蕴藏的智慧并非易事。医药卫生文物更具有特殊性，除文物的一般属性外，还承载着传统医学发展史迹与促进健康的信息。运用历史唯物主义观察发掘文物信息，善于从生活文物中领悟卫生信息，才能准确解读其功能，也才能诠释其在民生健康中的历史作用，收到以古鉴今之效果。"历史是现实的根源"，任何一个民族都不能割断历史，史料都包含在文化中。"文化是民族的血脉，是人民的精神家园"，文化繁荣才能实现中华民族的伟大复兴。值本《图典》付梓之际，用"梳理文化之脉，必获健康之果"作为序言并和作者、读者共勉！

中央文史研究馆馆员
中国工程院院士　王永炎
丁酉年仲夏

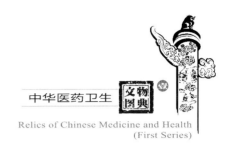

中华医药卫生 文物图典

Relics of Chinese Medicine and Health
(First Series)

前 言

　　文化是相对自然的概念，是考古界常用词汇。文物是文化的重要组成部分，既是文明的物证，又是物化的历史。狭义医药卫生文物是疾病防治模式语境下的解读，而广义医药卫生文物则是躯体、心态、环境适应三维健康模式下的诠释。中华民族是 56 个民族组成的多元一体大家庭，中华医药卫生文物当然包括各民族的健康文化遗存。

　　天地造化如造山、板块漂移、气候变迁、生物起源进化等形成自然。气化物生莫贵于人，即整个生物进化的最高成果是人类自身。广义而言，人类生存思维留下的痕迹即物质财富和精神财富总和构成文化，其一般的物化形式是视觉感知的文物、文献、胜迹等。其中质变标志明晰的文化如文字、文物、城市、礼仪等可称作文明。从唯物史观视角观察，狭义文化即精神财富，尤其体现人类精、气、神状态的事项，其本质也具有特殊物质属性，如量子也具有波粒二相性，这种粒子也是物质，无非运动方式特殊而已。现代所谓可重复验证的"科学"，事实上也是从文化中分离出来的事项，因此也是一种特殊文化形式。追求健康长寿是人类共同的夙愿。中华民族之所以繁衍昌盛，是因为健康文化异彩纷呈。中华优秀传统医药文化之所以博大精深，是因为其原创思维博大、格物致知精深，所以，习总书记说："中医药学是中国古代科学的瑰宝，也是打开中华文明宝库的钥匙"。

文化既反映时代、地域、民族分布、生产资料来源、技术水平等信息，又反映人类认知水平和生存智慧。发掘解读文物、文献中蕴藏的健康知识和灵动智慧，首先是从事健康工作者的责任和义务。《易经》设有"观"卦，人类作为观察者，不仅要积极收藏展陈文物，而且要善于捕捉文物倾诉的信息，汲取养分，启迪思维，收到古为今用之效果。墨子三表法，首先一表即"本之于古者圣王之事"，也是强调古代史实的重要性。"历史是现实的根源"，现实是未来的基础。任何一个国家、地区、民族都不能割断历史、忽略基础，这个基础就是文化。"文化是民族的血脉，是人民的精神家园"。文化繁荣才能驱动各项事业发展，才能实现中华民族的伟大复兴。

人类从类人猿分化出来。"禄丰古猿禄丰种"是云南禄丰发现的类人猿化石，距今七八百万年。距今 200 万年前人类进入旧石器时代，直立行走，打制石器产生工具意识，管理火种，是所谓"燧人氏"时代。中国留存有更新世早、中期的元谋、蓝田、北京人等遗址。距今 10 万—5 万年前，人类进入旧石器时代中期，即早期智人阶段，脑容量增加，和欧洲、非洲人种相比，原始蒙古人种颧骨前突等，是所谓"伏羲氏"时代。中国发现的马坝、长阳、丁村人等较典型。距今 5 万—1 万年前，人类进入旧石器时代晚期，即晚期智人阶段，细石器、骨角器等遍布全国，山顶洞、柳江、资阳人等较典型。

中石器时代距今约 1 万年，是旧石器时代向新石器时代的短暂过渡期，弓箭发明，狗被驯化。河南灵井、陕西沙苑遗址等作为代表。距今 1 万—公元前 2600 年前后，人类进入新石器时代，磨光石器、烧制陶器，出现农业村落并饲养家畜，是所谓"神农氏"时代。公元前 7000 年以来，在甲、骨、陶、石等载体上出现契刻符号、七音阶骨笛乐器等，反映出人文气息趋浓。公元前 6000—公元前 3500 年的老官台、裴李岗、河姆渡、马家浜、仰韶等文化遗址，彰显出先民围绕生存健康问题所做的各种努力。

公元前 4800 年以来，以关中、晋南、豫西为中心形成的仰韶文化，是中原史前文化的重要标志。以半坡、庙底沟类型为典型，自公元前 3500 年走向繁荣，属于锄耕粟黍稻兼营渔猎饲养猪鸡经济方式，彩陶尤其发达。公元前 4400—公元前 3300 年，长江中游的大溪文化，薄胎彩陶和白陶发达。公元前 4300—公元前 2500 年山东丰岛的大汶口文化，红陶为主。公元前 3500 年前后，辽东的红山文化原始宗教发展。公元前 3300 年以来，长江下游由河姆渡、马家浜文化衍续的良渚文化和陇西的马家窑文化、江淮间的薛家岗文化时趋发达。

公元前 2600—公元前 2000 年，黄河中下游龙山文化群形成，冶铸铜器，制作玉器，土坯、石灰、夯筑技术开始应用。公元前 2697 年，轩辕战败炎帝（有说其后裔）、蚩尤而为黄帝纪元元年。黄帝西巡访贤，"至岐见岐伯，引载而归，访于治道"。其引归地"溱洧襟带于前，梅泰环拱于后"，即今河南新密市古城寨。岐黄答问，构建《黄帝内经》健康知识体系，中华文明从关注民生健康起步。颛顼改革宗教，神职人员出现；帝喾修身节用，帝尧和合百国，舜同律度量衡，大禹疏导治水，中华民族不断繁衍昌盛。

公元前 2070 年，禹之子启以豫西晋南为中心建立夏王朝，二里头青铜文化为其特征，半地穴、窑洞、地面建筑并存。饮食卫生器具、酒器增多。朱砂安神作用在宫殿应用。公元前 1600 年，商灭夏。偃师商城设有铸铜作坊。公元前 1300 年，盘庚迁殷，使用甲骨文。武丁时期青铜浑铸、分铸并存。公元前 1056 年，相传周"文王被殷纣拘于羑里，演《周易》，成六十四卦"。公元前 1046 年，武王克商建周，定都镐京。青铜器始铸长篇铭文，周原发掘出微型甲骨文字。公元前 770 年，平王东迁。虢国铸铜柄铁剑。公元前 753 年，秦国设置史官。公元前 707 年出现蝗灾、公元前 613 年出现"哈雷彗星"，均被孔子载入《春秋》。公元前 221 年，秦始皇统一中国，多元一体民族大家庭形成，中华医药卫生文物异彩纷呈。

中国是治史大国，历来重视发展文化博物事业，1955 年成立卫生部中医研究院时就设置医史研究室，1982 年中国医史文献研究所成立时复建中国医史博物馆研究收藏展陈文物。2000—2003 年，经王永炎院士、姚乃礼院长等呼吁，科技部批准立项，由李经纬、梁峻为负责人的团队完成"国家重点医药卫生文物收集调研和保护"项目任务，受到科技部项目验收组专家的高度评价，获中华中医药学会科技进步二等奖。2013 年，在国家出版基金资助下，课题组对部分文物重新拍摄或必要置换、充实民族医药文物后，由西安交通大学出版社编辑、组聘国内一流翻译团队英译说明文字付梓，受到国家中医药博物馆筹备工作领导小组和办公室的高度重视。

"物以类聚"，《图典》主要依据文物质地、种类分为 9 卷，计有陶瓷，金属，纸质，竹木，玉石、织品及标本，壁画石刻及遗址，少数民族文物，其他，备考等卷。同卷下主要根据历史年代或小类分册设章。每卷下的历史时段不求统一。遵循上述规则将《图典》划分为 21 册，总计收载文物 5000 余件。对每件文物的描述，除质地、规格、馆藏等基本要素外，重点描述其在民生健康中的作用。对少数暂不明确的事项在括号中注明待考。对引自各博物馆的材料除在文物后列出馆藏外，还在书后再次统一列出馆名或参考书目，以充分尊重其馆藏权，也同时维护本典作者的引用权。

21 世纪，围绕人类健康的生命科学将飞速发展，但科学离不开文化，文化离不开文物。发掘文物承载的信息为现实服务，谨引用横渠先生四言之两语："为天地立心，为生民立命"，既作为编撰本《图典》之宗旨，也是我们践行国家"一带一路"倡议的具体努力。希冀通过本《图典》的出版发行，教育国人，提振中华民族精神；走向世界，为人类健康事业贡献力量。

李经纬　梁峻　刘学春

2017 年 6 月于北京

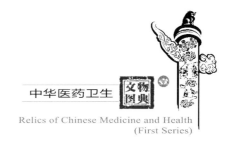

中华医药卫生 文物图典 ◎

Relics of Chinese Medicine and Health
(First Series)

目 录

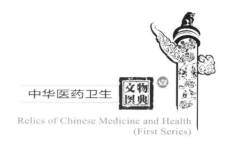

中华医药卫生 文物图典

Relics of Chinese Medicine and Health
(First Series)

Contents

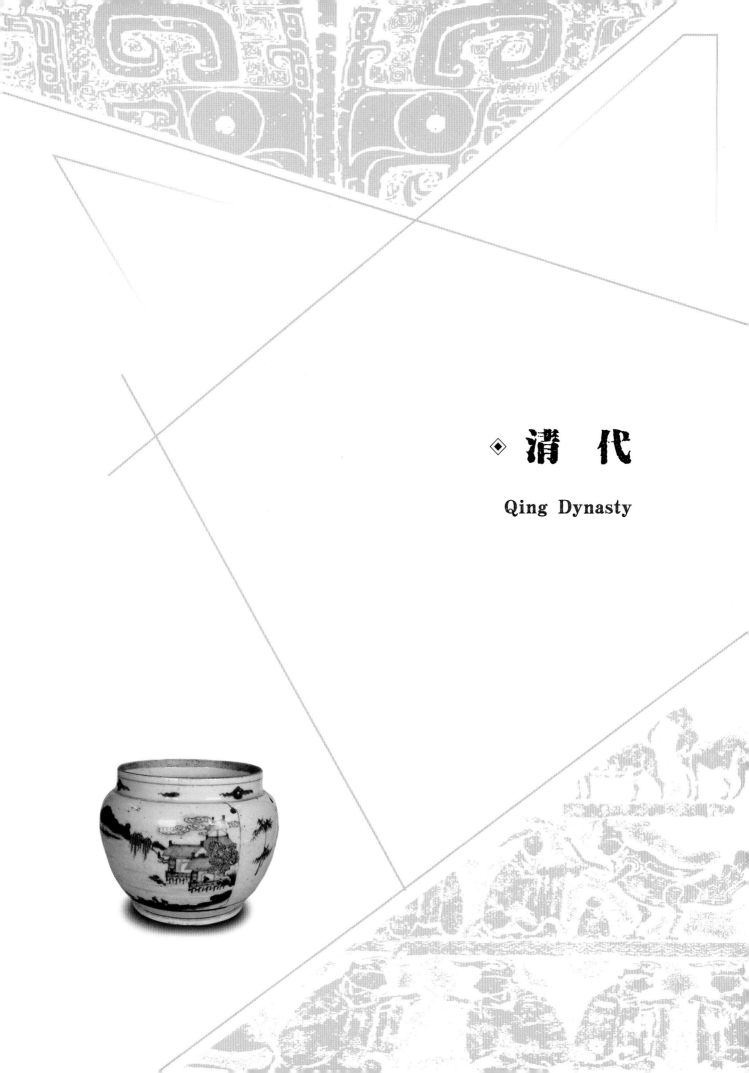

◆ 清 代

Qing Dynasty

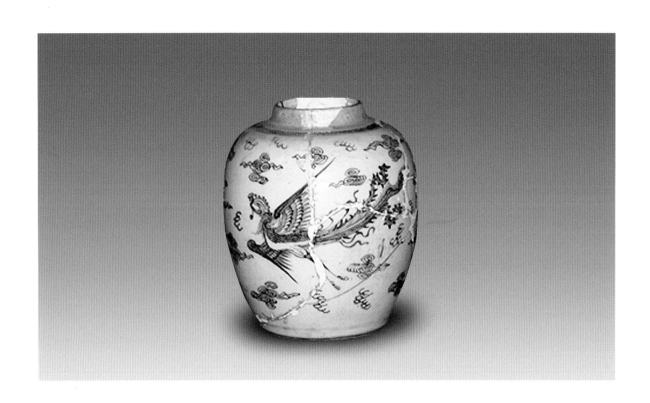

青花药罐

清

瓷质

口径 7.5 厘米，底径 11 厘米，通高 19 厘米，
重 1250 克

子母口，圆腹，圈足，图案为龙凤云火纹饰。贮
药器具。腹有修补。

陕西医史博物馆藏

Blue-and-white Medicine Jar

Qing Dynasty

Porcelain

Mouth Diameter 7.5 cm/ Bottom Diameter 11 cm/ Height
19 cm/ Weight 1,250 g

This jar has a snap lid, a rounded belly and a ring foot.
The jar is decorated with the design of a dragon and a
phoenix striding amidst flaming clouds. It was used as a
medicine storage container with the belly repaired.

Preserved in Shaanxi Museum of Medical History

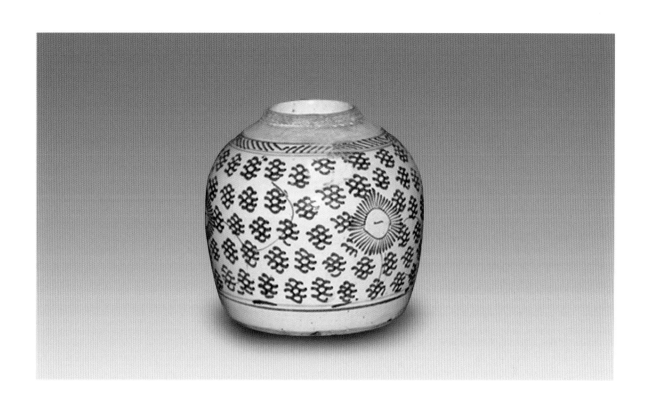

青花药罐

清

瓷质

口径 7 厘米，底径 13 厘米，通高 15.5 厘米，
重 1200 克

子母口，圆腹，圈足，图案为三菊变形图案。贮
药器具。完整无损。江苏省扬州市征集。

陕西医史博物馆藏

Blue-and-white Medicine Jar

Qing Dynasty

Porcelain

Mouth Diameter 7 cm/ Bottom Diameter 13 cm/ Height
15.5 cm/ Weight 1,200 g

This jar, featuring a snap lid, a rounded belly and a
ring foot, is adorned with chrysanthemum designs and
transmuted patterns. It was used as a medicine container
and remains intact. The object was collected from
Yangzhou City in Jiangsu Province.

Preserved in Shaanxi Museum of Medical History

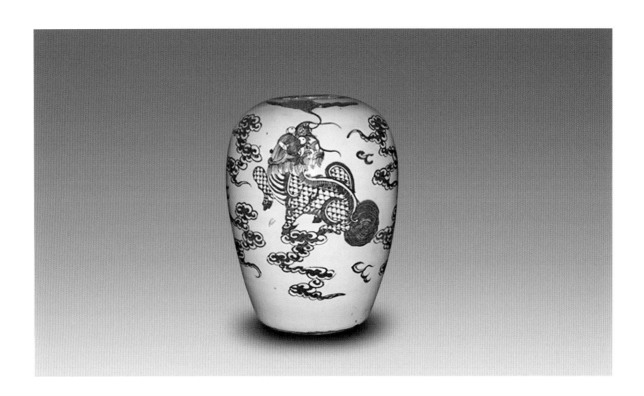

青花药罐

清

瓷质

口径 10 厘米，底径 14.5 厘米，通高 29 厘米，重 2500 克

Blue-and-white Medicine Jar

Qing Dynasty

Porcelain

Mouth Diameter 10 cm/ Bottom Diameter 14.5 cm/ Height 29 cm/ Weight 2,500 g

子母口，直腹，圈足，豆绿底，图案为狮子云火。贮药器具。完整无损。陕西省西安市藻露堂中药店征集。

陕西医史博物馆藏

Designed with a snap lid, a straight belly, a ring foot and a bottom in the colour of pea-green, this jar is decorated with the design of a lion striding amidst flaming clouds. The vessel was used as a medicine container and remains intact. It was collected from Zao Lu Tang Chinese Medicinal Herbs Store of Xi'an in Shaanxi Province.

Preserved in Shaanxi Museum of Medical History

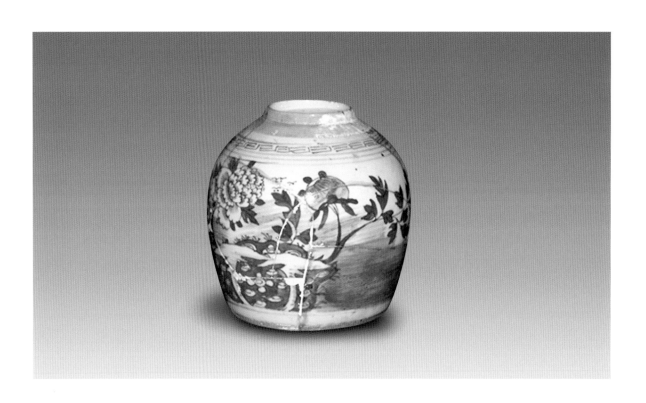

青花药罐

清

瓷质

口径 7.5 厘米，底径 13 厘米，通高 17.5 厘米，
重 1150 克

子母口，圆腹，圈足，图案为牡丹花，肩有云纹。
贮药器物。腹部有修补。江苏省扬州市征集。

陕西医史博物馆藏

Blue-and-white Medicine Jar

Qing Dynasty

Porcelain

Mouth Diameter 7.5 cm/ Bottom Diameter 13 cm/ Height
17.5 cm/ Weight 1,150 g

Adorned with peony designs, this jar has a snap lid, a
rounded belly, a ring foot and a shoulder with cloud
designs. The vessel was used as a medicine container
with the belly repaired. It was collected from Yangzhou
City in Jiangsu Province.

Preserved in Shaanxi Museum of Medical History

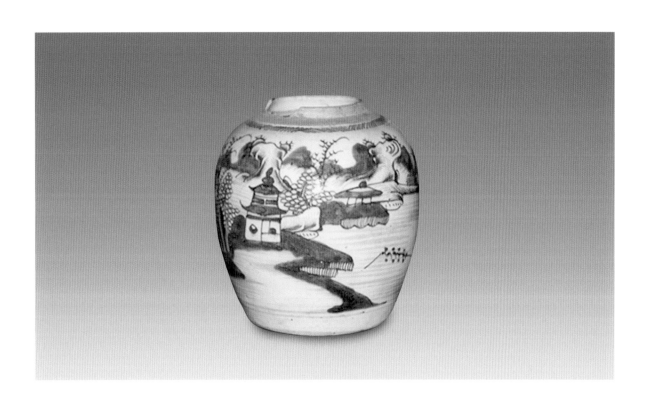

青花药罐

清

瓷质

口径 8 厘米，底径 13 厘米，通高 18 厘米，重 1200 克

子母口，圆腹，圈足，图案为山水垂钓。贮药器物。腹有修补，口沿残少许。江苏省扬州市征集。

陕西医史博物馆藏

Blue-and-white Medicine Jar

Qing Dynasty

Porcelain

Mouth Diameter 8 cm/ Bottom Diameter 13 cm/ Height 18 cm/ Weight 1,200 g

This jar has a snap lid, a rounded belly, and a ring foot. The body is adorned with designs of fishing by the river and mountain. It was used as a medicine container with the belly repatched and the mouth rim slightly damaged. The object was collected from Yangzhou City in Jiangsu Province.

Preserved in Shaanxi Museum of Medical History

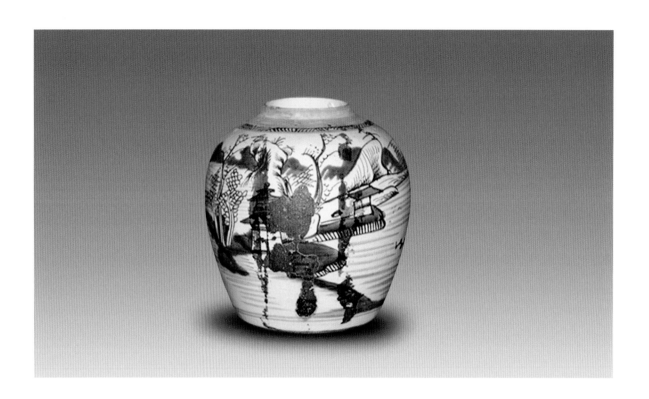

青花药罐

清

瓷质

口径 8 厘米，底径 12.5 厘米，通高 19 厘米，重 1100 克

Blue-and-white Medicine Jar

Qing Dynasty

Porcelain

Mouth Diameter 8 cm/ Bottom Diameter 12.5 cm/ Height 19 cm/ Weight 1,100 g

子母口，圆腹，圈足，图案为山水垂钓。贮
药器物。完整无损。陕西省西安市藻露堂中
药店征集。

陕西医史博物馆藏

This jar has a snap lid, a rounded belly, and a ring
foot. The body is adorned with designs of fishing by
the river and mountain. It was used as a medicine
container and remains intact. The object was
collected from Zao Lu Tang Chinese Medicinal
Herbs Store of Xi'an in Shaanxi Province.
Preserved in Shaanxi Museum of Medical History

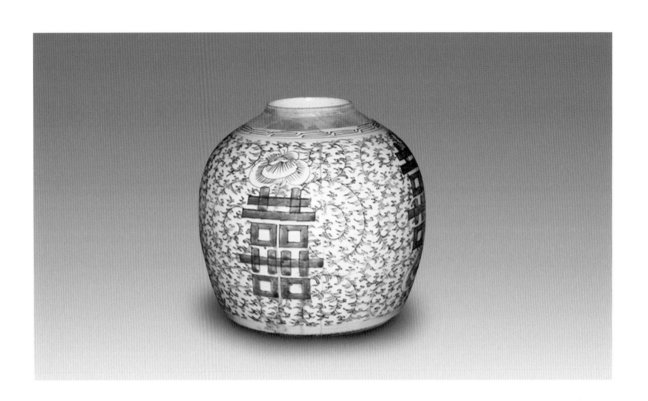

青花药罐

清

瓷质

口径 9.5 厘米，底径 20 厘米，通高 23 厘米，重 2550 克

Blue-and-white Medicine Jar

Qing Dynasty

Porcelain

Mouth Diameter 9.5 cm/ Bottom Diameter 20 cm/ Height 23 cm/ Weight 2,550 g

子母口，圆腹，圈足，表面饰四"喜"缠枝纹，

标签为"麦味丸"。盛贮器物。完整无损。

陕西省西安市藻露堂中药店征集。

陕西医史博物馆藏

This jar has a snap lid, a rounded belly, and a ring foot. The jar bears designs of four copies of the Chinese character "Xi" (happiness) and interlocking branches with a label of the name of the drug "Mai Wei Wan". It was used as a medicine container and remains intact. The object was collected from Zao Lu Tang Chinese Medicinal Herbs Store of Xi'an in Shaanxi Province.

Preserved in Shaanxi Museum of Medical History

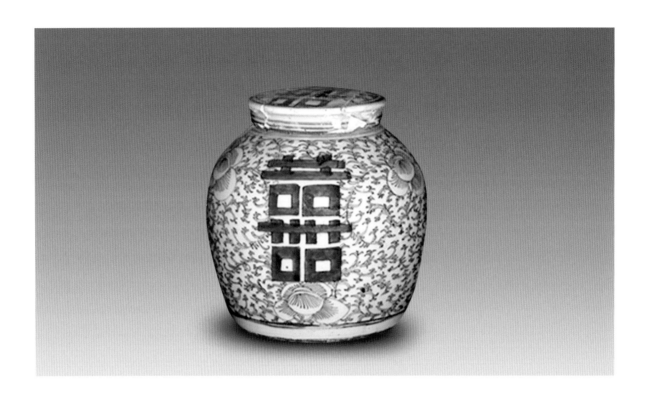

青花药罐

清

瓷质

口径 9.5 厘米，底径 16 厘米，通高 21 厘米，重 1800 克

Blue-and-white Medicine Jar

Qing Dynasty

Porcelain

Mouth Diameter 9.5 cm/ Bottom Diameter 16 cm/ Height 21 cm/ Weight 1,800 g

子母口，圆腹，圈足，带盖，表面饰三"喜"
缠枝兰花图。贮药器物。盖有修补。陕西省
西安市藻露堂中药店征集。

陕西医史博物馆藏

This jar has a snap lid, a rounded belly and a ring foot. The
body bears the designs of three copies of the Chinese
character "Xi" (happiness) and interlocking orchid
branches. It was used as a medicine container with
a repaired lid. The object was collected from Zao
Lu Tang Chinese Medicinal Herbs Store of Xi'an in
Shaanxi Province.

Preserved in Shaanxi Museum of Medical History

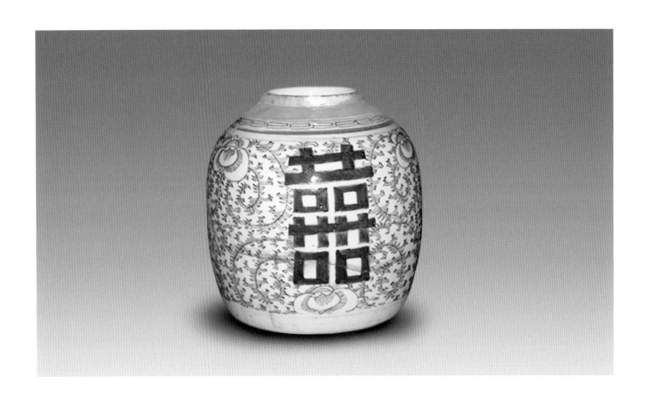

青花药罐

清

瓷质

口径 9.8 厘米，底径 17.5 厘米，通高 22 厘米，重 2100 克

子母口，溜肩，直腹，圈足，表面饰三"喜"缠枝纹。贮药器具。完整无损。江苏省扬州同松药店征集。

陕西医史博物馆藏

Blue-and-white Medicine Jar

Qing Dynasty

Porcelain

Mouth Diameter 9.8 cm/ Bottom Diameter 17.5 cm/ Height 22 cm/ Weight 2,100 g

This jar has a snap lid, a sloping shoulder, a straight belly, and a ring foot. The body bears the designs of three copies of the Chinese character "Xi" (happiness) and interlocking branches. It was used as a medicine container and remains intact. The jar was collected from Tongsong Drugstore of Yangzhou in Jiangsu Province. Preserved in Shaanxi Museum of Medical History

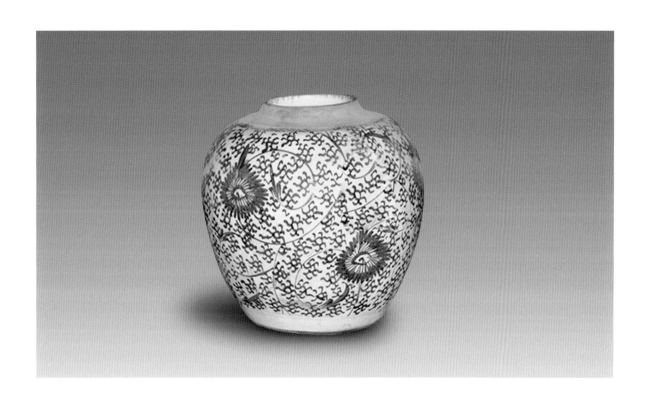

青花药罐

清

瓷质

口径 9 厘米，底径 14.2 厘米，通高 21 厘米，
重 2150 克

子母口，圆腹，圈足，表面饰缠枝菊花纹。贮药
器具。口沿有残。1983 年入藏，江苏省扬州同
松药店征集。

陕西医史博物馆藏

Blue-and-white Medicine Jar

Qing Dynasty

Porcelain

Mouth Diameter 9 cm/ Bottom Diameter 14.2 cm/ Height
21 cm/ Weight 2,150 g

This jar has a snap lid, a rounded belly, and a ring foot.
The body bears the designs of interlocking branches of
chrysanthemum. It was used as a medicine container
with the mouth rim cracked. The jar was collected from
Tongsong Drugstore of Yangzhou in Jiangsu Province in
the year 1983.

Preserved in Shaanxi Museum of Medical History

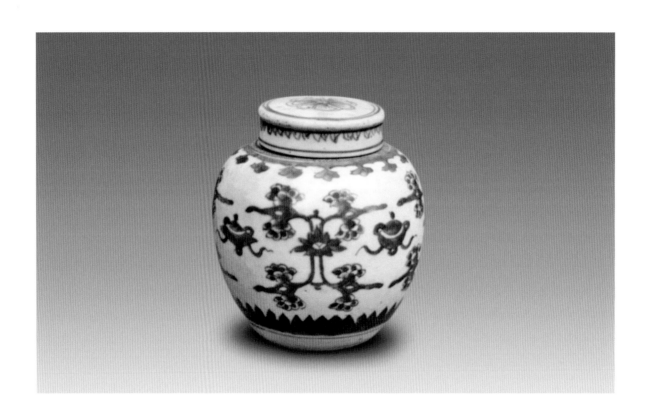

青花八宝曼陀罗花盖罐

清

瓷质

口外径 5.4 厘米，腹径 12.6 厘米，底径 8.15 厘米，带盖高 14.65 厘米，腹深 12 厘米，重 605 克

Blue-and-white Covered Jar with Eight Treasures and Mandala Designs

Qing Dynasty

Porcelain

Mouth Outer Diameter 5.4 cm/ Belly Diameter 12.6 cm/ Bottom Diameter 8.15 cm/ Height (with the lid) 14.65 cm/ Belly

Depth 12 cm/ Weight 605 g

子母口，溜肩，鼓腹，平底，圈足，表面绘
八宝曼陀罗花纹。用于存储药物。

广东中医药博物馆藏

This Jar has a snap lid, a sloping shoulder, a drum-like belly, a flat bottom, and a ring foot. On its lid and body are patterns of Mandala flowers. This jar was used to store medicine.

Preserved in Guangdong Chinese Medicine Museum

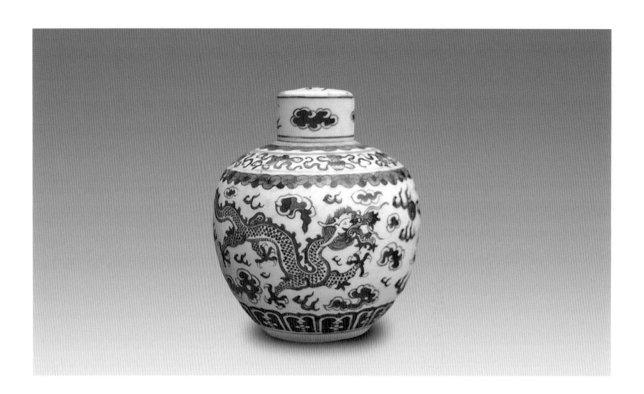

青花药罐

清

瓷质

口外径 4.85 厘米，腹径 13.8 厘米，底径 7.6 厘米，带盖高 17 厘米，腹深 14.3 厘米，重 700 克

Blue-and-white Medicine Jar

Qing Dynasty

Porcelain

Mouth Outer Diameter 4.85 cm/ Belly Diameter 13.8 cm/ Bottom Diameter 7.6 cm/ Height (with the lid) 17 cm/

Belly Depth 14.3 cm/ Weight 700 g

子母口，溜肩，鼓腹，平底，圈足，有盖，
腹部绘青花龙云纹。用于存放易受潮的药物。

广东中医药博物馆藏

This jar has a snap lid, a sloping shoulder, a drum-like belly, a flat bottom, and a ring foot. On its lid and body are blue-and-white patterns of clouds and dragons. The porcelain covered jar was used to store medicine that are inclined to get damp.

Preserved in Guangdong Chinese Medicine Museum

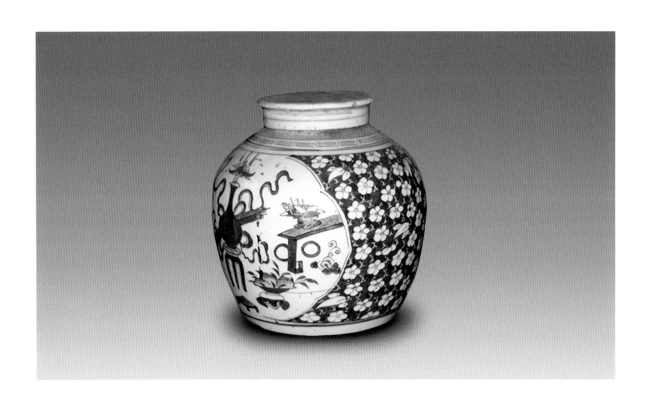

青花药罐

清

瓷质

口径 9 厘米，底径 14.5 厘米，通高 21.5 厘米，重 2300 克

Blue-and-white Medicine Jar

Qing Dynasty

Porcelain

Mouth Diameter 9 cm/ Bottom Diameter 14.5 cm/ Height 21.5 cm/ Weight 2,300 g

子母口，圆腹，圈足，表面饰博古图及小梅花，

带盖。贮药器物。腹有修补。陕西省西安市

藻露堂中药店征集。

陕西医史博物馆藏

This medicine jar has a snap lid, a rounded belly, a
ring foot and a lid. The body bears the designs of "Bo
Gu Tu" (pictures of assorted auspicious and precious
items) and small plum blossoms. It was used as a
medicine container with the belly mended. The jar
was collected from Zao Lu Tang Chinese Medicinal
Herbs Store of Xi'an in Shaanxi Province.

Preserved in Shaanxi Museum of Medical History

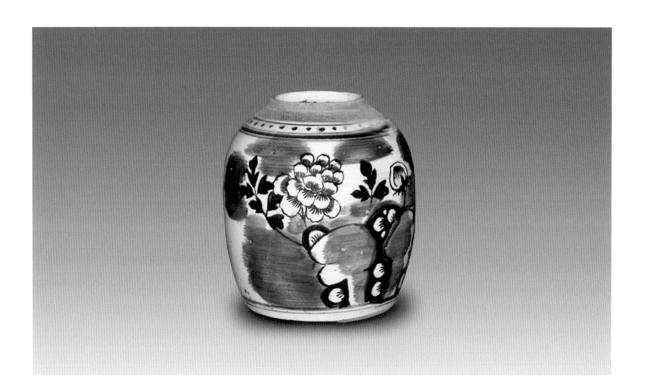

青花药罐

清

瓷质

口径 8.5 厘米，底径 14.5 厘米，通高 19.5 厘米，重 1600 克

Blue-and-white Medicine Jar

Qing Dynasty

Porcelain

Mouth Diameter 8.5 cm/ Bottom Diameter 14.5 cm/ Height 19.5 cm/ Weight 1,600 g

子母口，直腹，圈足，肩部一圈乳丁纹，腹
绘牡丹花图。贮药器具。完整无损。陕西省
西安市藻露堂中药店征集。

陕西医史博物馆藏

This medicine jar has a snap lid, a straight belly, a
ring foot and a shoulder surrounded by a band of
nipple patterns. The belly is adorned with peony
designs. It was used as a medicine container and
remains intact. The jar was collected from Zao Lu
Tang Chinese Medicinal Herbs Store of Xi'an in
Shaanxi Province.

Preserved in Shaanxi Museum of Medical History

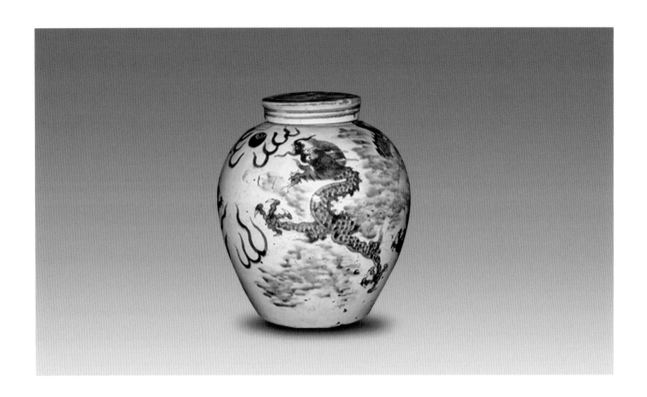

青花药罐

清

瓷质

口径 8.5 厘米，底径 14.5 厘米，通高 28 厘米，重 3700 克

Blue-and-white Medicine Jar

Qing Dynasty

Porcelain

Mouth Diameter 8.5 cm/ Bottom Diameter 14.5 cm/ Height 28 cm/ Weight 3,700 g

子母口，圆腹，平底，云火龙图，标签为"七制香腹丸"。贮药器物。完整无损。陕西省西安市藻露堂中药店征集。

陕西医史博物馆藏

The medicine jar is designed with a snap lid, a rounded belly and a flat bottom. The jar is adorned with designs of fire dragon among clouds, and bears a label of the name of the drug "Qi Zhi Xiang Fu Wan". It was used as a medicine container and remains intact. It was collected from Zao Lu Tang Chinese Medicinal Herbs Store of Xi'an in Shaanxi Province.

Preserved in Shaanxi Museum of Medical History

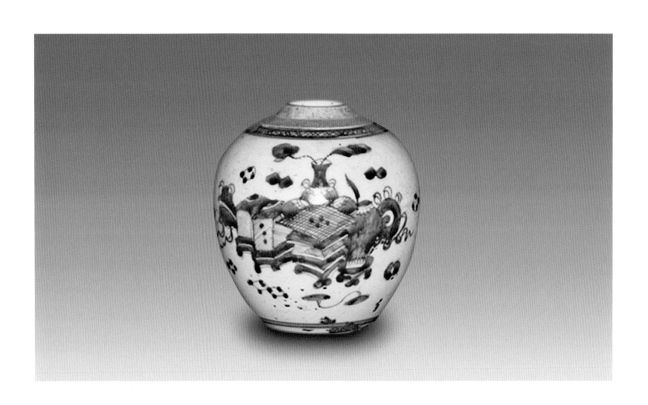

青花瓷药罐

清

瓷质

口径 3.5 厘米，底径 5.8 厘米，通高 12 厘米

子母口，圆肩，浅圈足。肩处有一圈棱纹，腹绘
博古图。贮药器具。完整无损。陕西省延安市征集。

陕西医史博物馆藏

Blue-and-white Porcelain Medicine Jar

Qing Dynasty

Porcelain

Mouth Diameter 3.5 cm/ Bottom Diameter 5.8 cm/
Height 12 cm

This medicine jar has a snap lid, a rounded shoulder, and a
shallow ring foot. The shoulder is surrounded by an edged
circle. and designs of "Bo Gu Tu" (pictures of assorted
auspicious and precious items). The jar was used as a
medicine container and remains intact. It was collected from
Yan'an City in Shaanxi Province.

Preserved in Shaanxi Museum of Medical History

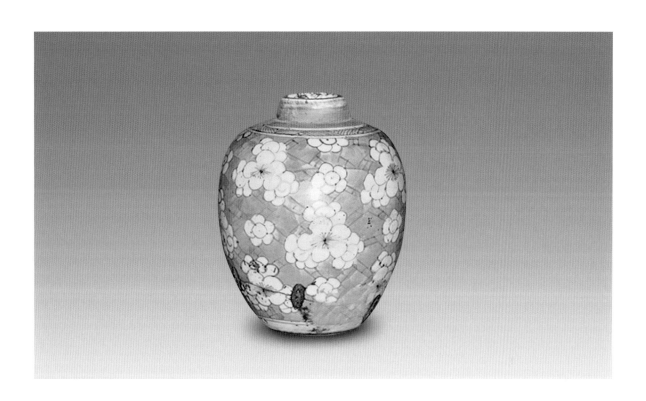

青花瓷药罐

清

瓷质

口径 3.8 厘米，底径 5.8 厘米，通高 12.5 厘米，
重 500 克

子母口，圆肩，圈足，表面绘冰梅图。贮药器具。
有修补。陕西省延安市征集。

陕西医史博物馆藏

Blue-and-white Porcelain Medicine Jar

Qing Dynasty

Porcelain

Mouth Diameter 3.8 cm/ Bottom Diameter 5.8 cm/
Height 12.5 cm/ Weight 500 g

This medicine jar is designed with a snap lid, a rounded
shoulder, and a ring foot. The body is adorned with patterns
of plum blossoms frozen in blocks of ice. It was used as
a medicine container which was mended. The object was
collected from Yan'an City in Shaanxi Province.

Preserved in Shaanxi Museum of Medical History

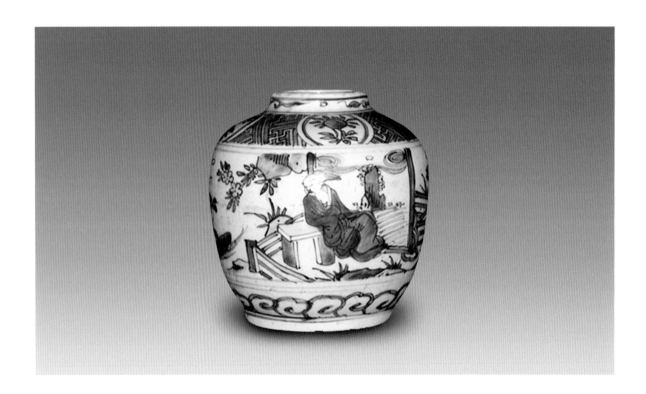

青花人物药罐

清

瓷质

口径 7.5 厘米，底径 11.5 厘米，通高 16.5 厘米，重 1250 克

Blue-and-white Medicine Jar with Portraiture Design

Qing Dynasty

Porcelain

Mouth Diameter 7.5 cm/ Bottom Diameter 11.5 cm/ Height 16.5 cm/ Weight 1,250 g

直口，圆肩，圈足，腹上有一人物观景图。贮药器具。口沿有残。三级文物。陕西省延安市征集。

陕西医史博物馆藏

This medicine jar has a straight mouth, a rounded shoulder, and a ring foot. The belly is decorated with a portrait of a figure who are enjoying the scenery. This jar, used as a medicine container, was rated as the national third-level cultural relic. The mouth rim of jar was incomplete. It was collected from Yan'an City in Shaanxi Province.

Preserved in Shaanxi Museum of Medical History

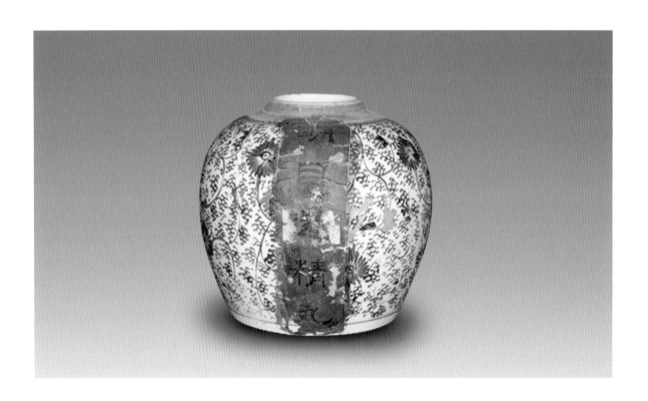

青花药罐

清

瓷质

口径 10 厘米，底径 18 厘米，通高 21 厘米，重 2700 克

Blue-and-white Medicine Jar

Qing Dynasty

Porcelain

Mouth Diameter 10 cm/ Bottom Diameter 18 cm/ Height 21 cm/ Weight 2,700 g

子母口，圆腹，圈足，通体施缠枝菊花纹，腹上标签名"明目还精丸"。贮药器具。完整无损。陕西省西安市藻露堂中药店征集。

陕西医史博物馆藏

This medicine jar has a snap lid, a rounded belly and a ring foot. The entire jar is decorated with designs of interlocking branches of chrysanthemum, with a label of the name of the drug "Ming Mu Huan Jing Wan" on the abdomen. It was used as a medicine storage container and remains intact. The object was collected from Zao Lu Tang Chinese Medicinal Herbs Store of Xi'an in Shaanxi Province.

Preserved in Shaanxi Museum of Medical History

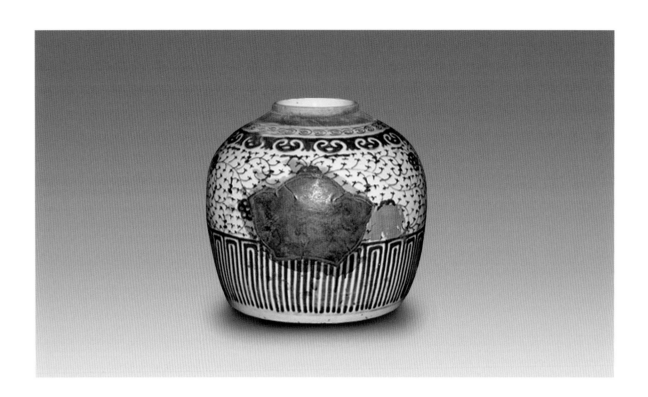

青花药罐

清

瓷质

口径 10 厘米，底径 21 厘米，通高 23 厘米，重 2450 克

Blue-and-white Medicine Jar

Qing Dynasty

Porcelain

Mouth Diameter 10 cm/ Bottom Diameter 21 cm/ Height 23 cm/ Weight 2,450 g

子母口，圆肩，圆腹，平底，腹上标签为"调经养荣丸"。贮药器具。完整无损。陕西省西安市藻露堂中药店征集。

陕西医史博物馆藏

This medicine jar has a snap lid, a rounded shoulder, a rounded belly, and a flat bottom. The entire jar is decorated with a label of the name of the drug "Tiao Jing Yang Rong Wan" on the belly. It was used as a medicine storage container and remains intact. The object was collected from Zao Lu Tang Chinese Medicinal Herbs Store of Xi'an in Shaanxi Province. Preserved in Shaanxi Museum of Medical History

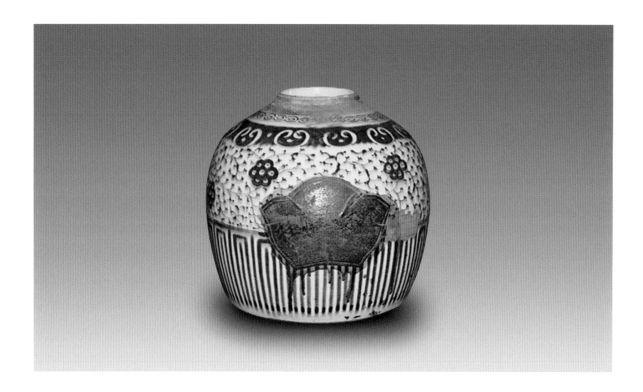

青花药罐

清

瓷质

口径 9.5 厘米，底径 21 厘米，通高 23.5 厘米，重 2300 克

Blue-and-white Medicine Jar

Qing Dynasty

Porcelain

Mouth Diameter 9.5 cm/ Bottom Diameter 21 cm/ Height 23.5 cm/ Weight 2,300 g

子母口，肩部有两道云纹，中腹为缠枝莲纹，贴有标签名"桂附八味丸"。贮药器具。完整无损。陕西省西安市藻露堂中药店征集。

陕西医史博物馆藏

This medicine jar has a snap lid. Around the shoulder are two bands of cloud patterns. In the middle of the belly are designs of interlocking lotus branches together with a label of the name of the drug "Gui Fu Ba Wei Wan". The jar was used as a medicine container and remains in good condition. It was collected from Zao Lu Tang Chinese Medicinal Herbs Store of Xi'an in Shaanxi Province.

Preserved in Shaanxi Museum of Medical History

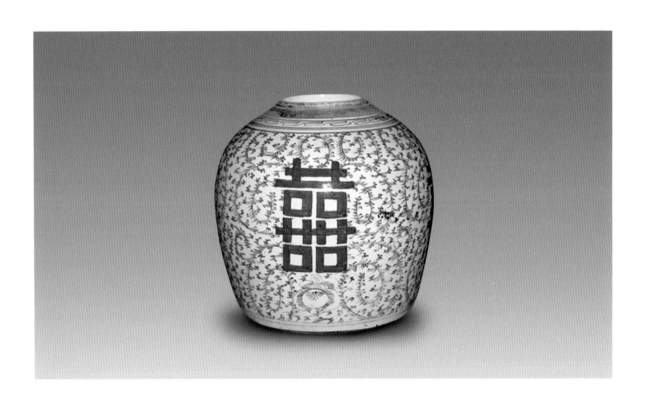

青花药罐

清

瓷质

口径 10.5 厘米，底径 20.5 厘米，通高 24.5 厘米，重 3100 克

Blue-and-white Medicine Jar

Qing Dynasty

Porcelain

Mouth Diameter 10.5 cm/ Bottom Diameter 20.5 cm/ Height 24.5 cm/ Weight 3,100 g

子母口，圆腹，圈足，表面饰四"喜"缠枝纹，肩部为一圈云纹。贮药器具。完整无损。陕西省西安市藻露堂中药店征集。

陕西医史博物馆藏

This medicine jar features a snap lid, a rounded belly, and a ring foot. The body of the jar is adorned with designs of interlocking branches and four copies of the Chinese character "Xi" (happiness). The shoulder is decorated with a band of cloud patterns. It was used as a medicine container which remains intact. The jar was collected from Zao Lu Tang Chinese Medicinal Herbs Store of Xi'an in Shaanxi Province.

Preserved in Shaanxi Museum of Medical History

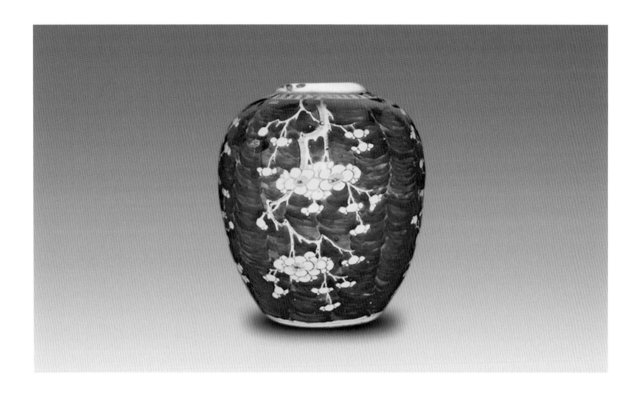

青花药罐

清

瓷质

口径 9.8 厘米，底径 14 厘米，通高 25.7 厘米，
重 2650 克

子母口，圈足，肩上饰一圈锯齿纹，腹部为干枝
梅图。贮药器具。有修补。陕西省西安市征集。

陕西医史博物馆藏

Blue-and-white Medicine Jar

Qing Dynasty

Porcelain

Mouth Diameter 9.8 cm/ Bottom Diameter 14 cm/ Height
25.7 cm/ Weight 2,650 g

This medicine jar has a snap lid and a ring foot. There
is a band of saw-tooth pattern around the shoulder with
paintings of plum branches on the belly. The jar was used
as medicine container which was mended. The object was
collected from Xi'an in Shaanxi Province.

Preserved in Shaanxi Museum of Medical History

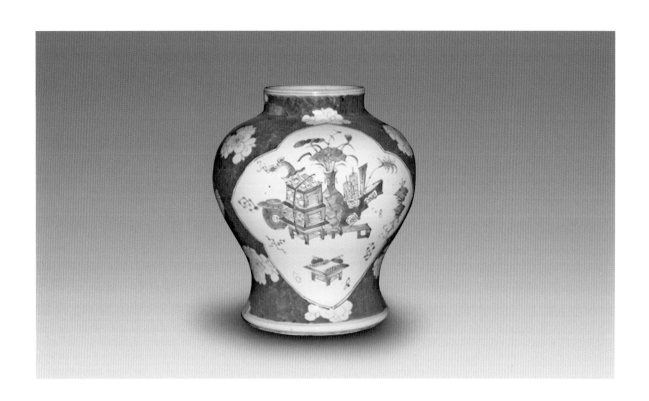

瓷药罐

清

瓷质

口径 8.6 厘米，底径 12 厘米，通高 19.5 厘米，
重 1150 克

直口，鼓腹，圈足，表面饰博古图，底有 "康熙
年制"。贮药器具。完整无损。

陕西医史博物馆藏

Porcelain Medicine Jar

Qing Dynasty

Porcelain

Mouth Diameter 8.6 cm/ Bottom Diameter 12 cm/ Height
19.5 cm/ Weight 1,150 g

This medicine jar features a straight mouth, a drum-like
belly, and a ring foot. The jar is decorated with "Bo Gu
Tu" (pictures of assorted auspicious and precious items)
and is stamped with the seal of "Kang Xi Nian Zhi" (Made
during the Reign of Kangxi) on the base. The jar was
utilized as a medicine container, and it remains intact.

Preserved in Shaanxi Museum of Medical History

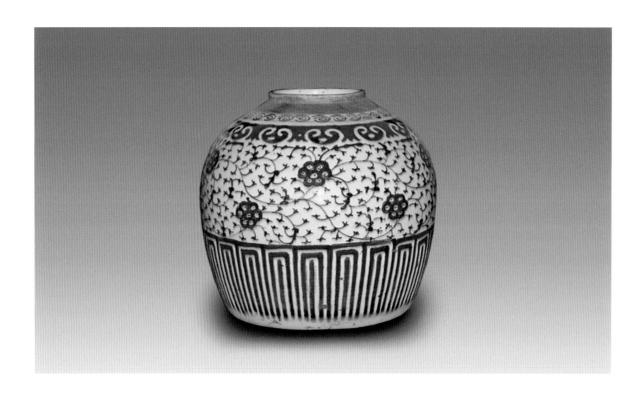

青花大药罐

清

瓷质

口径 9.5 厘米，底径 23 厘米，通高 20 厘米，重 2500 克

Big Blue-and-white Medicine Jar

Qing Dynasty

Porcelain

Mouth Diameter 9.5 cm/ Bottom Diameter 23 cm/ Height 20 cm/ Weight 2,500 g

子母口，圆腹，圈足，肩有两圈云纹，中腹
为缠枝纹，下为倒山字纹。贮药器具。完整
无损。陕西省西安市藻露堂中药店征集。

陕西医史博物馆藏

This medicine jar is designed with a snap lid, a
rounded belly, and a ring foot. Around the shoulder
are two bands of cloud patterns. In the middle of the
belly are designs of interlocking branches, under
which are inverted trident patterns. The jar was used
as a medicine container, and it remains intact. It
was collected from Zao Lu Tang Chinese Medicinal
Herbs Store of Xi'an in Shaanxi Province.

Preserved in Shaanxi Museum of Medical History

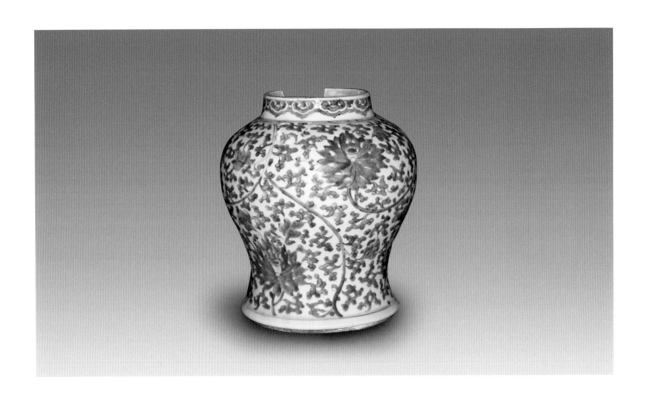

青花药罐

清

瓷质

口径 11 厘米，底径 16 厘米，通高 24 厘米，重 2700 克

Blue-and-white Medicine Jar

Qing Dynasty

Porcelain

Mouth Diameter 11 cm/ Bottom Diameter 16 cm/ Height 24 cm/ Weight 2,700 g

直口，口沿饰一圈云纹，圆肩，下撇底，圈足，

表面绘缠枝荷花图。贮药器物。口沿有残。

陕西省鄠邑区谢家店中药店征集。

　　　　　　　　　　陕西医史博物馆藏

This medicine jar is designed with a straight mouth

adorned with a band of cloud patterns, a rounded

shoulder, and an outwardly everted ring foot. The

whole jar is adorned with patterns of interlocking

lotus branches. It was used as a medicine container

with the mouth rim cracked. The jar was collected

from Xiejiadian Chinese Medicinal Herbs Store of

Huyi District in Shaanxi Province.

Preserved in Shaanxi Museum of Medical History

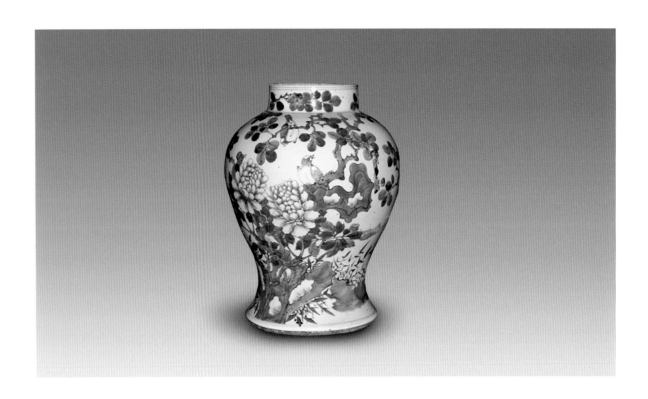

青花大药罐

清

瓷质

口径 12 厘米，底径 17 厘米，通高 32 厘米，重 3100 克

Big Blue-and-white Medicine Jar

Qing Dynasty

Porcelain

Mouth Diameter 12 cm/ Bottom Diameter 17 cm/ Height 32 cm/ Weight 3,100 g

直口，圆肩，圆腹，圈足，表面绘牡丹竹子鸟图，标签名"大胃丸"。贮药器物。完整无损。陕西省西安市藻露堂中药店征集。

陕西医史博物馆藏

The jar has a straight mouth, a rounded shoulder, a rounded belly, and a ring foot. The paintings on the jar comprise peonies, bamboos and birds. To the jar is attached a label of the name of the drug "Da Wei Wan". It was used as a medicine container which remains intact. The object was collected from Zao Lu Tang Chinese Medicinal Herbs Store of Xi'an in Shaanxi Province.

Preserved in Shaanxi Museum of Medical History

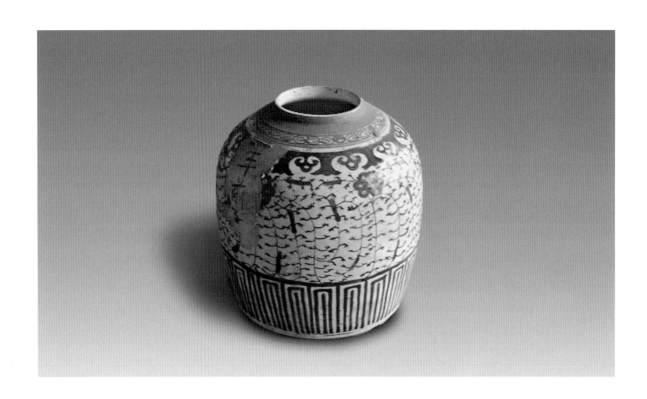

药罐

清

瓷质

口径 9 厘米，底径 18 厘米，高 21 厘米

鼓肩，直腹，浅圈足，器身饰青花草叶纹和回纹。由民间征集。

成都中医药大学中医药传统文化博物馆藏

Medicine Jar

Qing Dynasty

Porcelain

Mouth Diameter 9 cm/ Bottom Diameter 18 cm/ Height 21 cm

This medicine jar has a rounded shoulder, a straight belly, and a shallow ring foot. The jar is decorated with blue-and-white grass patterns and rectangular spiral patterns. The object was collected from a private owner.

Preserved in Museum of Traditional Chinese Medicine Culture, Chengdu University of Traditional Chinese Medicine

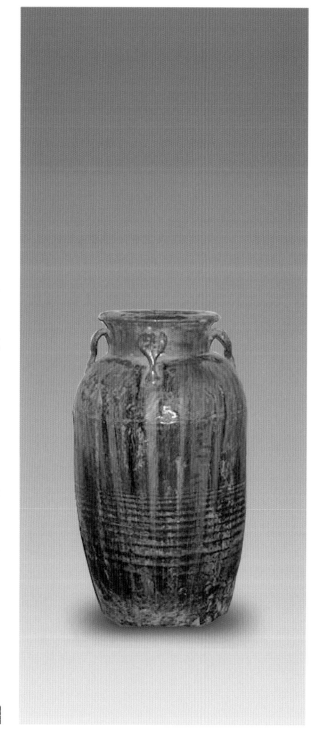

大瓷药罐

清

瓷质

口径 28 厘米，底径 29 厘米，通高 13 厘米

平敞口，直颈，直腹，平底，四耳，淡棕釉。贮药器具。完整无损。河南省征集。

陕西医史博物馆藏

Big Porcelain Medicine Jar

Qing Dynasty

Porcelain

Mouth Diameter 28 cm/ Bottom Diameter 29 cm/ Height 13 cm

This light-brown glazed jar is designed with a flat flared mouth, a straight neck, a straight belly, a flat bottom, and four ears. The vessel was used as a medicine storage container and remains intact. It was collected from Henan Province.

Preserved in Shaanxi Museum of Medical History

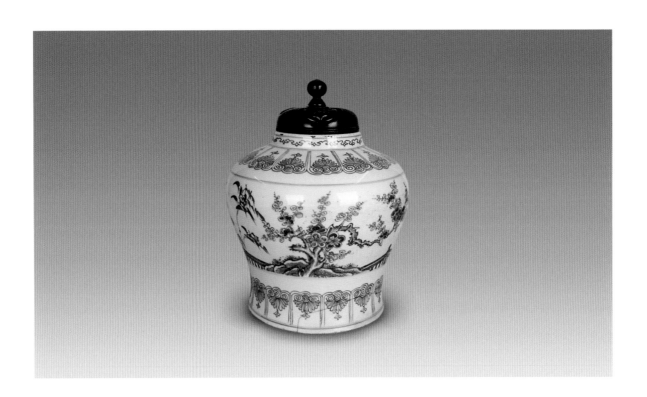

青花瓷药罐

清

瓷质

口径 9 厘米，底径 17 厘米，高 20 厘米

Blue-and-white Porcelain Medicine Jar

Qing Dynasty

Porcelain

Mouth Diameter 9 cm/ Bottom Diameter 17 cm/ Height 20 cm

敛口，短颈，溜肩，鼓腹，平底，圈足外撇，有盖。颈饰缠枝纹，肩和近底部绘菊花祥云纹，腹部绘梅竹图。由民间征集。

　　成都中医药大学中医药传统文化博物馆藏

This medicine jar has a lid, a contracted mouth, a short neck, a sloping shoulder, a drum-like belly, a flat bottom, and a flared ring foot. Interlocking branches are painted on the neck. Chrysanthemum and cloud patterns are decorated on its shoulder and lower part near the bottom. Its body is adorned with bamboos and plum blossoms. The object was collected from a private owner.

Preserved in Museum of Traditional Chinese Medicine Culture, Chengdu University of Traditional Chinese Medicine

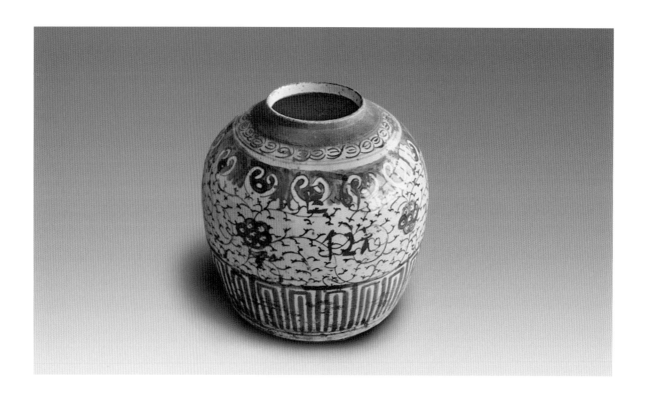

药罐

清

瓷质

口外径 5.9 厘米，口内径 5.1 厘米，腹径 13.1 厘米，底径 10 厘米，高 13.9 厘米

Medicine Jar

Qing Dynasty

Porcelain

Mouth Outer Diameter 5.9 cm/ Mouth Inner Diameter 5.1 cm/ Belly Diameter 13.1 cm/ Bottom Diameter 10 cm/ Height 13.9 cm

青花瓷，圆罐形，瓶身绘松、竹、梅图案，圈足，
底无款识，工艺精良。贮药器具。保存基本
完好。1959 年入藏。

　中华医学会 / 上海中医药大学医史博物馆藏

This blue-and-white porcelain jar, round in shape, is
decorated with designs of pine trees, bamboos and
plum blossoms. The jar has a ring foot and a bottom
without inscription. Used as a medicine container,
the jar is exquisite in craftsmanship. It was collected
in the year 1959 and remains intact.

Preserved in Chinese Medical Association/ Museum
of Chinese Medicine, Shanghai University of
Traditional Chinese Medicine

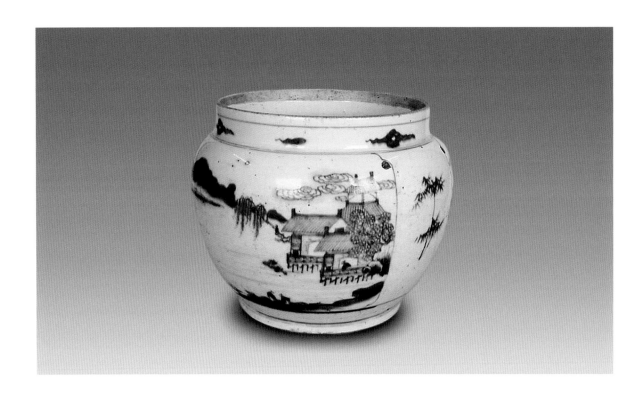

青花瓷药罐

清

瓷质

□外径 17.7 厘米，□内径 16.9 厘米，底径 14.5 厘米，通高 17.5 厘米

Blue-and-white Porcelain Medicine Jar

Qing Dynasty

Porcelain

Mouth Outer Diameter 17.7 cm/ Mouth Inner Diameter 16.9 cm/ Bottom Diameter 14.5 cm/ Height 17.5 cm

青花瓷，瓶身绘人物及动物风景画，圈足，
底无款识，工艺一般。盛药、酒器具。基本
完好。1959 年入藏。

　中华医学会 / 上海中医药大学医史博物馆藏

This blue-and-white glazed jar is decorated with a
landscape painting, along with human figures and
animals. It has a ring foot with no inscription on the
bottom. This jar, with average quality workmanship,
was used as a medicine and wine container. The
object was collected in the year 1959 and remains
intact.

Preserved in Chinese Medical Association/ Museum
of Chinese Medicine, Shanghai University of
Traditional Chinese Medicine

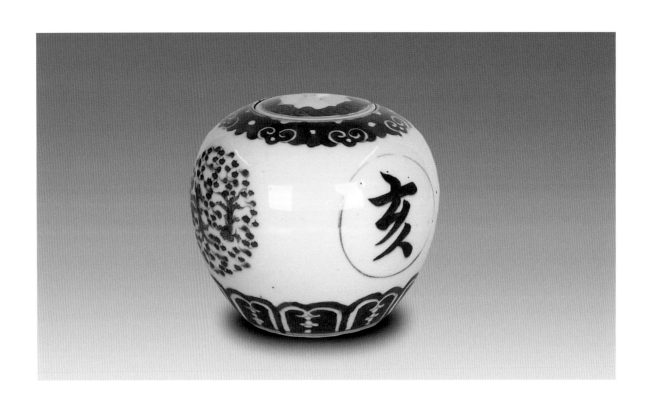

青花瓷药罐

清

瓷质

口外径 7.3 厘米，口内径 6.2 厘米，腹径 15.4 厘米，底径 9.5 厘米，高 16.3 厘米

Blue-and-white Porcelain Medicine Jar

Qing Dynasty

Porcelain

Mouth Outer Diameter 7.3 cm/ Mouth Inner Diameter 6.2 cm/ Belly Diameter 15.4 cm/ Bottom Diameter 9.5 cm/ Height 16.3 cm

青花瓷，圆罐形，瓶身绘双鱼团花图案，并
有"亥"字，配瓷盖，圈足，底有"养真局制"
款识，工艺精良。盛药器具。保存基本完好。
1958 年入藏。

中华医学会 / 上海中医药大学医史博物馆藏

This blue-and-white glazed jar has a bulging profile.
The body is adorned with double fish and posy
designs, along with a Chinese character "Hai". The
jar is designed with a porcelain lid, a ring foot with
an inscription of "Yang Zhen Ju Zhi" (Made by the
Bureau for Recuperation) on the bottom. This object,
which was used as a medicine container, enjoys a
high level of workmanship. It was collected in the
year 1958 and remains intact.
Preserved in Chinese Medical Association/ Museum
of Chinese Medicine, Shanghai University of
Traditional Chinese Medicine

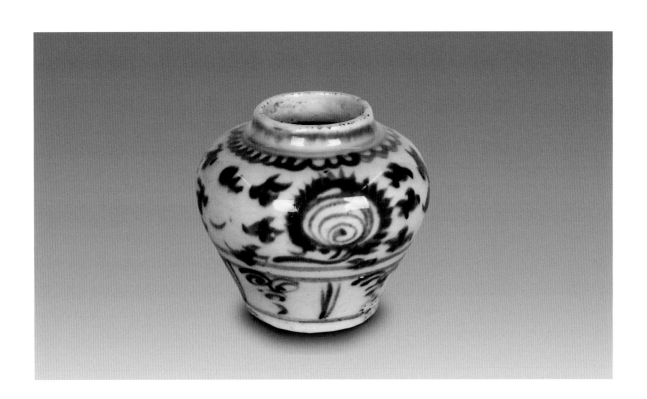

青花瓷药罐

清

瓷质

口外径 4.7 厘米，口内径 4.8 厘米，腹径 9.25 厘米，底径 5.6 厘米，通高 8.15 厘米

Blue-and-white Porcelain Medicine Jar

Qing Dynasty

Porcelain

Mouth Outer Diameter 4.7 cm/ Mouth Inner Diameter 4.8 cm/ Belly Diameter 9.25 cm/ Bottom Diameter 5.6 cm/ Height 8.15 cm

青花瓷，圆罐形，瓶身绘青花花鸟写意图，

瓶底无釉、无款识，工艺一般。贮药器具。

保存基本完好。1959 年入藏。

中华医学会 / 上海中医药大学医史博物馆藏

This blue-and-white glazed jar has a bulging
profile. The body is adorned with designs of blue-
and-white flowers and birds in a free style. There
is no inscription on the unglazed bottom. The jar
with average workmanship was used as a medicine
container, and it was collected in the year 1959 and
remains intact.
Preserved in Chinese Medical Association/ Museum
of Chinese Medicine, Shanghai University of
Traditional Chinese Medicine

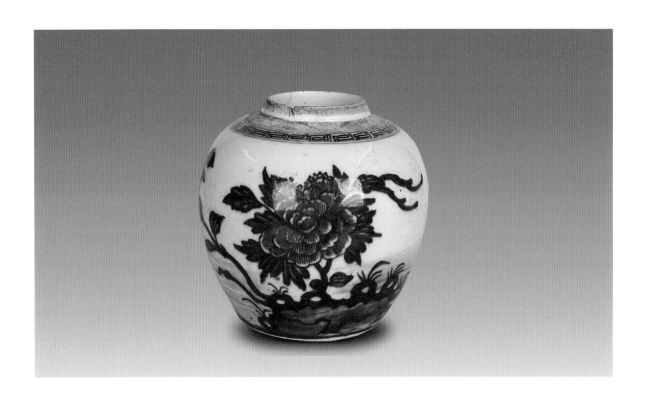

青花瓷药罐

清

瓷质

口外径 6.9 厘米，口内径 6.2 厘米，腹径 15.8 厘米，底径 11 厘米，通高 15.4 厘米

Blue-and-white Porcelain Medicine Jar

Qing Dynasty

Porcelain

Mouth Outer Diameter 6.9 cm/ Mouth Inner Diameter 6.2 cm/ Belly Diameter 15.8 cm/ Bottom Diameter 11 cm/

Height 15.4 cm

青花瓷，圆罐形，瓶身绘花卉枝叶，底无款识，

工艺一般。盛药器具。有残。1959 年入藏。

中华医学会 / 上海中医药大学医史博物馆藏

This blue-and-white glazed jar has a bulging profile. The body is adorned with designs of flowers along with branches and leaves. There is no inscription on the bottom. With average workmanship, the jar was used as a medicine container. It was collected in the year 1959 and was slightly damaged.
Preserved in Chinese Medical Association/ Museum of Chinese Medicine, Shanghai University of Traditional Chinese Medicine

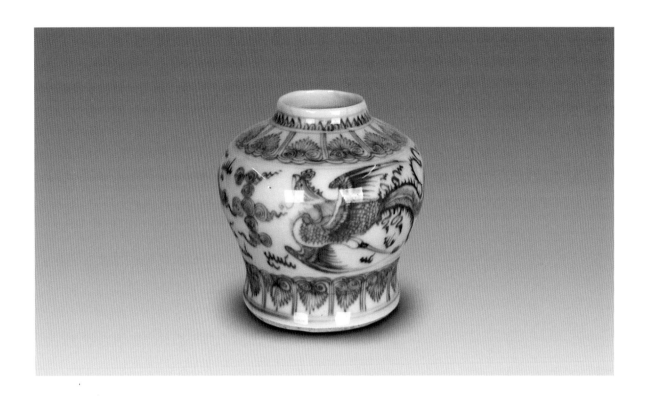

青花瓷药罐

清

瓷质

口外径 4.4 厘米，口内径 3:8 厘米，腹径 13 厘米，底径 8.2 厘米，通高 9 厘米

Blue-and-white Porcelain Medicine Jar

Qing Dynasty

Porcelain

Mouth Outer Diameter 4.4 cm/ Mouth Inner Diameter 3.8 cm/ Belly Diameter 13 cm/ Bottom Diameter 8.2 cm/ Height 9 cm

青花瓷，圆罐形，通身施釉，瓶身绘青花双凤祥云，瓶底有一青花"天"字，工艺较好。盛药器具。保存基本完好。1957 年入藏。

中华医学会 / 上海中医药大学医史博物馆藏

This object is blue-and-white porcelain ware in the shape of a jar. Glazed entirely, the jar shows good workmanship. The body is adorned with designs of a pair of phoenixes flying amidst auspicious clouds in blue and white. There is a Chinese character "Tian" (sky) inscribed on the bottom. The jar was used as a medicine container which remains intact. It was collected in the year 1957.

Preserved in Chinese Medical Association/ Museum of Chinese Medicine, Shanghai University of Traditional Chinese Medicine

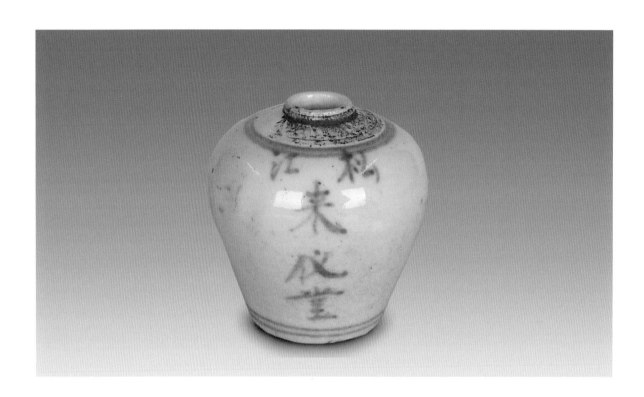

青花瓷药罐

清

瓷质

口外径 2.1 厘米，口内径 1.45 厘米，腹径 6.8 厘米，底径 4.1 厘米，通高 7.15 厘米

Blue-and-white Porcelain Medicine Jar

Qing Dynasty

Porcelain

Mouth Outer Diameter 2.1 cm/ Mouth Inner Diameter 1.45 cm/ Belly Diameter 6.8 cm/ Bottom Diameter 4.1 cm/ Height 7.15 cm

青花瓷，圆罐形，除肩颈部外通身施釉，罐表面有胎疤，罐身有兽形图案，并书"松江来仪堂"字样，罐底无款识，工艺一般。盛药器具。保存基本完好。1959 年入藏。

中华医学会 / 上海中医药大学医史博物馆藏

This object is blue-and-white porcelain ware in the shape of a jar. It is covered entirely with the glaze except for the shoulder and the neck. The jar shows average workmanship with scars on the surface. The body is adorned with animal patterns and on its belly is inscribed the name of the pharmacy "Song Jiang Lai Yi Tang". The bottom of the jar bears no reign mark or other inscription. The jar was used as a medicine container, and is kept in good condition. It was collected in the year 1959.

Preserved in Chinese Medical Association/ Museum of Chinese Medicine, Shanghai University of Traditional Chinese Medicine

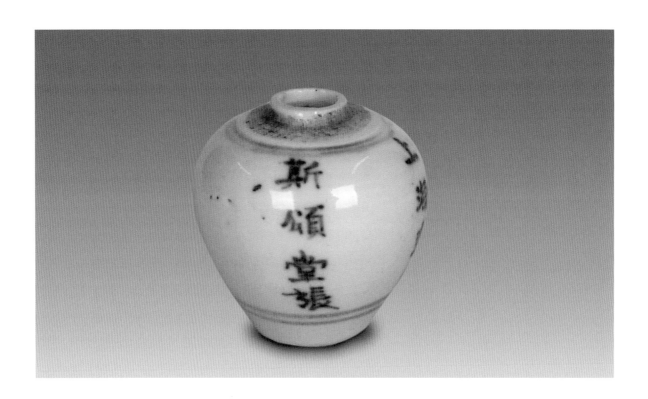

青花瓷药罐

清

瓷质

口外径 2.3 厘米，口内径 1.6 厘米，腹径 6.6 厘米，底径 3.05 厘米，通高 6.7 厘米

Blue-and-white Porcelain Medicine Jar

Qing Dynasty

Porcelain

Mouth Outer Diameter 2.3 cm/ Mouth Inner Diameter 1.6 cm/ Belly Diameter 6.6 cm/ Bottom Diameter 3.05 cm/ Height 6.7 cm

青花瓷，圆罐形，除肩颈部外通身施釉，罐
身书"上海东街斯颂堂张"字样，罐底无款识，
工艺一般。盛药器具。保存基本完好。1959 年
入藏。

中华医学会 / 上海中医药大学医史博物馆藏

This blue-and-white porcelain ware of average
workmanship is in the shape of a jar. It is covered
entirely with glaze except the shoulder and the neck.
On the body of the jar is inscribed the name of the
pharmacy together with its address "Shang Hai Dong
Jie Si Song Tang Zhang". The bottom of the jar bears
no reign mark or inscription. Used as a medicine
container, the object is kept in good condition. It was
collected in the year 1959.

Preserved in Chinese Medical Association/ Museum
of Chinese Medicine, Shanghai University of
Traditional Chinese Medicine

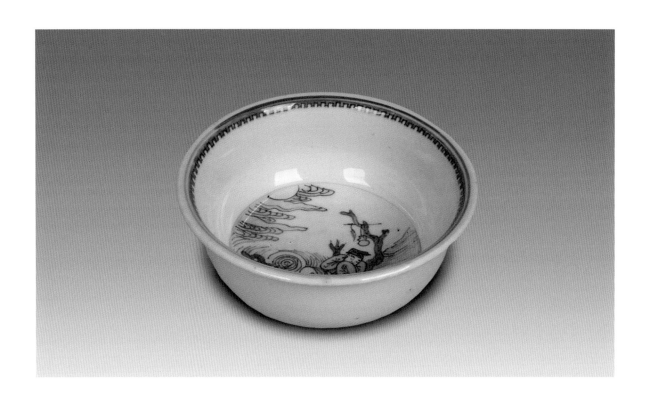

青花瓷药碗

清

瓷质

口径 13.9 厘米，底径 7.9 厘米，通高 5.8 厘米

Blue-and-white Porcelain Medicine Bowl

Qing Dynasty

Porcelain

Mouth Diameter 13.9 cm/ Bottom Diameter 7.9 cm/ Height 5.8 cm

碗形，碗内绘人物故事青花图案，碗外壁施

纯青灰色釉，底无款，工艺较好。制药工具。

保存基本完好。1957 年入藏。

　中华医学会／上海中医药大学医史博物馆藏

In the shape of a bowl, this blue-and-white bowl is

adorned with a portrait of narrative scenes on the

interior wall, while the exterior is coated entirely

with pale glaze. Without reign mark or inscription on

the bottom, the bowl shows good craftsmanship. The

bowl was used for pharmaceutical use which remains

intact. It was collected in the year 1957.

Preserved in Chinese Medical Association/ Museum

of Chinese Medicine, Shanghai University of

Traditional Chinese Medicine

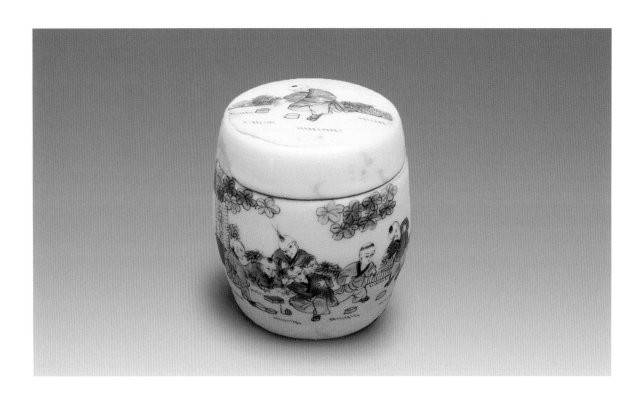

药缸

清

瓷质

口径 6.5 厘米，高 9 厘米

表面饰五彩童子嬉戏图，器身成圆筒状，深盘形盖。由民间征集。

成都中医药大学中医药传统文化博物馆藏

Medicine Jar

Qing Dynasty

Porcelain

Mouth Diameter 6.5 cm/ Height 9 cm

Adorned with polychrome portraiture designs featuring little children playing around, the body of the jar is in cylinder shape, covered with a deep plate-shaped lid. The object was collected from a private owner.

Preserved in Museum of Traditional Chinese Medicine Culture, Chengdu University of Traditional Chinese Medicine

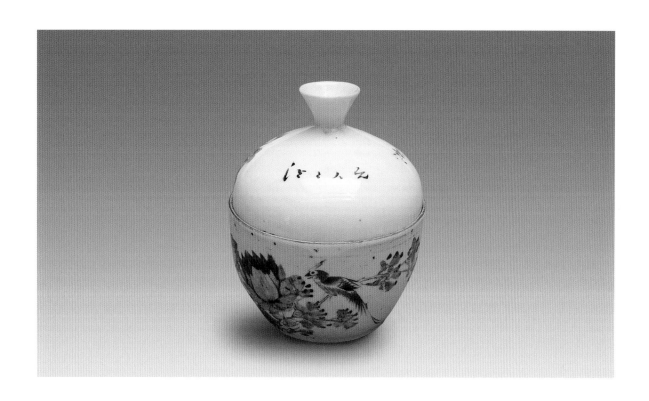

药缸

清

瓷质

口径 10.5 厘米，高 12 厘米

整器成圆鼓形，盖与器身由子母口衔接，鼓腹，平底，饰五彩人物和树枝纹。盛装药物的工具。由民间征集。

成都中医药大学中医药传统文化博物馆藏

Medicine Jar

Qing Dynasty

Porcelain

Mouth Diameter 10.5 cm/ Height 12 cm

The jar, in the shape of a round drum, features a snap lid, a drum-like belly, and a flat bottom. The jar is adorned with polychrome designs of portraiture and tree branches. It was used for storing medicine and was collected from a private owner.

Preserved in Museum of Traditional Chinese Medicine Culture, Chengdu University of Traditional Chinese Medicine

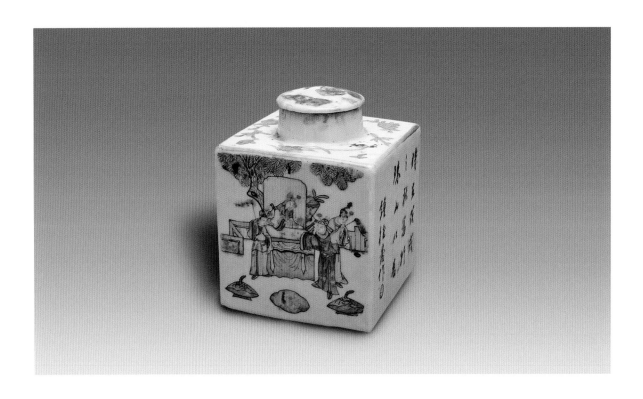

药缸

清

瓷质

口径 4.5 厘米，宽 9 厘米，高 12 厘米

器形成正方形，上有圆井形口，口上有纽扣形盖，饰有彩绘人物图案和墨书文字。盛放药物的用具。保存完好。由民间征集。

成都中医药大学中医药传统文化博物馆藏

Medicine Jar

Qing Dynasty

Porcelain

Mouth Diameter 4.5 cm/ Width 9 cm/ Height 12 cm

The square-shaped vessel has a well-shaped mouth, covered by a button-shaped lid. The body is adorned with painted portraiture designs and ink inscriptions. It was used as a medicine container and is kept intact. The object was collected from a private owner.

Preserved in Museum of Traditional Chinese Medicine Culture, Chengdu University of Traditional Chinese Medicine

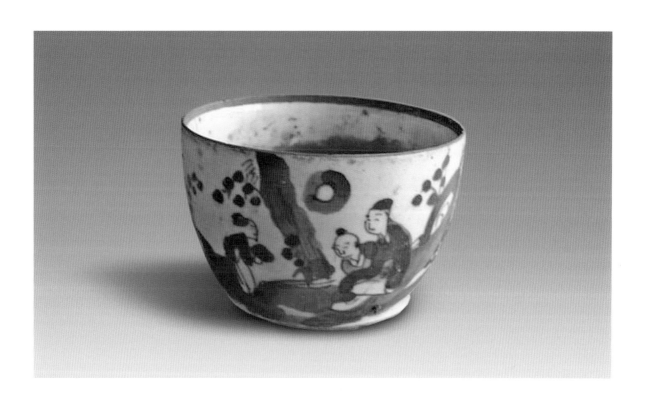

药缸

清

瓷质

口径 10.5 厘米，高 6 厘米

敞口，平底，表面饰青花人物、枝叶等纹饰。原
应有盖，已失。由民间征集。

成都中医药大学中医药传统文化博物馆藏

Medicine Jar

Qing Dynasty

Porcelain

Mouth Diameter 10.5 cm/ Height 6 cm

Adorned with designs of portraiture, branches and leaves,
this blue-and-white porcelain jar features a flared mouth
and a flat bottom. The lid is missing. The object was
collected from a private owner.

Preserved in Museum of Traditional Chinese Medicine
Culture, Chengdu University of Traditional Chinese
Medicine

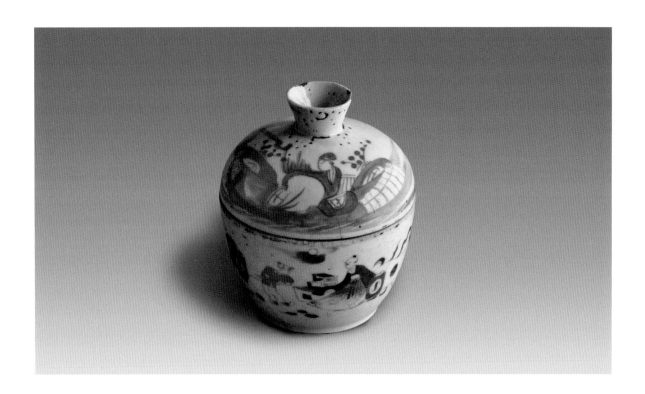

药缸

清

瓷质

口径 10.5 厘米，底径 6.8 厘米，高 11.5 厘米

Medicine Jar

Qing Dynasty

Porcelain

Mouth Diameter 10.5 cm/ Bottom Diameter 6.8 cm/ Height 11.5 cm

平底，腹内收，杯形盖，上有圈足形钮，盖
与身有子母口相合，盖、身上分别饰有青花
人物图案，色泽淡雅，线条流畅。盛装药物
用品。保存完好。由民间征集。

成都中医药大学中医药传统文化博物馆藏

This jar has a flat bottom, a belly which is inwardly
concaved, and a domed lid with a ring-shaped knob.
The lid can be buckled with the body of the jar.
Both the lid and the body are adorned with simple
and elegant blue-and-white portraiture designs
with smooth lines. The jar was used as a medicine
container, and is kept in good shape. It was collected
from a private owner.

Preserved in Museum of Traditional Chinese Medicine
Culture, Chengdu University of Traditional Chinese
Medicine

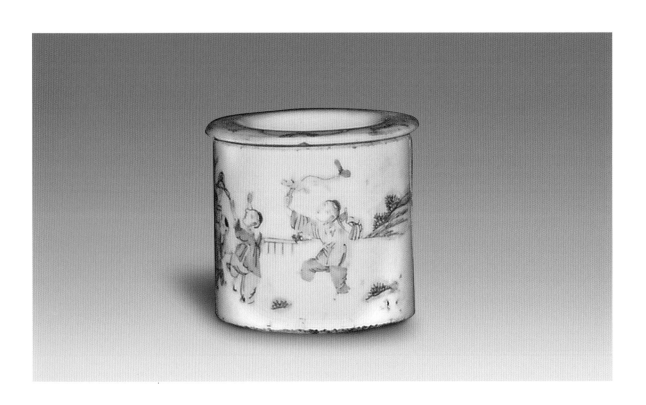

瓷药盒

清

瓷质

口径 5 厘米，底径 5 厘米，通高 4.5 厘米，重 100 克

子母口，直腹，圈足，盖呈盘状，腹上有五人嬉戏图。贮药器具。完整无损。

陕西医史博物馆藏

Porcelain Medicine Case

Qing Dynasty

Porcelain

Mouth Diameter 5 cm/ Bottom Diameter 5 cm/ Height 4.5 cm/ Weight 100 g

The case has a snap lid in the shape of a plate, a straight belly, and a ring foot. The belly is adorned with a portrait of five figures who are teasing one another. The case was used as a medicine container, and is kept intact.

Preserved in Shaanxi Museum of Medical History

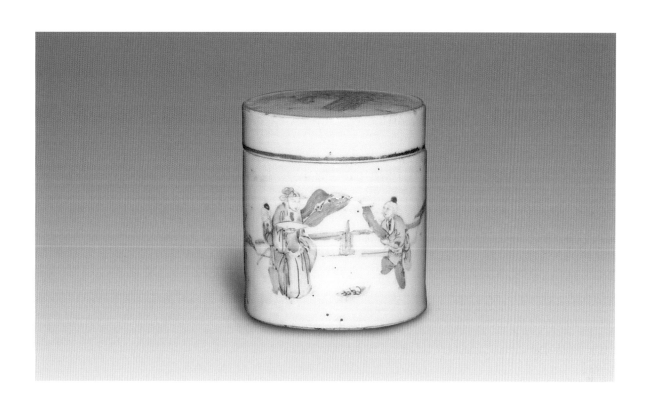

人物瓷药盒

清

瓷质

口径 7.5 厘米，底径 7.3 厘米，通高 8.5 厘米，
重 250 克

白瓷，子母口，直腹，盖顶有父子两人，腹上有
"三口之家"图。贮药器具。完整无损。

陕西医史博物馆藏

Porcelain Medicine Case with Portraiture Design

Qing Dynasty

Porcelain

Mouth Diameter 7.5 cm/ Bottom Diameter 7.3 cm/
Height 8.5 cm/ Weight 250 g

This white porcelain case features a snap lid and a
straight belly. On the top of the lid is an image of father
and son, while on the belly is a drawing of "A Family of
Three". The case was used as a medicine container, and is
kept intact.

Preserved in Shaanxi Museum of Medical History

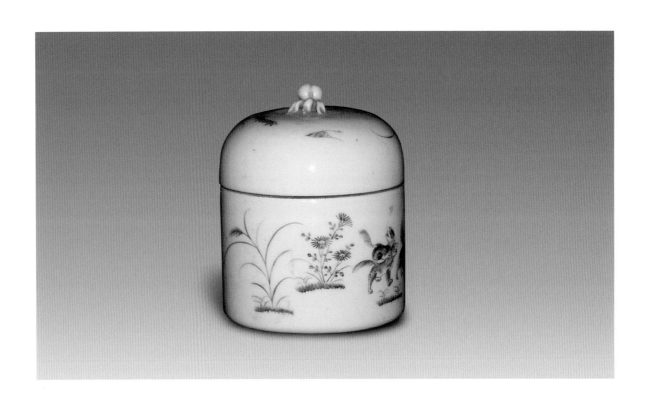

瓷药盒

清

瓷质

口径 8 厘米，底径 8 厘米，通高 6.5 厘米，重 150 克

Porcelain Medicine Case

Qing Dynasty

Porcelain

Mouth Diameter 8 cm/ Bottom Diameter 8 cm/ Height 6.5 cm/ Weight 150 g

白瓷，子母口，直腹，平底，带盖，腹有彩绘狗尾草、菊花、竹子、小动物图，底有印章"同治年制"。贮药器具。

陕西医史博物馆藏

This white porcelain case features a snap lid, a straight belly, and a flat bottom. Designs of green bristlegrass, chrysanthemum, bamboos and little animals were painted on the belly. The bottom was inscribed with a reign mark "Tong Zhi Nian Zhi" (Made during the Reign of Tongzhi). It was used as a medicine container.

Preserved in Shaanxi Museum of Medical History

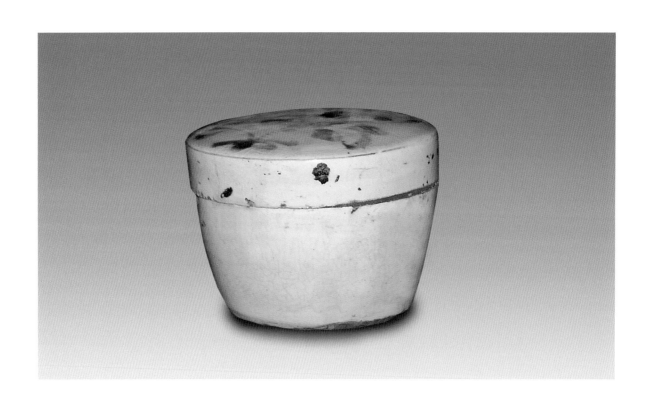

青花带盖小药盒

清

瓷质

口径 8.5 厘米，底径 7.5 厘米，通高 7.5 厘米，重 300 克

Blue-and-white Medicine Case with Lid

Qing Dynasty

Porcelain

Mouth Diameter 8.5 cm/ Bottom Diameter 7.5 cm/ Height 7.5 cm/ Weight 300 g

白釉，子母口，斜腹，圈足，小兰花，盒内无釉，

药签名为"烦赭石"。贮存器具。完整无损。

陕西省西安市藻露堂中药店征集。

陕西医史博物馆藏

This white glaze case has a snap lid, an oblique belly,

and a ring foot. It is decorated with designs of little

blue flowers. The interior of the case is unglazed. It

has a medicine label named "Fan Zhe Shi "(ochre).

It is a container, intact. It was collected from Zao

Lu Tang Chinese Medical Herbs Store of Xi'an in

Shaanxi Province.

Preserved in Shaanxi Museum of Medical History

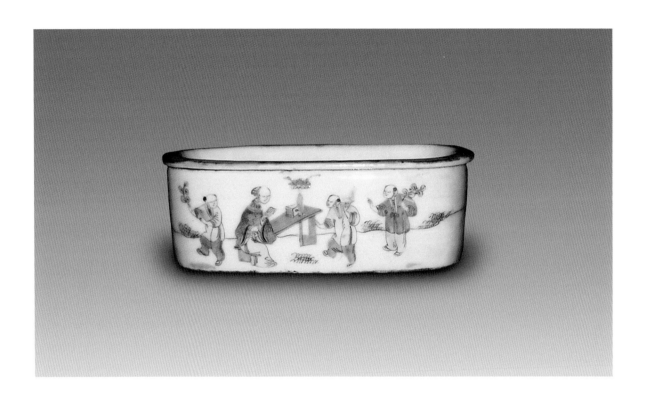

长形瓷药盒

清

瓷质

口径 13 厘米，底径 6.5 厘米，通高 4.5 厘米，重 250 克

Long Porcelain Medicine Case

Qing Dynasty

Porcelain

Mouth Diameter 13 cm/ Bottom Diameter 6.5 cm/ Height 4.5 cm/ Weight 250 g

椭圆状，子母口，直腹，盖内凹有两个麻钱
状孔并有彩绘，腹有八个人物。贮药器具。
完整无损。

陕西医史博物馆藏

This oval-shaped case features a snap lid and a
straight belly. Two holes shaped in ancient Chinese
coins are found on the painted lid which is inwardly
concaved. The belly is adorned with portraits of eight
figures. The case was used as a medicine container,
which is kept intact.

Preserved in Shaanxi Museum of Medical History

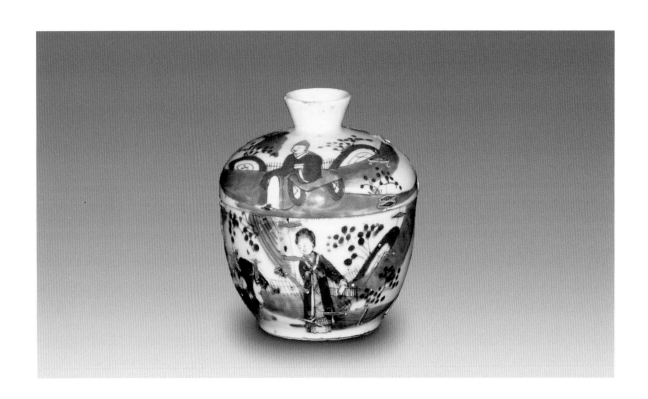

青花带盖小药盒

清

瓷质

口径 10.2 厘米，底径 7 厘米，通高 12 厘米，重 300 克

Small Blue-and-white Medicine Case with Lid

Qing Dynasty

Porcelain

Mouth Diameter 10.2 cm/ Bottom Diameter 7 cm/ Height 12 cm/ Weight 300 g

子母口，直斜腹，圈足，表面绘母子玩耍图案。
贮药器具。有修补。陕西省西安市藻露堂中
药店征集。

陕西医史博物馆藏

The case features a snap lid, a straight and oblique
belly, and a ring foot. On the case is a drawing of
"Mother Playing with Her child". The case was used
as a medicine container with some parts repaired. It
was collected from Zao Lu Tang Chinese Medicinal
Herbs Store of Xi'an in Shaanxi Province.
Preserved in Shaanxi Museum of Medical History

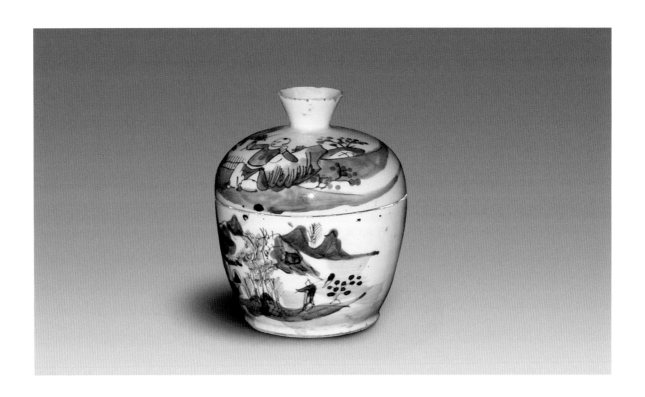

青花带盖小药盒

清

瓷质

口径 10.2 厘米，底径 7 厘米，通高 12 厘米，重 300 克

Small Blue-and-white Medicine Case with Lid

Qing Dynasty

Porcelain

Mouth Diameter 10.2 cm/ Bottom Diameter 7 cm/ Height 12 cm/ Weight 300 g

子母口，直斜腹，圈足，表面绘山水垂钓图案。
贮药器具。完整无损。陕西省西安市藻露堂
中药店征集。

陕西医史博物馆藏

The case features a snap lid, a straight and oblique
belly, and a ring foot. On the case is a scene of
"Fishing by Mountains and Rivers". The case was
used as a medicine container which remains intact. It
was collected from Zao Lu Tang Chinese Medicinal
Herbs Store of Xi'an in Shaanxi Province.
Preserved in Shaanxi Museum of Medical History

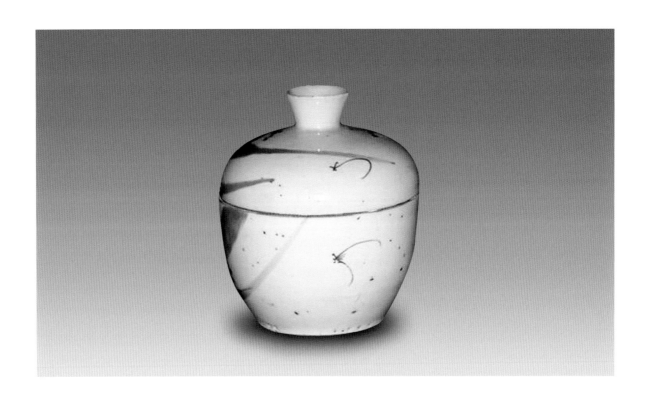

青花带盖小药盒

清

瓷质

口径 10.2 厘米，底径 7 厘米，通高 12 厘米，重 300 克

Small Blue-and-white Medicine Case with Lid

Qing Dynasty

Porcelain

Mouth Diameter 10.2 cm/ Bottom Diameter 7 cm/ Height 12 cm/ Weight 300 g

子母口，直斜腹，圈足，表面绘两个小马驹

图案。贮药器具。完整无损。陕西省西安市

藻露堂中药店征集。

陕西医史博物馆藏

This blue-and-white medicine case has a snap lid, a
straight and oblique belly, and a ring foot. The case
is adorned with designs of two colts. This medicine
storage utensil remains intact. It was collected from
Zao Lu Tang Chinese Medicinal Herbs Store of Xi'an
in Shaanxi Province.

Preserved in Shaanxi Museum of Medical History

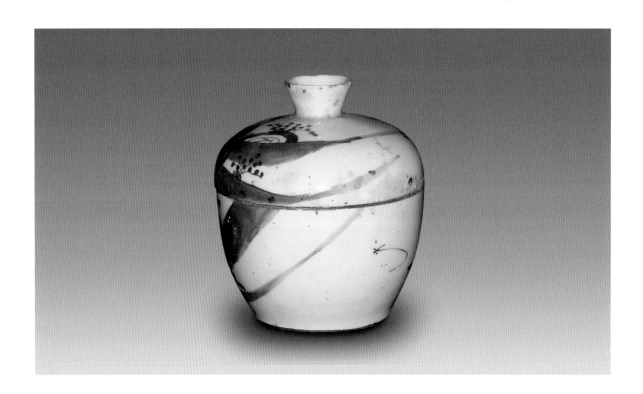

青花带盖小药盒

清

瓷质

口径 10.2 厘米，底径 7 厘米，通高 12 厘米，重 300 克

Small Blue-and-white Medicine Case with Lid

Qing Dynasty

Porcelain

Mouth Diameter 10.2 cm/ Bottom Diameter 7 cm/ Height 12 cm/ Weight 300 g

子母口，直斜腹，圈足，表面绘两人读书图案。
贮药器具。完整无损。陕西省西安市藻露堂
中药店征集。

陕西医史博物馆藏

This blue-and-white medicine case has a snap lid, a
straight and oblique belly, and a ring foot. The case
is adorned with the design of two persons who are
reading. This medicine storage utensil remains in
good condition. It was collected from Zao Lu Tang
Chinese Medicinal Herbs Store of Xi'an in Shaanxi
Province.

Preserved in Shaanxi Museum of Medical History

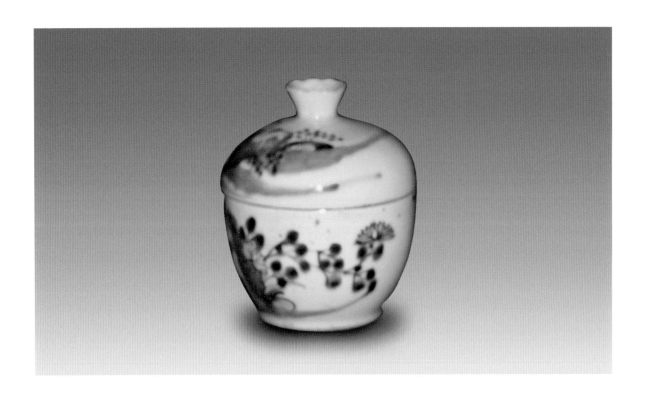

青花带盖小药盒

清

瓷质

口径 10 厘米，底径 7 厘米，通高 12.2 厘米，重 300 克

Small Blue-and-white Medicine Case with Lid

Qing Dynasty

Porcelain

Mouth Diameter 10 cm/ Bottom Diameter 7 cm/ Height 12.2 cm/ Weight 300 g

子母口，直斜腹，圈足，表面饰菊花图案。
贮药器具。完整无损。陕西省西安市藻露堂
中药店征集。

陕西医史博物馆藏

This blue-and-white medicine case has a snap lid, a
straight and oblique belly, and a ring foot. The case is
adorned with chrysanthemum motifs on the exterior
surface. This medicine storage utensil remains in
good condition. It was collected from Zao Lu Tang
Chinese Medicinal Herbs Store of Xi'an in Shaanxi
Province.

Preserved in Shaanxi Museum of Medical History

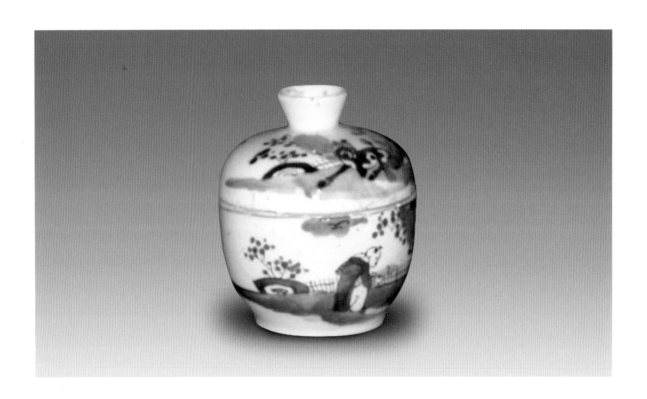

带盖小药盒

清

瓷质

口径 10.5 厘米，底径 7 厘米，通高 12 厘米，重 300 克

子母口，直斜腹，圈足，表面绘两小孩戏耍图案。贮药器具。完整无损。陕西省西安市藻露堂中药店征集。

陕西医史博物馆藏

Small Medicine Case with Lid

Qing Dynasty

Porcelain

Mouth Diameter 10.5 cm/ Bottom Diameter 7 cm/ Height 12 cm/ Weight 300 g

This blue-and-white medicine case has a snap lid, a straight and oblique belly, and a ring foot. The case is adorned with designs of two playing kids. This medicine storage utensil is kept in good condition. It was collected from Zao Lu Tang Chinese Medicinal Herbs Store of Xi'an in Shaanxi Province.

Preserved in Shaanxi Museum of Medical History

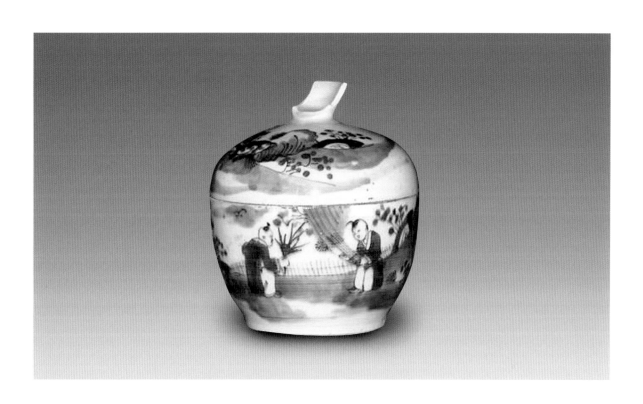

青花瓷药盒

清

瓷质

口径 10 厘米，底径 7 厘米，通高 12 厘米，重 250 克

子母口，直斜腹，圈足，带盖，表面绘两小孩戏耍图。贮药器具。盖把残。陕西省西安市藻露堂中药店征集。

陕西医史博物馆藏

Blue-and-white Porcelain Medicine Case

Qing Dynasty

Porcelain

Mouth Diameter 10 cm/ Bottom Diameter 7 cm/ Height 12 cm/ Weight 250 g

This blue-and-white medicine case has a snap lid, a straight and oblique belly, and a ring foot. The case is adorned with designs of two playing kids. This case was used as a medicine storage container. The knob on the case lid was broken. It was collected from Zao Lu Tang Chinese Medicinal Herbs Store of Xi'an in Shaanxi Province. Preserved in Shaanxi Museum of Medical History

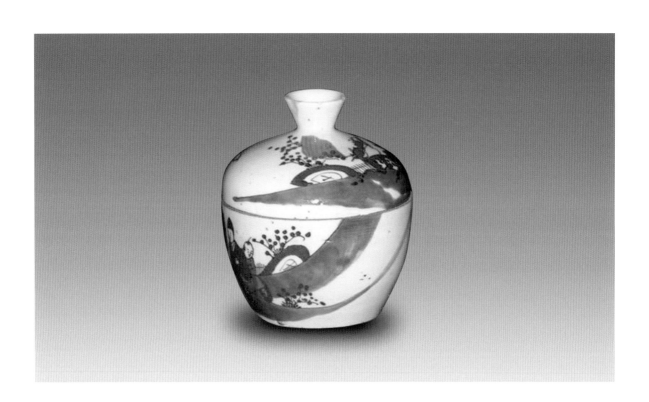

青花带盖小药盒

清

瓷质

口径 10.5 厘米，底径 7 厘米，通高 12 厘米，重 300 克

Small Blue-and-white Medicine Case with Lid

Qing Dynasty

Porcelain

Mouth Diameter 10.5 cm/ Bottom Diameter 7 cm/ Height 12 cm/ Weight 300 g

子母口，直斜腹，圈足，表面绘三人读书图案。

贮药器具。盖有修补。陕西省西安市藻露堂

中药店征集。

陕西医史博物馆藏

This blue-and-white medicine case has a snap lid, a
straight and oblique belly, and a ring foot. The case
is adorned with designs of three persons who are
reading. This case was used as a medicine storage
utensil with a repaired lid. It was collected from Zao
Lu Tang Chinese Medicinal Herbs Store of Xi'an in
Shaanxi Province.

Preserved in Shaanxi Museum of Medical History

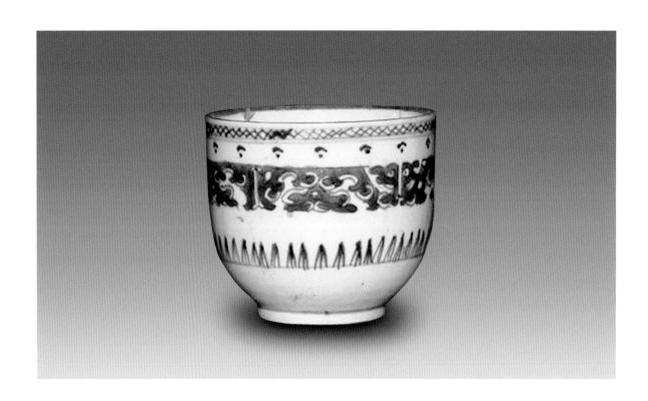

青花瓷药盒

清

瓷质

口径 10 厘米，底径 5.5 厘米，通高 8.5 厘米，重 200 克

Porcelain Medicine Case with Blue-and-white Motifs

Qing Dynasty

Porcelain

Mouth Diameter 10 cm/ Bottom Diameter 5.5 cm/ Height 8.5 cm/ Weight 200 g

子母口，直腹，圈足，腹上三圈花纹，上为菱纹，中为云纹，下为草纹。贮药器具。无盖，有修补。陕西省鄠邑区谢家店中药店贮药用具。

陕西医史博物馆藏

This medicine case has a snap lid, a straight belly, and a ring foot. The belly is decorated with three bands of motifs, including diamond patterns on the top, cloud motifs in the middle and grass patterns at the bottom. This restored case with no lid was used to store medicine at Xiejiadian Chinese Medicinal Herbs Store of Huyi District in Shaanxi Province. Preserved in Shaanxi Museum of Medical History

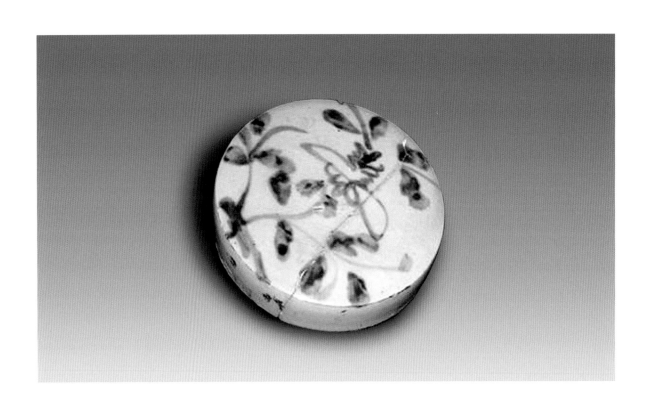

蓝花白瓷药盒盖

清

瓷质

口径 10.2 厘米，高 2.1 厘米，重 150 克

白瓷，青花，子母盖。医药器具。有残。陕西省西安市藻露堂中药店征集。

陕西医史博物馆藏

White Porcelain Medicine Case Lid with Blue Floral Designs

Qing Dynasty

Porcelain

Mouth Diameter 10.2 cm/ Height 2.1 cm/ Weight 150 g

This is a snap lid featuring white porcelain and blue floral designs. This cracked lid is a part of medicine container, and it was collected from Zao Lu Tang Chinese Medicinal Herbs Store of Xi'an in Shaanxi Province.

Preserved in Shaanxi Museum of Medical History

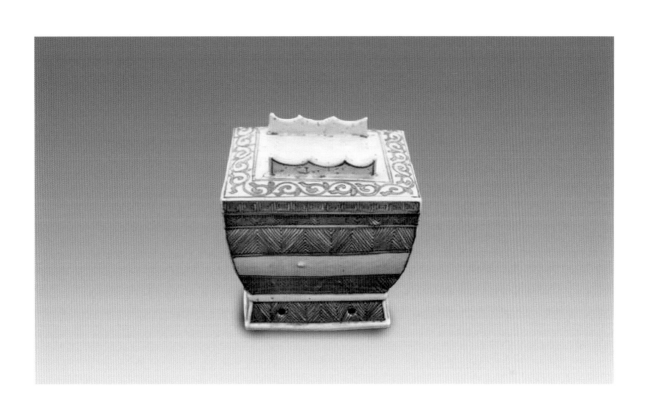

青花梯形药用瓷盒

清

瓷质

口外径 17.9 厘米，底径 16.8 厘米，带盖高 19.5 厘米，
重 2750 克

梯形瓷质药盒。用于存放易潮药物。

广东中医药博物馆藏

Ladder-type Blue-and-white Porcelain Case for Medicinal Purpose

Qing Dynasty

Porcelain

Mouth Outer Diameter 17.9 cm/ Bottom Diameter 16.8 cm/
Height (with the lid) 19.5 cm/ Weight 2,750 g

This ladder-type porcelain medicine case was used for storing the medicines which are easily affected by moisture.

Preserved in Guangdong Chinese Medicine Museum

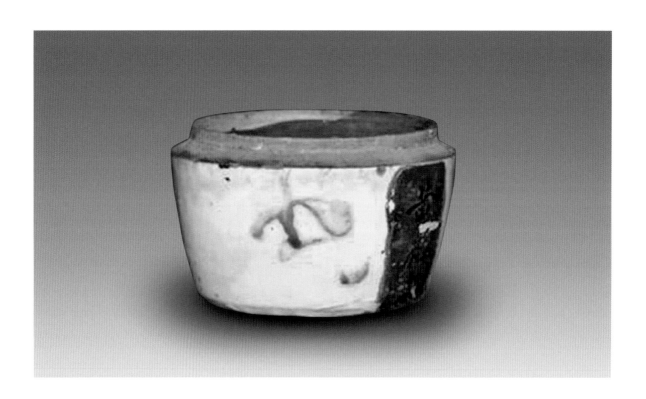

白瓷药盒

清

瓷质

口径 8.5 厘米，底径 7.5 厘米，通高 0.6 厘米，重 200 克

White Porcelain Medicine Case

Qing Dynasty

Porcelain

Mouth Diameter 8.5 cm/ Bottom Diameter 7.5 cm/ Height 0.6 cm/ Weight 200 g

白粗瓷，子母口，斜腹，圈足，腹绘小兰花图，药签名为"黄柏麦面"，无盖。贮药器具。陕西省西安市藻露堂中药店征集。

陕西医史博物馆藏

This grit white porcelain case has a snap lid, an oblique belly, and a ring foot. The body is adorned with motifs of tiny orchids and carries a label with the name of the drug "Huang Bai Mai Mian". This medicine container without a lid was collected from Zao Lu Tang Chinese Medicinal Herbs Store of Xi'an in Shaanxi Province.

Preserved in Shaanxi Museum of Medical History

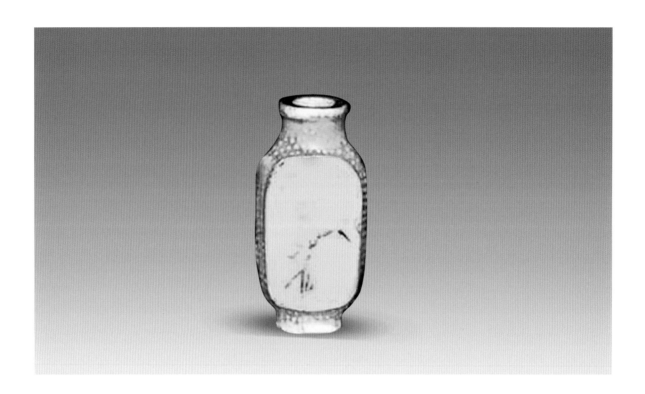

绿釉瓷药瓶

清

瓷质

口径 1.5 厘米，底径 1.5 厘米 ×1.1 厘米，高 5.3 厘米，重 20 克

Porcelain Medicine Bottle with Green Glaze

Qing Dynasty

Porcelain

Mouth Diameter 1.5 cm/ Bottom Diameter 1.5 cm×1.1cm/ Height 5.3 cm/ Weight 20 g

平口沿，扁腹，浅圈足，腹两侧为绿点釉，
腹面有彩色图案。药具。底略残。陕西省西
安市古玩市场征集。

陕西医史博物馆藏

This porcelain medicine bottle features a flat mouth
rim, an oblate belly, and a shallow ring foot. Green
spotted glaze are applied to both sides of the belly
and colourful patterns are painted on the front sides.
This medicine container with a slightly damaged
bottom was collected from the Antique Market in
Xi'an, Shaanxi Province.

Preserved in Shaanxi Museum of Medical History

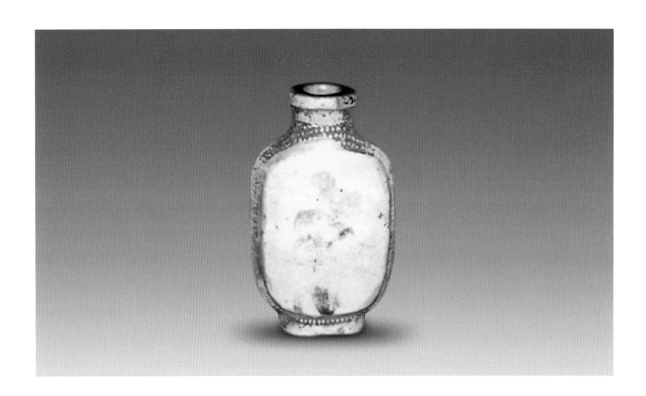

瓷药瓶

清

瓷质

口径 1.6 厘米，底径 1.9 厘米 ×1.3 厘米，高 5.7 厘米，重 23 克

Porcelain Medicine Bottle

Qing Dynasty

Porcelain

Mouth Diameter 1.6 cm/ Bottom Diameter 1.9 cm×1.3 cm/ Height 5.7 cm/ Weight 23 g

平口沿，扁腹，椭圆圈足，腹两侧为绿点釉，
腹两面有彩色图案。药具。底略残。陕西省
西安市古玩市场征集。

陕西医史博物馆藏

This porcelain medicine bottle features a flat mouth
rim, an oblate belly, and an oval ring foot. Green
spotted glaze are applied to both sides of the belly,
while colourful patterns are painted on the front
sides. This medicine container with a slightly
damaged bottom was collected from the Antique
Market in Xi'an, Shaanxi Province.

Preserved in Shaanxi Museum of Medical History

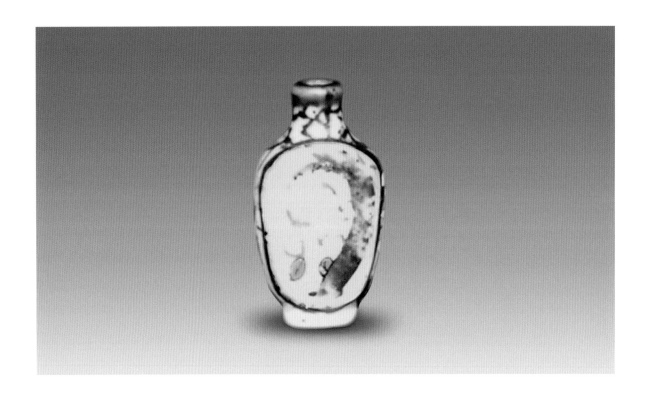

小瓷药瓶

清

瓷质

口径 1.6 厘米，底径 2 厘米，通高 6.8 厘米，重 50 克

直口，扁腹，圈足，两肩为青花缠枝纹，腹为釉里红。贮药器具。完整无损。

陕西医史博物馆藏

Small Porcelain Medicine Bottle

Qing Dynasty

Porcelain

Mouth Diameter 1.6 cm/ Bottom Diameter 2 cm/ Height 6.8 cm/ Weight 50 g

This small porcelain medicine bottle has a straight mouth, an oblate belly, and a ring foot. The shoulder is decorated with blue-and-white designs of interlocking branches, while the belly is coated with underglaze red. This medicine storage utensil is kept in good condition.

Preserved in Shaanxi Museum of Medical History

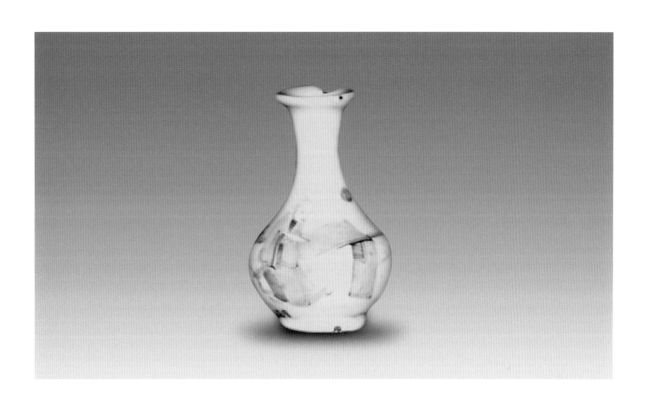

小瓷药瓶

清

瓷质

口径 2.8 厘米，底径 2.7 厘米，通高 7.5 厘米，

重 50 克

喇叭口，长颈，垂腹，圈足，腹上有一人物图案。

贮药器具。口沿小残。

陕西医史博物馆藏

Small Porcelain Medicine Bottle

Qing Dynasty

Porcelain

Mouth Diameter 2.8 cm/ Bottom Diameter 2.7 cm/

Height 7.5 cm/ Weight 50 g

This small porcelain medicine bottle has a trumpet mouth,

a long neck, a droop belly with portraiture designs, and a

ring foot. It was used as a medicine storage container and

the mouth rim was slightly damaged.

Preserved in Shaanxi Museum of Medical History

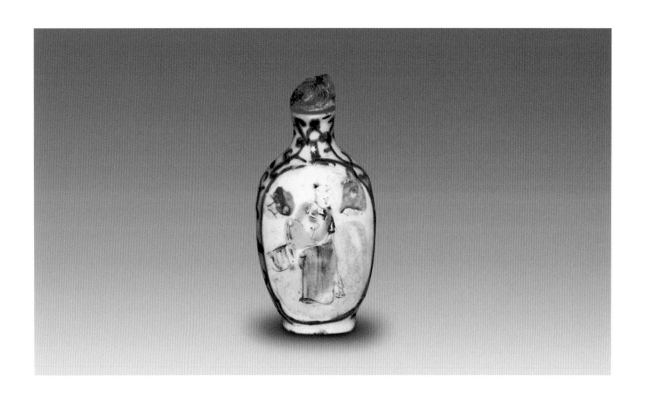

瓷药瓶

清

瓷质

口径 1.5 厘米，底径 1.8 厘米 ×2.6 厘米，高 7.6 厘米，重 40 克

Porcelain Medicine Bottle

Qing Dynasty

Porcelain

Mouth Diameter 1.5 cm/ Bottom Diameter 1.8 cm×2.6 cm/ Height 7.6 cm/ Weight 40 g

平口沿，扁腹，椭圆圈足，腹两侧为青花缠枝纹，腹两面为彩色人物图。药具。底略残。2001 年 9 月入藏，陕西省西安市古玩市场征集。

陕西医史博物馆藏

This porcelain medicine bottle features a flat mouth rim, an oblate belly, and an oval ring foot. Both sides of the belly are decorated with blue-and-white motifs of interlocking branches, while the front sides of the bottle are adorned with a colourful portraiture design. This medicine container with a slightly damaged bottom was collected from the Antique Market in Xi'an, Shaanxi Province, in September 2001.

Preserved in Shaanxi Museum of Medical History

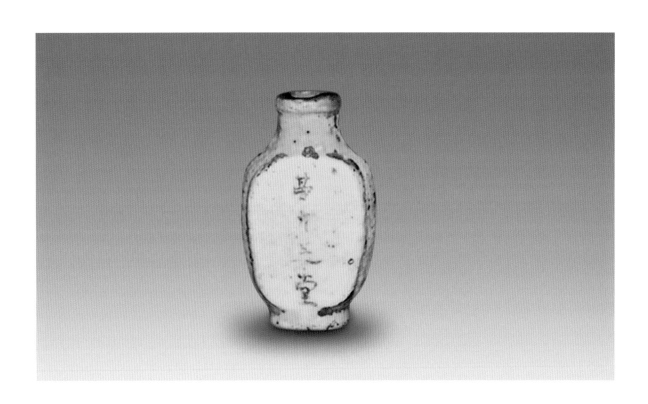

瓷药瓶

清

瓷质

口径 1.6 厘米，底径 1.9 厘米 ×1.4 厘米，高 5.5 厘米，重 25 克

Porcelain Medicine Bottle

Qing Dynasty

Porcelain

Mouth Diameter 1.6 cm/ Bottom Diameter 1.9 cm×1.4 cm/ Height 5.5 cm/ Weight 25 g

平口沿，扁腹，圈足，瓶颈和腹两侧施黄釉，

腹为白釉，一面有"□九芝堂"，一面有"□□

丹"字样。药具。口沿略残。2001年9月入藏，

陕西省西安市古玩市场征集。

陕西医史博物馆藏

This porcelain medicine bottle has a flat mouth rim,
an oblate belly, and a ring foot. The neck and lateral
sides of the belly are coated with yellow glaze while
the two front sides are white-glazed, one side of
which carries the name of the pharmacy " □ Jiu Zhi
Tang", with the name of the drug on the other side.
This medicine container with a slightly damaged
mouth rim was collected from the Antique Market in
Xi'an, Shaanxi Province, in September 2001.

Preserved in Shaanxi Museum of Medical History

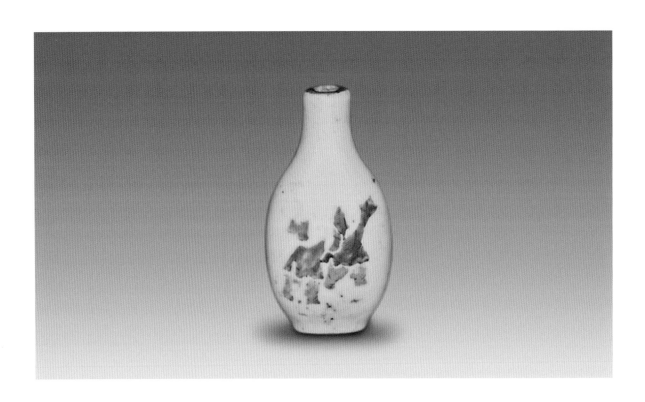

瓷药瓶

清

瓷质

口径 1.3 厘米，底径 1.1 厘米 ×2 厘米，高 6.5 厘米，重 41 克

Porcelain Medicine Bottle

Qing Dynasty

Porcelain

Mouth Diameter 1.3 cm/ Bottom Diameter 1.1 cm×2 cm/ Height 6.5 cm/ Weight 41 g

白瓷，直口，扁腹，椭圆圈足，腹有彩色人物图。
药具。完整无损。2001 年 9 月入藏，陕西省西
安市古玩市场征集。

陕西医史博物馆藏

This white porcelain medicine bottle has a straight mouth,
an oblate belly with colourful portraiture designs，
and an oval ring foot. This well-kept bottle was used as
a medical utensil, and was collected from the Antique
Market in Xi'an, Shaanxi Province, in September 2001.
Preserved in Shaanxi Museum of Medical History

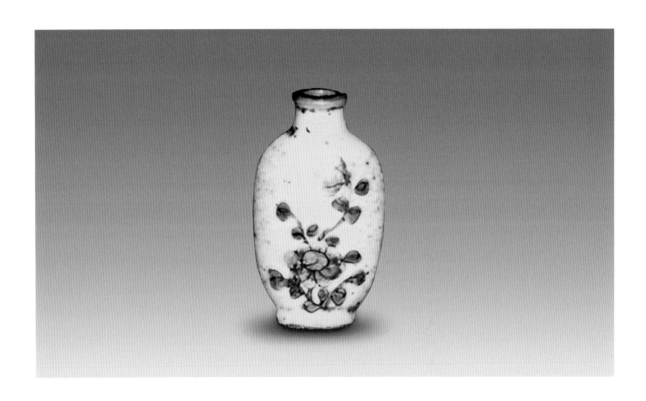

粉彩瓷药瓶

清

瓷质

口径 1.1 厘米，底径 2 厘米 × 1.2 厘米，高 5.6 厘米，重 23 克

Porcelain Medicine Bottle with Famille Rose Decoration

Qing Dynasty

Porcelain

Mouth Diameter 1.1 cm/ Bottom Diameter 2 cm×1.2 cm/ Height 5.6 cm/ Weight 23 g

平口沿，扁腹，浅圈足，腹一面有花卉图案，另一面有"只在此山中，言医不知处"，口沿施黄釉。药具。完整无损。2001年9月入藏，陕西省西安市古玩市场征集。

陕西医史博物馆藏

This porcelain medicine bottle has a yellow-glazed flat mouth rim, an oblate belly, and a shallow ring foot. One side of the belly is adorned with floral motifs, while on the other side are inscribed two lines of a verse. This well-kept bottle was used as a medical utensil, and it was collected from the Antique Market in Xi'an, Shaanxi Province, in September 2001.

Preserved in Shaanxi Museum of Medical History

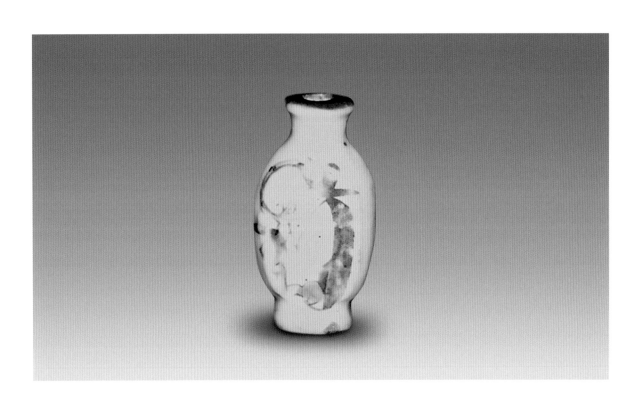

人物瓷药瓶

清

瓷质

口径 1.5 厘米，底径 1.8 厘米，高 5.3 厘米，重 22 克

平口沿，扁腹，浅圈足，腹部有一人物图案。药具。完整无损。2001 年 9 月入藏，陕西省西安市古玩市场征集。

陕西医史博物馆藏

Porcelain Medicine Bottle with Portraiture Design

Qing Dynasty

Porcelain

Mouth Diameter 1.5 cm/ Bottom Diameter 1.8 cm/ Height 5.3 cm/ Weight 22 g

This porcelain medicine bottle has a flat mouth rim, an oblate belly with a portraiture design, and a shallow ring foot. This well-kept bottle was used as a medical utensil, and it was collected from the Antique Market in Xi'an, Shaanxi Province, in September 2001.

Preserved in Shaanxi Museum of Medical History

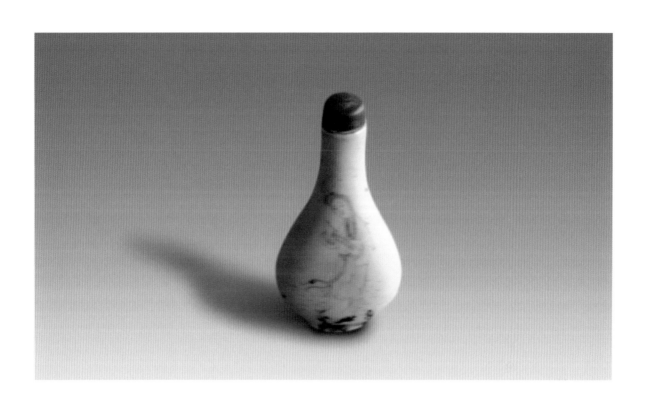

药瓶

清

瓷质

高 8.5 厘米

瓶身扁平呈葫芦状，白瓷上有刻画的人物图案，圈足。由民间征集。

成都中医药大学中医药传统文化博物馆藏

Medicine Bottle

Qing Dynasty

Porcelain

Height 8.5 cm

This white porcelain gourd-shaped bottle has an oblate belly incised with portraiture designs and a ring foot. The object was collected from a private owner.

Preserved in Museum of Traditional Chinese Medicine Culture, Chengdu University of Traditional Chinese Medicine

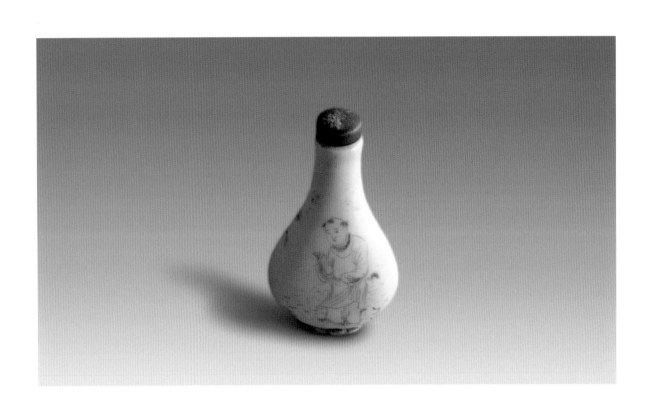

药瓶

清

瓷质

高 8.5 厘米

瓶身扁平呈葫芦状，直口，长颈，鼓腹，平底，圈足，白瓷上刻画着人物图案。由民间征集。

成都中医药大学中医药传统文化博物馆藏

Medicine Bottle

Qing Dynasty

Porcelain

Height 8.5cm

This bottle is oblate and in the shape of gourd. It has a straight mouth, a long neck, a drum-like belly, a flat bottom, and a ring foot. On the porcelain whiteware is carved a human figure pattern. It was collected from a private owner.

Preserved in Museum of Traditional Chinese Medicine Culture, Chengdu University of Traditional Chinese Medicine

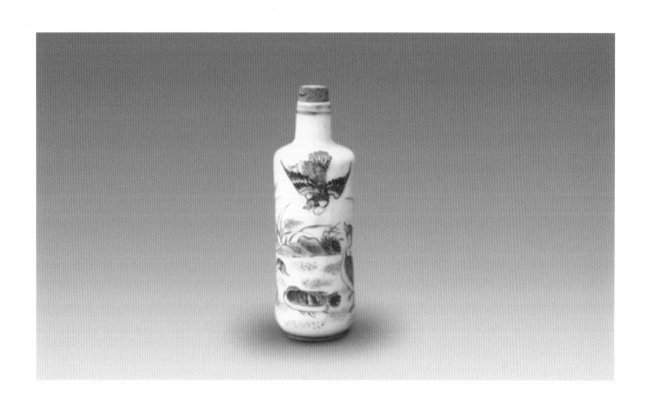

小药瓶

清

瓷质

口外径 1.2 厘米，腹径 2.7 厘米，底径 2.1 厘米，

通高 7.2 厘米

圆柱形，直口，长颈，溜肩，平底，圈足，瓶身

彩绘野鸭嬉戏图。用于装药。

广东中医药博物馆藏

Small Medicine Bottle

Qing Dynasty

Porcelain

Mouth Outer Diameter 1.2 cm/ Belly Diameter 2.7 cm/

Bottom Diameter 2.1 cm/ Height 7.2 cm

This small cylindrical bottle has a straight mouth, a long

neck, a sloping shoulder, a flat bottom, and a ring foot.

Patterns of ducks playing in the water decorates the body

of it. It was used for storing medicine.

Preserved in Guangdong Chinese Medicine Museum

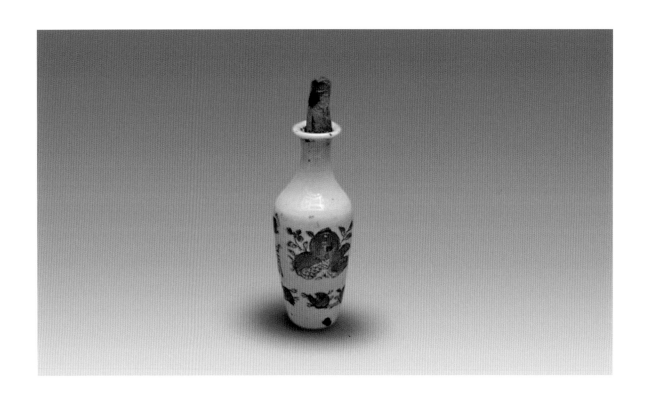

药瓶

清

瓷质

口径 4.5 厘米，高 12 厘米

Medicine Bottle

Qing Dynasty

Porcelain

Mouth Diameter 4.5 cm/ Height 12 cm

盘形口，细长颈，鼓肩，斜直腹，平底，施白釉，瓶身饰红色花果纹和寿字纹。盛装较小或粉状药物的用具。由民间征集。

成都中医药大学中医药传统文化博物馆藏

This white-glazed medicine bottle has a dish-shaped mouth, a long and thin neck, a drum-like shoulder, an oblique and straight belly, and a flat bottom. The body is adorned with red floral and fruit motifs, as well as the Chinese character "Shou" (longevity). The bottle was used for storing small-grained drugs or drug powder. It was collected from a private owner.

Preserved in Museum of Traditional Chinese Medicine Culture, Chengdu University of Traditional Chinese Medicine

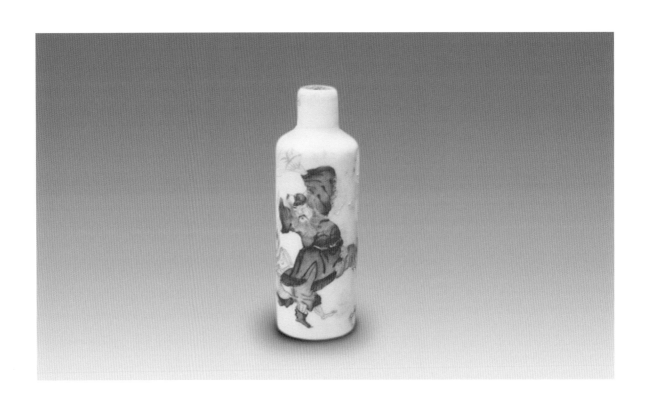

粉彩人物药瓶

清

瓷质

口径 1.36 厘米，底径 2.63 厘米，通高 7.45 厘米，

瓶身高 5.94 厘米，重 25 克

圆形，小口，绘粉彩一人物。装药用。

广东中医药博物馆藏

Medicine Bottle with Famille Rose Decoration of Portraiture

Qing Dynasty

Porcelain

Mouth Diameter 1.36 cm/ Bottom Diameter 2.63 cm/ Height 7.45 cm/ Body Height 5.94 cm/ Weight 25 g

This narrow-mouthed round bottle is adorned with a figure rendered in the famille rose colour. The bottle was used for storage of medicines.

Preserved in Guangdong Chinese Medicine Museum

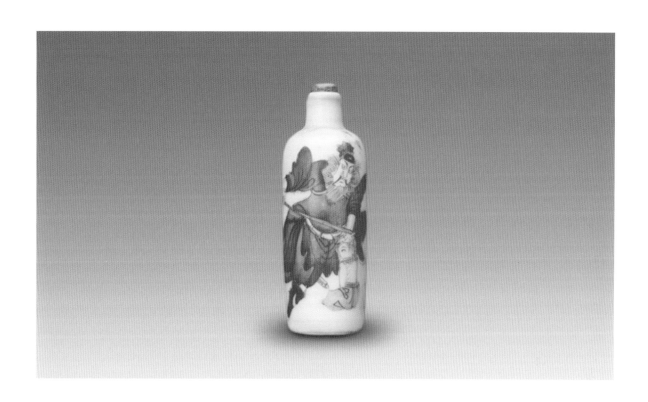

小药瓶

清

瓷质

口外径 1.1 厘米，腹径 2.4 厘米，底径 2.2 厘米，

通高 6.45 厘米，重 14 克

圆柱形，直口，长颈，溜肩，直腹，平底，圈足，

瓶身彩绘人像。用于装药。

广东中医药博物馆藏

Small Medicine Bottle

Qing Dynasty

Porcelain

Mouth Outer Diameter 1.1 cm/ Belly Diameter 2.4 cm/
Bottom Diameter 2.2 cm/ Height 6.45 cm/ Weight 14 g

This cylindrical small bottle with a painted figure has a straight mouth, a long neck, a sloping shoulder, a straight belly, a flat bottom, and a ring foot. It was used for storing medicine.

Preserved in Guangdong Chinese Medicine Museum

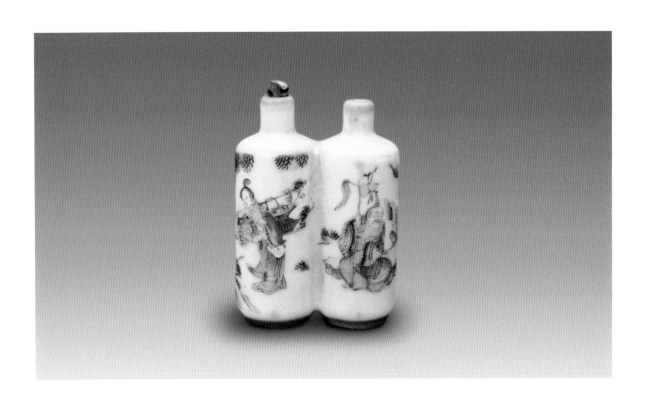

粉彩人物联珠药瓶

清

瓷质

口外径 1.05 厘米，腹径 2.66 厘米，通高 6.9 厘米，
腹深 6.2 厘米，重 75 克

圆柱形，细直颈，圈足，瓶身彩绘人物像。用于
装药。

广东中医药博物馆藏

A Pair of Medicine Bottle with Famille Rose Decoration of Portraiture

Qing Dynasty

Porcelain

Mouth Outer Diameter 1.05 cm/ Belly Diameter 2.66 cm/
Height 6.9 cm/ Belly Depth 6.2 cm/ Weight 75 g

This pair of cylindrical bottles feature straight and thin
necks, bellies adorned with painted figures and ring feet.
They were used for storing medicine.

Preserved in Guangdong Chinese Medicine Museum

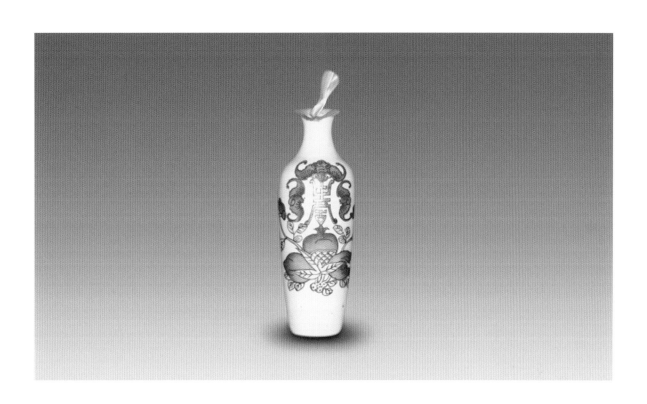

瓷药瓶

清

瓷质

口径 3 厘米，底径 3.5 厘米，通高 15 厘米，重 200 克

白瓷，喇叭口，长颈，斜腹，圈足，腹饰红花寿桃奉寿图。贮药器具。口沿有残。

陕西医史博物馆藏

Porcelain Medicine Bottle

Qing Dynasty

Porcelain

Mouth Diameter 3 cm/ Bottom Diameter 3.5 cm/ Height 15 cm/ Weight 200 g

This white porcelain medicine bottle has a trumpet-shaped mouth, a long neck, an oblique belly, and a ring foot. The belly is adorned with patterns of red flowers and peaches commonly given as birthday gifts to the elderly. It was used as a medicine storage container with the mouth rim cracked.

Preserved in Shaanxi Museum of Medical History

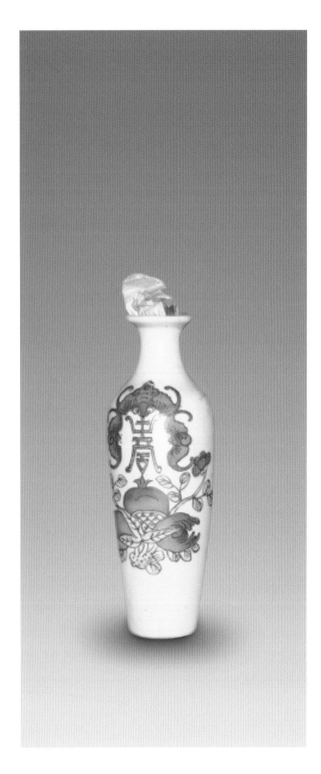

瓷药瓶

清

瓷质

口径 3 厘米，底径 3.5 厘米，通高 15 厘米，重
200 克

白瓷，喇叭口，斜腹，圈足，腹饰红花寿桃奉寿
图。贮药器具。完整无损。

陕西医史博物馆藏

Porcelain Medicine Bottle

Qing Dynasty

Porcelain

Mouth Diameter 3 cm/ Bottom Diameter 3.5 cm/ Height
15 cm/ Weight 200 g

This white porcelain medicine bottle has a trumpet-
shaped mouth, an oblique belly, and a ring foot. The
belly is adored with patterns of red flowers and peaches
commonly given as birthday gifts to the elderly. It was
used as a medicine storage container. It is kept in good
condition.

Preserved in Shaanxi Museum of Medical History

瓷药瓶

清

瓷质

口径 3.6 厘米，底径 3.2 厘米，通高 12 厘米，
重 100 克

喇叭口，圆肩，斜腹，圈足，腹饰母子两人乘凉
图。贮药器具。完整无损。

陕西医史博物馆藏

Porcelain Medicine Bottle

Qing Dynasty

Porcelain

Mouth Diameter 3.6 cm/ Bottom Diameter 3.2 cm/
Height 12 cm/ Weight 100 g

This medicine bottle has a trumpet-shaped mouth, a
rounded shoulder, an oblique belly, and a ring foot. The
belly is adorned with a portrait of a mother and her son
resting under the shade of the trees. The bottle was used
as a medicine storage container, and is kept in good
condition.

Preserved in Shaanxi Museum of Medical History

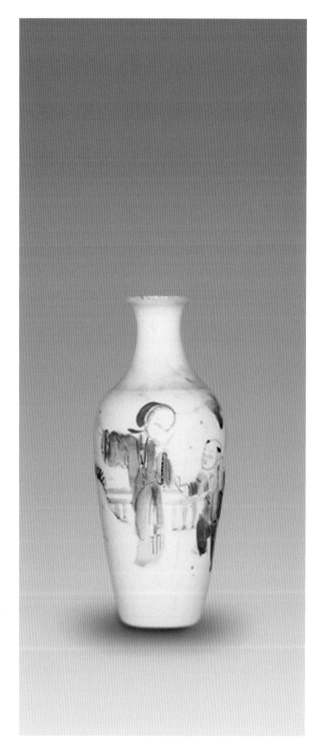

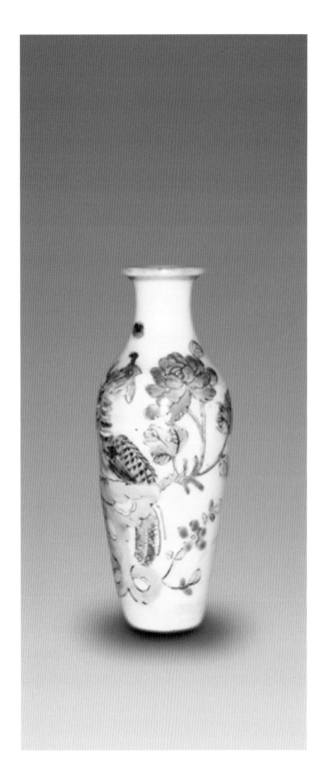

瓷药瓶

清

瓷质

口径 3.5 厘米，底径 3 厘米，通高 12 厘米，重
150 克

白瓷，喇叭口，圆肩，斜腹，圈足，表面饰彩绘
凤鸟、牡丹纹。贮药器具。完整无损。

陕西医史博物馆藏

Porcelain Medicine Bottle

Qing Dynasty

Porcelain

Mouth Diameter 3.5 cm/ Bottom Diameter 3 cm/ Height
12 cm/ Weight 150 g

This white porcelain bottle has a trumpet-shaped mouth,
a rounded shoulder, an oblique belly, and a ring foot. The
bottle is patterned with birds and peonies. The bottle was
used as a medicine storage container, and is kept in good
condition.

Preserved in Shaanxi Museum of Medical History

瓷药瓶

清

瓷质

口径 3.5 厘米，底径 2.8 厘米，通高 11.5 厘米，
重 150 克

白瓷，喇叭口，圆肩，斜腹，圈足，彩绘中有"喜"
字。贮药器具。完整无损。

陕西医史博物馆藏

Porcelain Medicine Bottle

Qing Dynasty

Porcelain

Mouth Diameter 3.5 cm/ Bottom Diameter 2.8 cm/
Height 11.5 cm/ Weight 150 g

This white porcelain bottle has a trumpet-shaped mouth,
a rounded shoulder, an oblique belly, and a ring foot.
The bottle is adorned with painted designs and a Chinese
character "Xi" (happiness). The bottle was used as a
medicine storage container, and is kept in good condition.

Preserved in Shaanxi Museum of Medical History

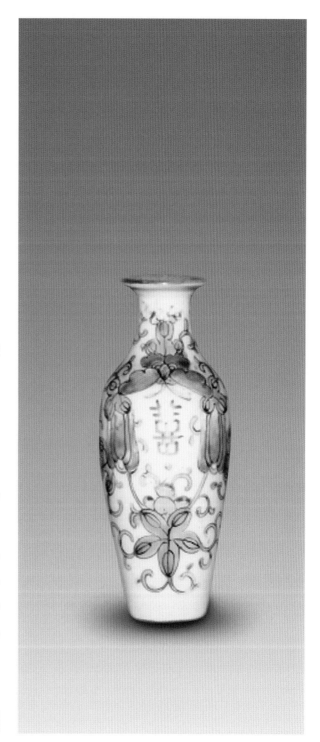

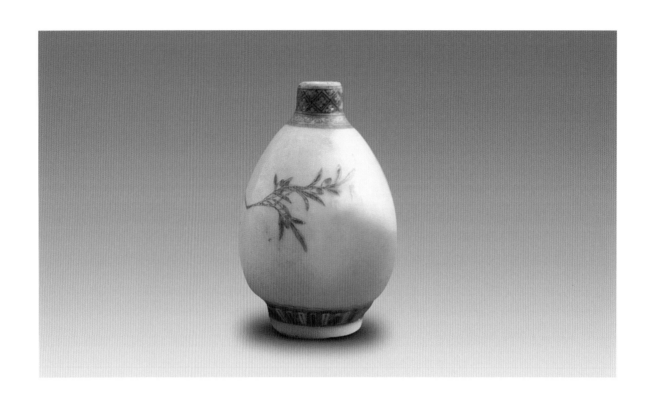

小药瓶

清

瓷质

口外径 1.1 厘米，腹径 4.15 厘米，底径 2.4 厘米，通高 6.3 厘米，重 55 克

Small Medicine Bottle

Qing Dynasty

Porcelain

Mouth Outer Diameter 1.1 cm/ Belly Diameter 4.15 cm/ Bottom Diameter 2.4 cm/ Height 6.3 cm/ Weight 55 g

直口，平沿，竖颈，颈部绘菱形纹，内绘四瓣小花，溜肩，肩上绘卷云纹，鼓腹，腹部绘植物一枝，腹渐收至底，平底，圈足。用于装药。

广东中医药博物馆藏

This small porcelain medicine bottle has a straight mouth, a flat mouth rim, a straight neck, a sloping shoulder, a drum-like belly, a flat bottom, and a ring foot. Its neck is patterned with rhombus, within which are painted flowers with four petals. Circus clouds are painted on its shoulder. A branch of plant is on its belly, which narrows down to the bottom. It was used for storing medicine.

Preserved in Guangdong Chinese Medicine Museum

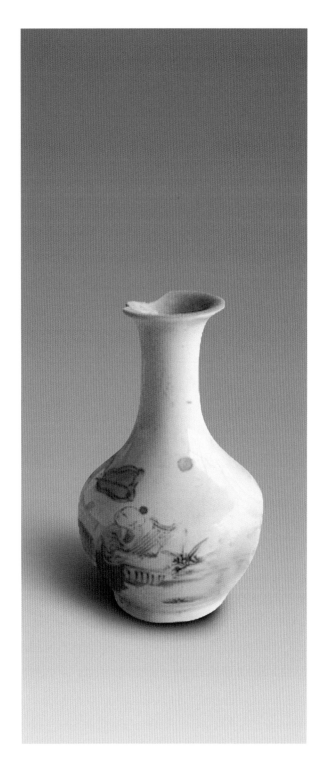

药瓶

清

瓷质

口径 4 厘米，底径 4.5 厘米，高 12 厘米

Medicine Bottle

Qing Dynasty

Porcelain

Mouth Diameter 4 cm/ Bottom Diameter 4.5 cm/

Height 12 cm

颈较长，圆鼓腹，浅圈足，腹饰五彩童子踏
青图。口部残。由民间征集。

　　成都中医药大学中医药传统文化博物馆藏

This medicine bottle featuring a long neck, a round
and drum-like belly, and a shallow ring foot, is
adorned with polychrome motifs showing a child
hiking. The bottle with the mouth broken was
collected from a private owner.

Preserved in Museum of Traditional Chinese
Medicine Culture, Chengdu University of Traditional
Chinese Medicine

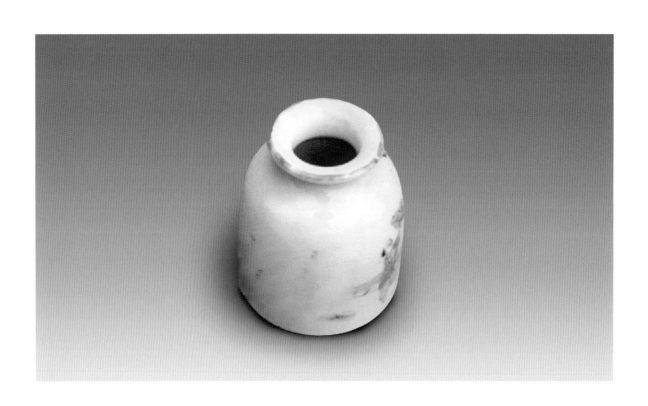

小药瓶

清

瓷质

口外径 3.4 厘米，底径 5.4 厘米，通高 5.9 厘米，

腹深 5.4 厘米，重 77 克

粉彩，盘口，口沿绘金色圈，束颈，腹部近似圆

柱形，上稍窄，小圈足。盛细碎物品容器。

广东中医药博物馆藏

Small Medicine Bottle

Qing dynasty

Porcelain

Mouth Outer Diameter 3.4 cm/ Bottom Diameter 5.4 cm/
Height 5.9 cm/ Belly Depth 5.4 cm/ Weight 77 g

This famille-rose bottle features a dish-shaped mouth, a
mouth rim painted in gold, a contracted neck, a cylinder-
shaped belly which is narrower at the top, and a small ring
foot. The bottle was used for storing small items.

Preserved in Guangdong Chinese Medicine Museum

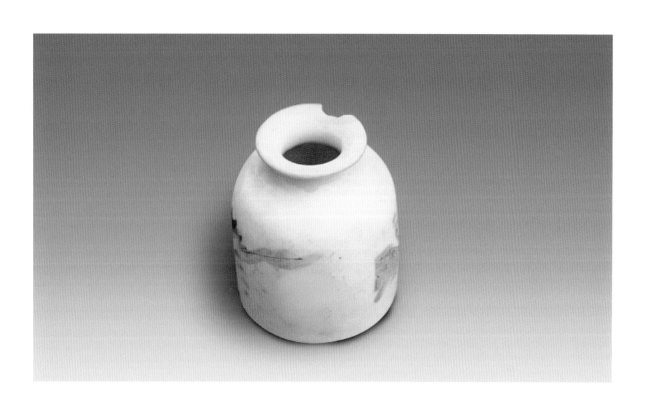

小药瓶

清

瓷质

口外径 3.9 厘米，底径 6.5 厘米，通高 7.5 厘米，
腹深 6.8 厘米，重 132 克

粉彩，盘口，束颈，腹部近似圆柱形，腹上部稍
收，小圈足。盛细碎药物容器。口沿有残。

广东中医药博物馆藏

Small Medicine Bottle

Qing Dynasty

Porcelain

Mouth Outer Diameter 3.9 cm/ Bottom Diameter 6.5 cm/
Height 7.5 cm/ Belly Depth 6.8 cm/ Weight 132 g

This famille-rose bottle features a dish-shaped mouth
with one part broken, a contracted neck, a cylinder-
shaped belly which is narrower at the top, and a small
ring foot. It was used for storing small-grained medicine.

Preserved in Guangdong Chinese Medicine Museum

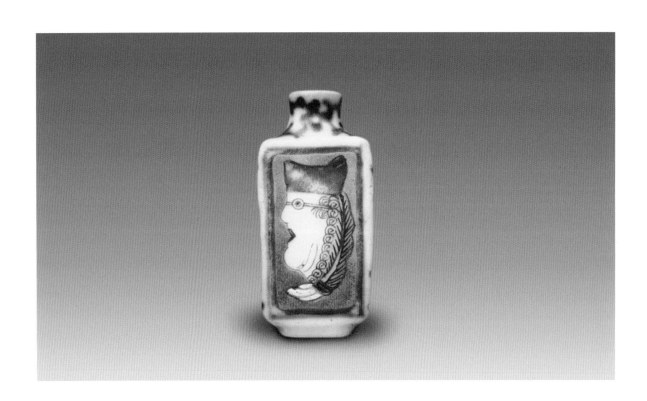

小药瓶

清

瓷质

口外径 1.35 厘米，腹径 2.2 厘米，底径 1.8 厘米，通高 5 厘米，重 22 克

Small Medicine Bottle

Qing Dynasty

Porcelain

Mouth Outer Diameter 1.35 cm/ Belly Diameter 2.2 cm/ Bottom Diameter 1.8 cm/ Height 5 cm/ Weight 22 g

长方体，直口，平沿，溜肩，平底，腹绘彩
色人头像。用于装药。

广东中医药博物馆藏

This medicine bottle has a straight mouth, a flat
mouth rim, a sloping shoulder, and a flat bottom. It
is rectangular and adorned with a portrait of a human
face. It was used for storing medicine.

Preserved in Guangdong Chinese Medicine Museum

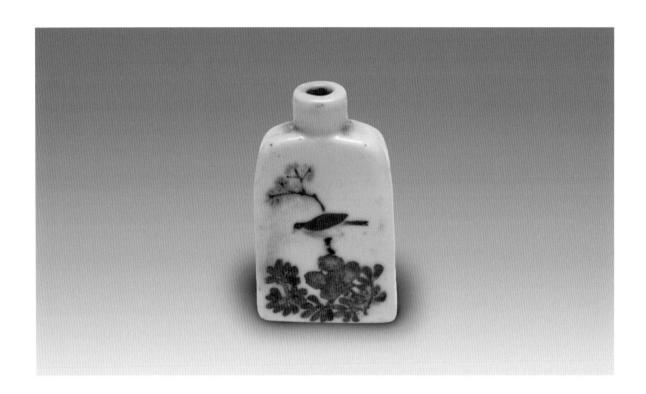

药瓶

清

瓷质

口径 1.5 厘米，宽 4.2 厘米，厚 1.9 厘米，高 7 厘米

Medicine Bottle

Qing Dynasty

Porcelain

Mouth Diameter 1.5 cm/ Width 4.2 cm/ Thickness 1.9 cm/ Height 7 cm

器形呈扁平状，圆井形口，腹部为上小下大的梯形，平底，腹饰有彩绘花鸟图案，颜色较暗，腹侧有墨书文字，造型匀称，线条流畅。盛装小型药物的用具。保存完好。

成都中医药大学中医药传统文化博物馆藏

This oblate bottle has a well-shaped round mouth, a ladder-shaped belly which is narrow at the top and wide at the flat bottom. The belly is decorated with painted flowers and birds patterns in dark colour. Some Chinese characters are found on the side of the belly. This well-proportioned bottle with smooth lines was used as a container for small pills. It is kept in good condition.

Preserved in Museum of Traditional Chinese Medicine Culture, Chengdu University of Traditional Chinese Medicine

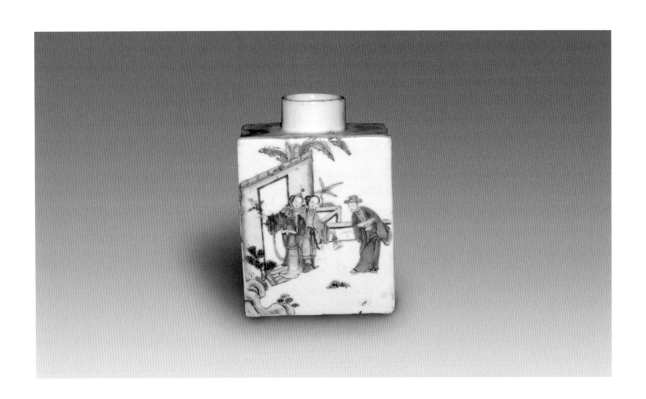

方瓷瓶

清

瓷质

口径 4 厘米，底径 9.1 厘米，通高 12.5 厘米，重 400 克

Rectangular Porcelain Bottle

Qing Dynasty

Porcelain

Mouth Diameter 4 cm/ Bottom Diameter 9.1 cm/ Height 12.5 cm/ Weight 400 g

直口，长方形腹，平底，四面彩绘，正面为
人物图。贮药器具。完整无损。

陕西医史博物馆藏

This rectangular porcelain bottle has a straight mouth,
a rectangular belly, and a flat bottom. This bottle has
designs painted on four sides and portraiture designs
on the front side. The bottle was used as a storage
utensil, and is kept in good condition.

Preserved in Shaanxi Museum of Medical History

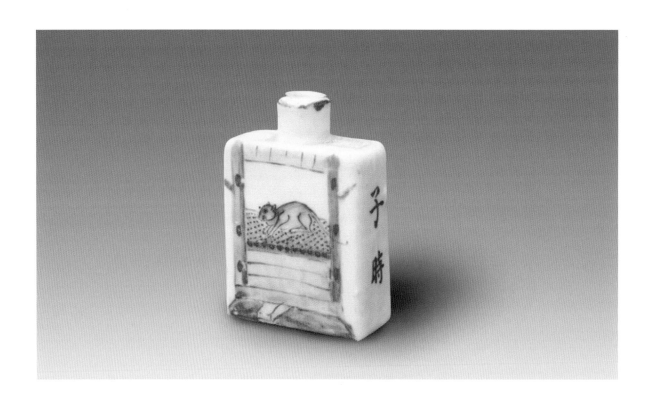

十二时辰方形小药瓶（子时）

清

瓷质

口外径 1.59 厘米，通高 6.66 厘米，瓶身长 4.67 厘米，瓶身宽 2.23 厘米，瓶身高 5.37 厘米，重 65 克

Small Rectangular Medicine Bottle (Zi Shi)

Qing Dynasty

Porcelain

Mouth Outer Diameter 1.59 cm/ Height 6.66 cm/ Body Length 4.67 cm/ Body Width 2.23 cm/ Body Height 5.37 cm/ Weight 65 g

一套十二件，长方形，平口，细颈，平底，

侧面书有"子时"，正面绘子鼠像。盛药用。

广东中医药博物馆藏

This medicine bottle is one piece of a medicine

bottle set, which has twelve pieces. It is rectangular

and has a flat mouth, a thin neck and a flat bottom.

On the side surface are inscribed Chinese characters

"Zi Shi" (or midnight time, which is the first of the

twelve time periods, i.e. from 23∶00 to 01∶00) and

the front side is adorned with a rat design (one of the

twelve zodiacs). It was used for storing medicine.

Preserved in Guangdong Chinese Medicine Museum

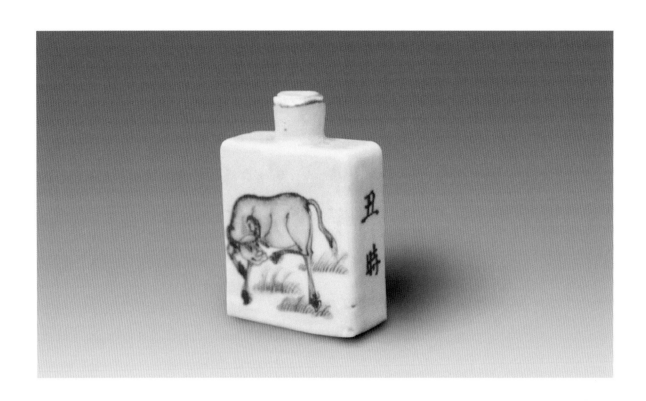

十二时辰方形小药瓶（丑时）

清

瓷质

口外径 1.55 厘米，通高 6.69 厘米，瓶身长 4.69 厘米，瓶身宽 2.02 厘米，瓶身高 5.4 厘米，重 60 克

Small Rectangular Medicine Bottle (Chou Shi)

Qing Dynasty

Porcelain

Mouth Outer Diameter 1.55 cm/ Height 6.69 cm/ Body Length 4.69 cm/ Body Width 2.02 cm/ Body Height 5.4 cm/ Weight 60 g

一套十二件，长方形，平口，细颈，平底，
侧面书有"丑时"，正面绘丑牛像。盛药用。

广东中医药博物馆藏

This medicine bottle is one piece of a medicine bottle
set, which has twelve pieces. It is rectangular and has
a flat mouth, a thin neck and a flat bottom. On the
side surface are inscribed Chinese characters "Chou
Shi" (which is the second time segment of the twelve
time periods, i.e. from 01 : 00 to 03 : 00 am) and the
front side is adorned with an ox design (one of the
twelve zodiacs). It was used for storing medicine.
Preserved in Guangdong Chinese Medicine Museum

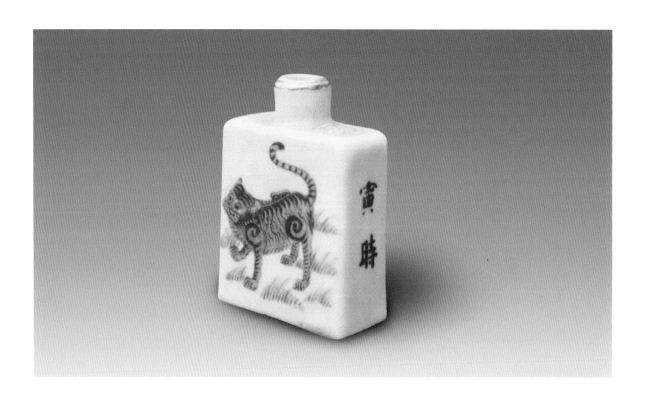

十二时辰方形小药瓶（寅时）

清

瓷质

口外径 1.52 厘米，通高 6.6 厘米，瓶身长 4.52 厘米，瓶身宽 2.2 厘米，瓶身高 5.35 厘米，重 65 克

Small Rectangular Medicine Bottle (Yin Shi)

Qing Dynasty

Porcelain

Mouth Outer Diameter 1.52 cm/ Height 6.6 cm/ Body Length 4.52 cm/ Body Width 2.2 cm/ Body Height 5.35 cm/ Weight 65 g

一套十二件，长方形，平口，细颈，平底，

侧面书有"寅时"，正面绘寅虎像。盛药用。

广东中医药博物馆藏

This medicine bottle is one piece of a medicine bottle

set, which has twelve pieces. It is rectangular and has

a flat mouth, a thin neck and a flat bottom. On the

side surface are inscribed Chinese characters "Yin

Shi" (which is the third time segment of the twelve

time periods, i.e. from 03 : 00 to 05 : 00 am) and the

front side is adorned with a tiger design (one of the

twelve zodiacs). It was used for storing medicine.

Preserved in Guangdong Chinese Medicine Museum

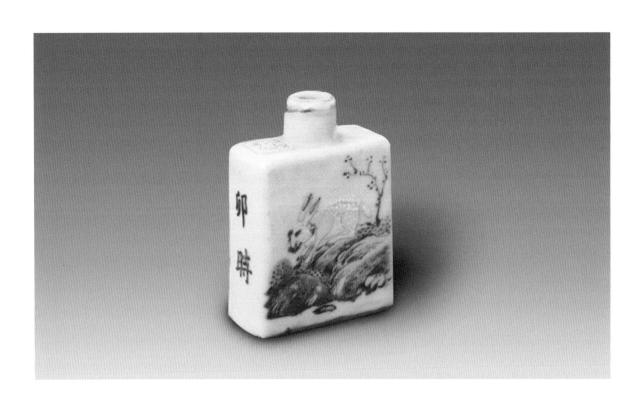

十二时辰方形小药瓶（卯时）

清

瓷质

口外径 1.55 厘米，通高 6.64 厘米，瓶身长 4.57 厘米，瓶身宽 2.14 厘米，瓶身高 5.35 厘米，重 62.5 克

Small Rectangular Medicine Bottle (Mao Shi)

Qing Dynasty

Porcelain

Mouth Outer Diameter 1.55 cm/ Height 6.64 cm/ Body Length 4.57 cm/ Body Width 2.14 cm/ Body Height 5.35 cm/ Weight 62.5 g

一套十二件，长方形，平口，细颈，平底，

侧面书有"卯时"，正面绘卯兔像。盛药用。

广东中医药博物馆藏

This medicine bottle is one piece of a medicine bottle
set, which has twelve pieces. It is rectangular and has
a flat mouth, a thin neck and a flat bottom. On the
side surface are inscribed Chinese characters "Mao
Shi" (which is the fourth time segment of the twelve
time periods, i.e. from 05：00 to 07：00 am) and the
front side is adorned with a rabbit design (one of the
twelve zodiacs). It was used for storing medicine.

Preserved in Guangdong Chinese Medicine Museum

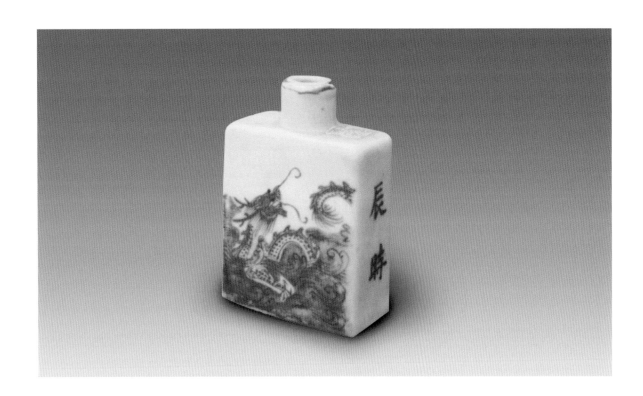

十二时辰方形小药瓶（辰时）

清

瓷质

口外径 1.55 厘米，通高 6.62 厘米，瓶身长 4.59 厘米，瓶身宽 2.14 厘米，瓶身高 5.32 厘米，重 62.5 克

Small Rectangular Medicine Bottle (Chen Shi)

Qing Dynasty

Porcelain

Mouth Outer Diameter 1.55 cm/ Height 6.62 cm/ Body Length 4.59 cm/ Body Width 2.14 cm/ Body Height 5.32 cm/ Weight 62.5 g

一套十二件，长方形，平口，细颈，平底，
侧面书有"辰时"，正面绘辰龙像。盛药用。

广东中医药博物馆藏

This medicine bottle is one piece of a medicine bottle
set, which has twelve pieces. It is rectangular and has
a flat mouth, a thin neck and a flat bottom. On the
side surface are inscribed Chinese characters "Chen
Shi" (which is the fifth time segment of the twelve
time periods, i.e. from 07:00 to 09:00 am) and the
front side is adorned with a dragon design (one of the
twelve zodiacs). It was used for storing medicine.

Preserved in Guangdong Chinese Medicine Museum

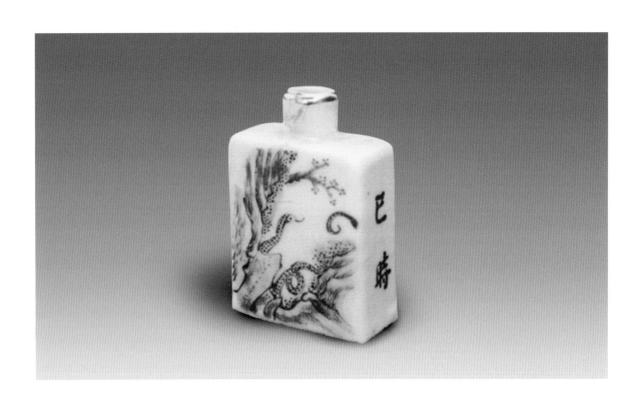

十二时辰方形小药瓶（巳时）

清

瓷质

口外径 1.62 厘米，通高 6.63 厘米，瓶身长 4.59 厘米，瓶身宽 2.19 厘米，瓶身高 5.42 厘米，重 62.5 克

Small Rectangular Medicine Bottle (Si Shi)

Qing Dynasty

Porcelain

Mouth Outer Diameter 1.62 cm/ Height 6.63 cm/ Body Length 4.59 cm/ Body Width 2.19 cm/ Body Height 5.42 cm/ Weight 62.5 g

一套十二件，长方形，平口，细颈，平底，

侧面书有"巳时"，正面绘巳蛇像。盛药用。

广东中医药博物馆藏

This medicine bottle is one piece of a medicine bottle set, which has twelve pieces. It is rectangular and has a flat mouth, a thin neck and a flat bottom. On the side surface are inscribed Chinese characters "Si Shi" (which is the sixth time segment of the twelve time periods, i.e. from 09∶00 to 11∶00 am) and the front side is adorned with a snake design (one of the twelve zodiacs). It was used for storing medicine.

Preserved in Guangdong Chinese Medicine Museum

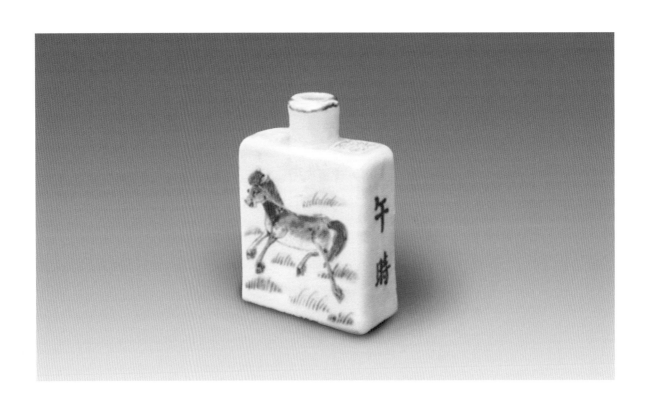

十二时辰方形小药瓶（午时）

清

瓷质

口外径 1.61 厘米，通高 6.24 厘米，瓶身长 4.61 厘米，瓶身宽 2.05 厘米，瓶身高 5.43 厘米，重 60 克

Small Rectangular Medicine Bottle (Wu Shi)

Qing Dynasty

Porcelain

Mouth Outer Diameter 1.61 cm/ Height 6.24 cm/ Body Length 4.61 cm/ Body Width 2.05 cm/ Body Height 5.43 cm/
Weight 60 g

一套十二件，长方形，平口，细颈，平底，

侧面书有"午时"，正面绘午马像。盛药用。

广东中医药博物馆藏

This medicine bottle is one piece of a medicine

bottle set, which has twelve pieces. It is rectangular

and has a flat mouth, a thin neck and a flat bottom.

On the side surface are inscribed Chinese characters

"Wu Shi" (which is the seventh time segment of the

twelve time periods, i.e. from 11 : 00 to 13 : 00) and

the front side is adorned with a horse design (one of

the twelve zodiacs). It was used for storing medicine.

Preserved in Guangdong Chinese Medicine Museum

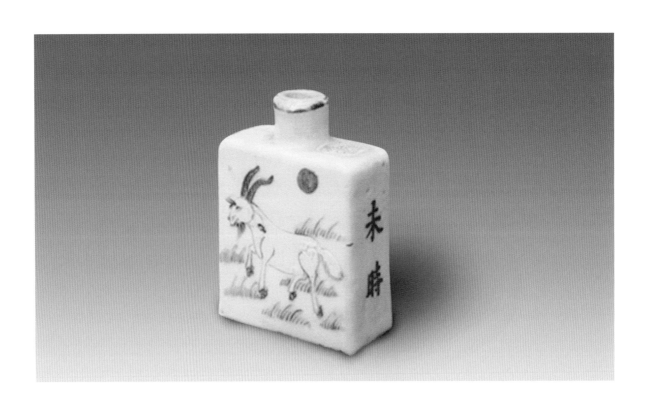

十二时辰方形小药瓶（未时）

清

瓷质

口外径 1.6 厘米，通高 6.51 厘米，瓶身长 4.55 厘米，瓶身宽 2.15 厘米，瓶身高 5.33 厘米，重 65 克

Small Rectangular Medicine Bottle (Wei Shi)

Qing Dynasty

Porcelain

Mouth Outer Diameter 1.6 cm/ Height 6.51 cm/ Body Length 4.55 cm/ Body Width 2.15 cm/ Body Height 5.33 cm/ Weight 65 g

一套十二件，长方形，平口，细颈，平底，

侧面书有"未时"，正面绘未羊像。盛药用。

广东中医药博物馆藏

This medicine bottle is one piece of a medicine bottle set, which has twelve pieces. It is rectangular and a flat mouth, a thin neck and a flat bottom. On the side surface are inscribed Chinese characters "Wei Shi" (which is the eighth time segment of the twelve time periods, i.e. from 13:00 to 15:00) and the front side is adorned with a sheep design (one of the twelve zodiacs). It was used for storing medicine.

Preserved in Guangdong Chinese Medicine Museum

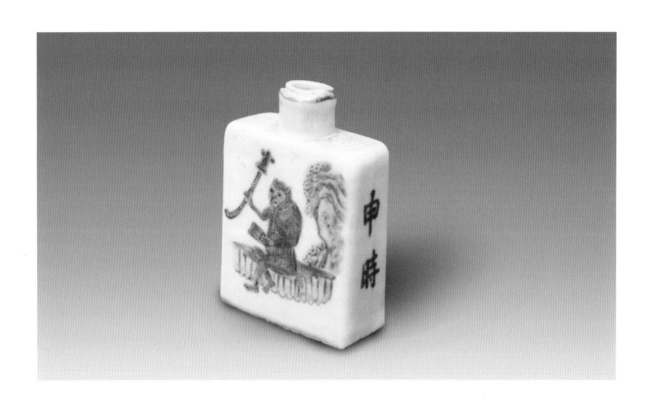

十二时辰方形小药瓶（申时）

清

瓷质

口外径 1.51 厘米，通高 6.59 厘米，瓶身长 4.56 厘米，瓶身宽 2.01 厘米，瓶身高 5.32 厘米，重 62.5 克

Small Rectangular Medicine Bottle (Shen Shi)

Qing Dynasty

Porcelain

Mouth Outer Diameter 1.51 cm/ Height 6.59 cm/ Body Length 4.56 cm/ Body Width 2.01 cm/ Body Height 5.32 cm/ Weight 62.5 g

一套十二件，长方形，平口，细颈，平底，

侧面书有"申时"，正面绘申猴像。盛药用。

广东中医药博物馆藏

This medicine bottle is one piece of a medicine bottle

set, which has twelve pieces. It is rectangular and a

flat mouth, a thin neck and a flat bottom. On the side

surface are inscribed Chinese characters "Shen Shi"

(which is the ninth time segment of the twelve time

periods, i.e. from 15：00 to 17：00) and the front side

is adorned with a monkey design (one of the twelve

zodiacs). It was used for storing medicine.

Preserved in Guangdong Chinese Medicine Museum

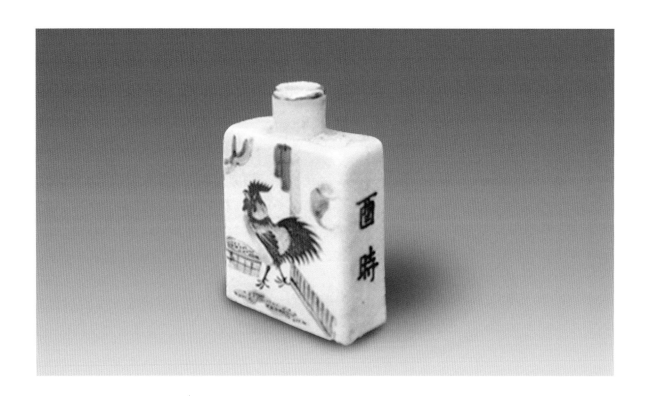

十二时辰方形小药瓶（酉时）

清

瓷质

口外径 1.64 厘米，通高 6.64 厘米，瓶身长 4.73 厘米，瓶身宽 2.04 厘米，瓶身高 5.44 厘米，重 60 克

Small Rectangular Medicine Bottle (You Shi)

Qing Dynasty

Porcelain

Mouth Outer Diameter 1.64 cm/ Height 6.64 cm/ Body Length 4.73 cm/ Body Width 2.04 cm/ Body Height 5.44 cm/

Weight 60 g

一套十二件，长方形，平口，细颈，平底，
侧面书有"酉时"，正面绘酉鸡像。盛药用。

广东中医药博物馆藏

This medicine bottle is one piece of a medicine bottle set, which has twelve pieces. It is rectangular and has a flat mouth, a thin neck and a flat bottom. On the side surface are inscribed Chinese characters "You Shi" (which is the tenth time segment of the twelve time periods, i.e. from 17:00 to 19:00) and the front side is adorned with a rooster design (one of the twelve zodiacs). It was used for storing medicine.

Preserved in Guangdong Chinese Medicine Museum

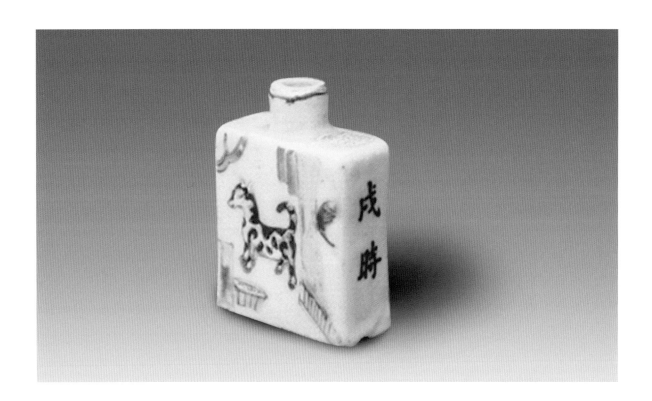

十二时辰方形小药瓶 (戌时)

清

瓷质

口外径 1.62 厘米，通高 6.59 厘米，瓶身长 4.57 厘米，瓶身宽 2.2 厘米，瓶身高 5.42 厘米，重 60 克

Small Rectangular Medicine Bottle (Xu Shi)

Qing Dynasty

Porcelain

Mouth Outer Diameter 1.62 cm/ Height 6.59 cm/ Body Length 4.57 cm/ Body Width 2.2 cm/ Body Height 5.42 cm/ Weight 60 g

一套十二件，长方形，平口，细颈，平底，侧面书有"戌时"，正面绘戌狗像。盛药用。

广东中医药博物馆藏

This medicine bottle is one piece of a medicine bottle set, which has twelve pieces. It is rectangular and has a flat mouth, a thin neck and a flat bottom. On the side surface are inscribed Chinese characters "Xu Shi" (which is the eleventh time segment of the twelve time periods, i.e. from 19:00 to 21:00) and the front side is adorned with a dog design (one of the twelve zodiacs). It was used for storing medicine. Preserved in Guangdong Chinese Medicine Museum

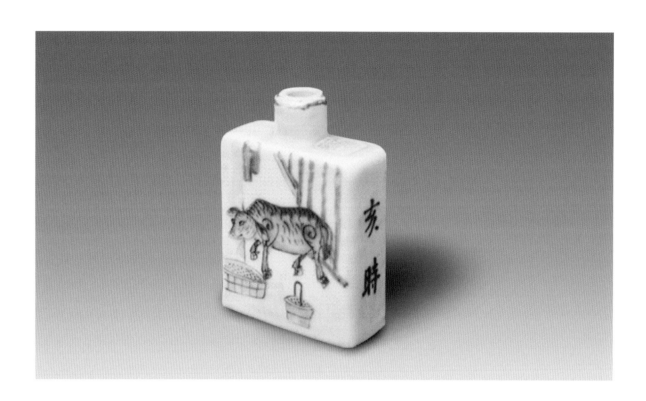

十二时辰方形小药瓶（亥时）

清

瓷质

口外径 1.51 厘米，通高 6.53 厘米，瓶身长 4.54 厘米，瓶身宽 1.96 厘米，瓶身高 5.35 厘米，重 60 克

Small Rectangular Medicine Bottle (Hai Shi)

Qing Dynasty

Porcelain

Mouth Outer Diameter 1.51 cm/ Height 6.53 cm/ Body Length 4.54 cm/ Body Width 1.96 cm/ Body Height 5.35 cm/ Weight 60 g

一套十二件，长方形，平口，细颈，平底，

侧面书有"亥时"，正面绘亥猪像。盛药用。

广东中医药博物馆藏

This medicine bottle is one piece of a medicine bottle set, which has twelve pieces. It is rectangular and has a flat mouth, a thin neck and a flat bottom. On the side surface are inscribed Chinese characters "Hai Shi" (which is the last time segment of the twelve time periods, i.e. from 21:00 to 23:00) and the front side is adorned with a pig design (one of the twelve zodiacs). It was used for storing medicine.

Preserved in Guangdong Chinese Medicine Museum

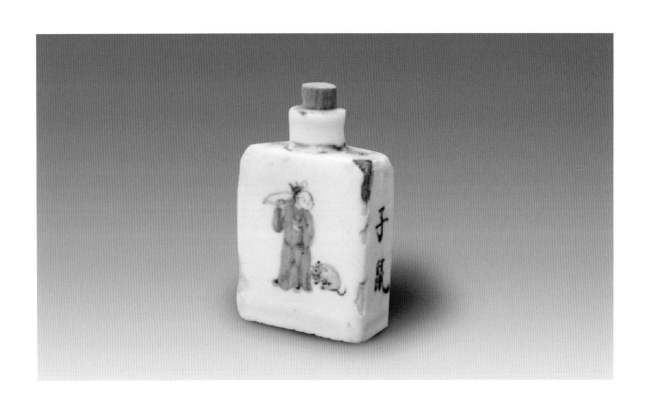

十二生肖方形瓷药瓶（子鼠）

清

瓷质

口外径 1.78 厘米，通高 6.64 厘米，瓶身长 4.3 厘米，瓶身宽 2.05 厘米，瓶身高 5.33 厘米，重 55 克

Rectangular Porcelain Medicine Bottle with Zodiac Design (Rat)

Qing Dynasty

Porcelain

Mouth Outer Diameter 1.78 cm/ Height 6.64 cm/ Body Length 4.3 cm/ Body Width 2.05 cm/ Body Height 5.33 cm/ Weight 55 g

一套十二件，上绘生肖鼠像，书有"子鼠"二字。用于装药。

广东中医药博物馆藏

This medicine bottle is one piece of a medicine bottle set, which has twelve pieces. It is rectangular and is adorned with an image of a rat and on the side of its body are inscribed two Chinese characters "Zi Shu" (Rat, the first of the twelve zodiacs). It was used for storing medicine.

Preserved in Guangdong Chinese Medicine Museum

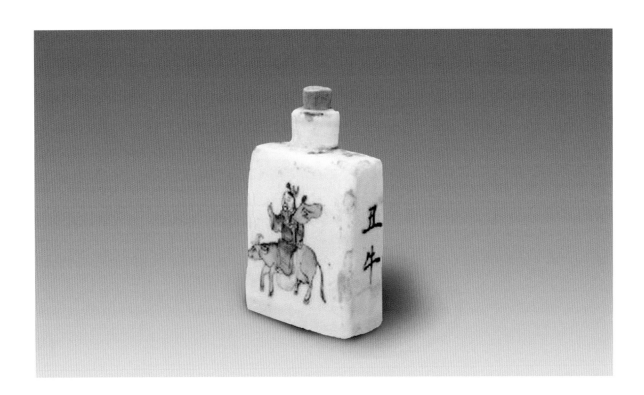

十二生肖方形瓷药瓶（丑牛）

清

瓷质

口外径 1.65 厘米，通高 6.52 厘米，瓶身长 4.34 厘米，瓶身宽 2.05 厘米，瓶身高 5.28 厘米，重 56 克

Rectangular Porcelain Medicine Bottle with Zodiac Design (Ox)

Qing Dynasty

Porcelain

Mouth Outer Diameter 1.65 cm/ Height 6.52 cm/ Body Length 4.34 cm/ Body Width 2.05 cm/ Body Height 5.28 cm/

Weight 56 g

一套十二件，上绘生肖丑牛像，书有"丑牛"

二字。用于盛药。

广东中医药博物馆藏

This medicine bottle is one piece of a medicine bottle

set, which has twelve pieces. It is rectangular and is

adorned with an image of an ox and on the side of

its body are inscribed two Chinese characters "Chou

Niu" (Ox, the second of the twelve zodiacs). It was

used for storing medicine.

Preserved in Guangdong Chinese Medicine Museum

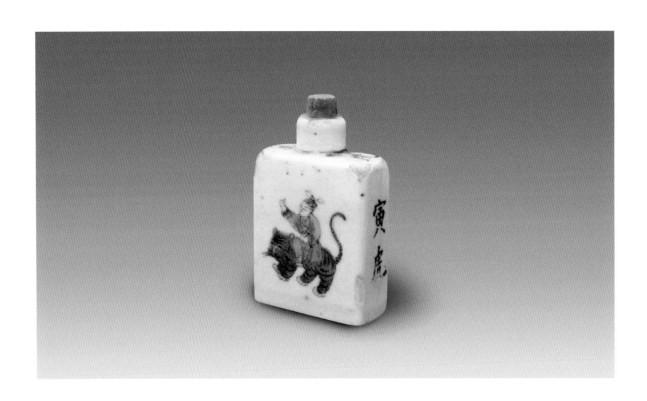

十二生肖方形瓷药瓶（寅虎）

清

瓷质

口外径 1.74 厘米，通高 6.4 厘米，瓶身长 4.35 厘米，瓶身宽 2.05 厘米，瓶身高 5.21 厘米，重 55 克

Rectangular Porcelain Medicine Bottle with Zodiac Design (Tiger)

Qing Dynasty

Porcelain

Mouth Outer Diameter 1.74 cm/ Height 6.4 cm/ Body Length 4.35 cm/ Body Width 2.05 cm/ Body Height 5.21 cm/ Weight 55 g

一套十二件，上绘生肖寅虎像，书有"寅虎"二字。用于盛药。

广东中医药博物馆藏

This medicine bottle is one piece of a medicine bottle set, which has twelve pieces. It is rectangular and is adorned with an image of a tiger and on the side of its body are inscribed two Chinese characters "Yin Hu" (Tiger, the third of the twelve zodiacs). It was used for storing medicine.

Preserved in Guangdong Chinese Medicine Museum

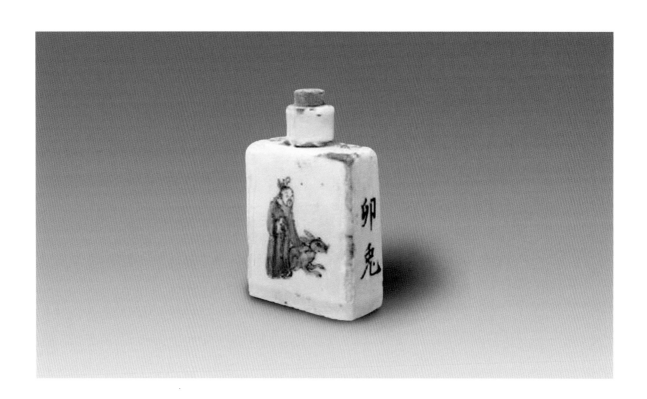

十二生肖方形瓷药瓶（卯兔）

清

瓷质

口外径 1.71 厘米，通高 6.5 厘米，瓶身长 4.36 厘米，瓶身宽 2.04 厘米，瓶身高 5.28 厘米，重 56 克

Rectangular Porcelain Medicine Bottle with Zodiac Design (Rabbit)

Qing Dynasty

Porcelain

Mouth Outer Diameter 1.71 cm/ Height 6.5 cm/ Body Length 4.36 cm/ Body Width 2.04 cm/ Body Height 5.28 cm/ Weight 56 g

一套十二件，上绘生肖卯兔，书有"卯兔"
二字。用于盛药。

广东中医药博物馆藏

This medicine bottle is one piece of a medicine bottle
set, which has twelve pieces. It is rectangular and is
adorned with an image of a rabbit and on the side of
its body are inscribed two Chinese characters "Mao
Tu" (Rabbit, the fourth of the twelve zodiacs). It was
used for storing medicine.

Preserved in Guangdong Chinese Medicine Museum

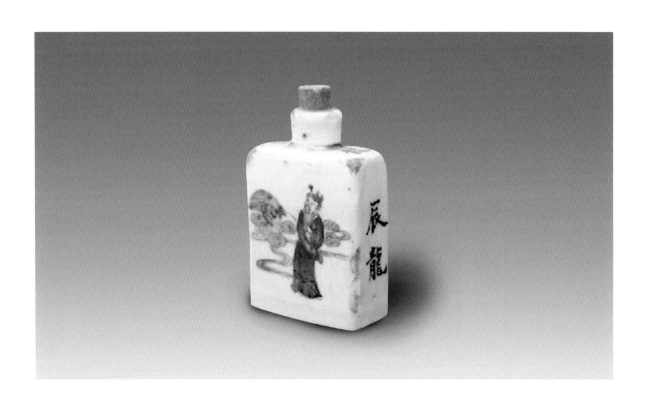

十二生肖方形瓷药瓶（辰龙）

清

瓷质

口外径 1.76 厘米，通高 6.39 厘米，瓶身长 4.32 厘米，瓶身宽 2.06 厘米，瓶身高 5.2 厘米，重 53 克

Rectangular Porcelain Medicine Bottle with Zodiac Design (Dragon)

Qing Dynasty

Porcelain

Mouth Outer Diameter 1.76 cm/ Height 6.39 cm/ Body Length 4.32 cm/ Body Width 2.06 cm/ Body Height 5.2 cm/ Weight 53 g

一套十二件，上绘生肖辰龙，书有"辰龙"
二字。用于盛药。

广东中医药博物馆藏

This medicine bottle is one piece of a medicine bottle
set, which has twelve pieces. It is rectangular and is
adorned with an image of a dragon and on the side of
its body are inscribed two Chinese characters "Chen
Long" (Dragon, the fifth of the twelve zodiacs). It
was used for storing medicine.
Preserved in Guangdong Chinese Medicine Museum

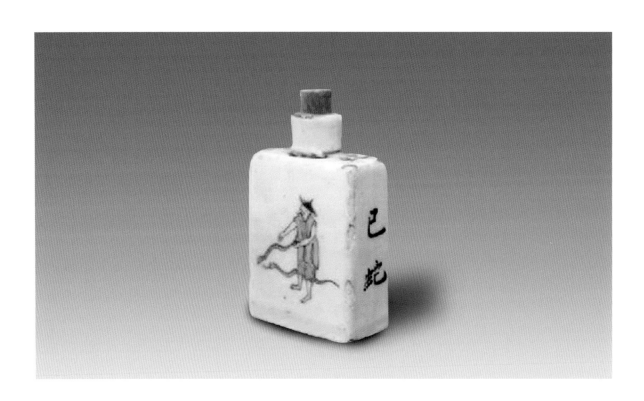

十二生肖方形瓷药瓶（巳蛇）

清

瓷质

口外径 1.69 厘米，通高 6.56 厘米，瓶身长 4.36 厘米，瓶身宽 2.03 厘米，瓶身高 5.37 厘米，重 56 克

Rectangular Porcelain Medicine Bottle with Zodiac Design (Snake)

Qing Dynasty

Porcelain

Mouth Outer Diameter 1.69 cm/ Height 6.56 cm/ Body Length 4.36 cm/ Body Width 2.03 cm/ Body Height 5.37 cm/

Weight 56 g

一套十二件，上绘生肖巳蛇图案，书有"巳蛇"二字，用于盛药。

广东中医药博物馆藏

This medicine bottle is one piece of a medicine bottle set, which has twelve pieces. It is rectangular and is adorned with an image of a snake and on the side of its body are inscribed two Chinese characters "Si She" (Snake, the sixth of the twelve zodiacs). It was used for storing medicine.

Preserved in Guangdong Chinese Medicine Museum

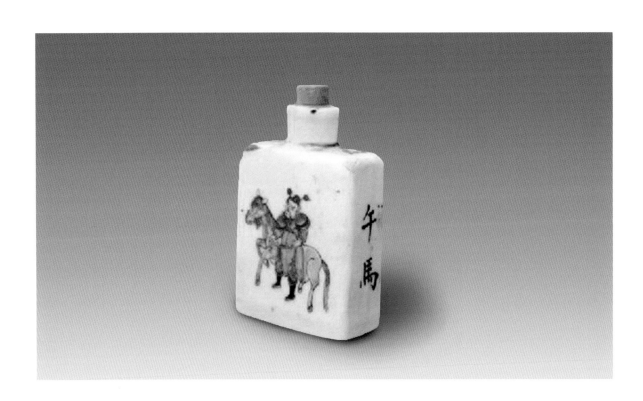

十二生肖方形瓷药瓶（午马）

清

瓷质

口外径 1.73 厘米，通高 6.42 厘米，瓶身长 4.36 厘米，瓶身宽 2.03 厘米，瓶身高 5.19 厘米，重 53 克

Rectangular Porcelain Medicine Bottle with Zodiac Design (Horse)

Qing Dynasty

Porcelain

Mouth Outer Diameter 1.73 cm/ Height 6.42 cm/ Body Length 4.36 cm/ Body Width 2.03 cm/ Body Height 5.19 cm/

Weight 53 g

一套十二件，上绘生肖午马像，书有"午马"二字。用于盛药。

广东中医药博物馆藏

This medicine bottle is one piece of a medicine bottle set, which has twelve pieces.It is rectangular and is adorned with an image of a horse and on the side of its body are inscribed two Chinese characters "Wu Ma" (Horse, the seventh of the twelve zodiacs). It was used for storing medicine.

Preserved in Guangdong Chinese Medicine Museum

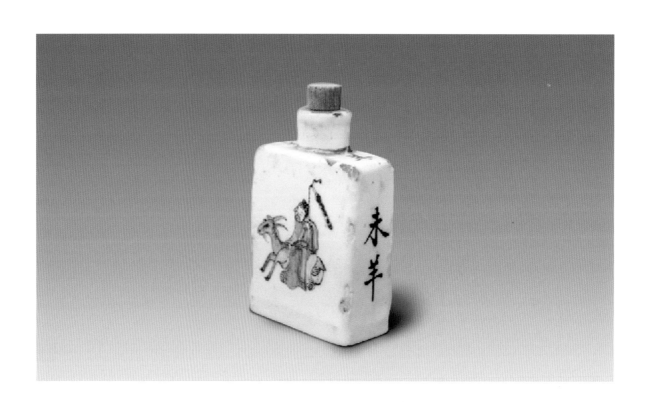

十二生肖方形瓷药瓶（未羊）

清

瓷质

口外径 1.73 厘米，通高 6.5 厘米，瓶身长 4.3 厘米，瓶身宽 2.03 厘米，瓶身高 5.31 厘米，重 55 克

Rectangular Porcelain Medicine Bottle with Zodiac Design (Sheep)

Qing Dynasty

Porcelain

Mouth Outer Diameter 1.73 cm/ Height 6.5 cm/ Body Length 4.3 cm/ Body Width 2.03 cm/ Body Height 5.31 cm/ Weight 55 g

一套十二件，上绘生肖未羊像，上书有"未羊"

二字。用于盛药。

广东中医药博物馆藏

This medicine bottle is one piece of a medicine bottle

set, which has twelve pieces. It is rectangular and is

adorned with an image of a sheep and on the side of

its body are inscribed two Chinese characters "Wei

Yang" (Sheep, the eighth of the twelve zodiacs). It

was used for storing medicine.

Preserved in Guangdong Chinese Medicine Museum

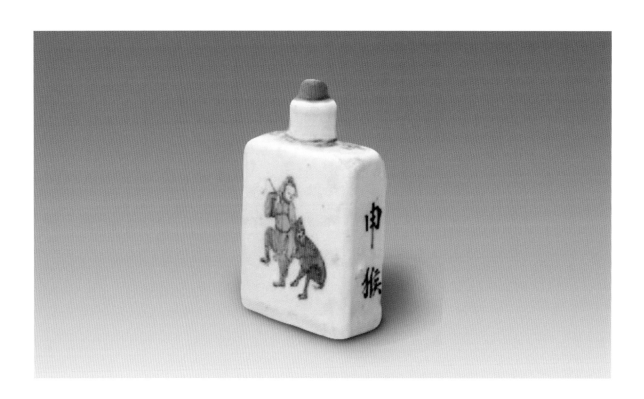

十二生肖方形瓷药瓶（申猴）

清

瓷质

口外径 1.72 厘米，通高 6.49 厘米，瓶身长 4.34 厘米，瓶身宽 2.04 厘米，瓶身高 5.28 厘米，重 56 克

Rectangular Porcelain Medicine Bottle with Zodiac Design (Monkey)

Qing Dynasty

Porcelain

Mouth Outer Diameter 1.72 cm/ Height 6.49 cm/ Body Length 4.34 cm/ Body Width 2.04 cm/ Body Height 5.28 cm/

Weight 56 g

一套十二件，上绘生肖申猴像，书有"申猴"
二字。用于盛药。

广东中医药博物馆藏

This medicine bottle is one piece of a medicine bottle set, which has twelve pieces. It is rectangular and is adorned with an image of a monkey and on the side of its body are inscribed two Chinese characters "Shen Hou" (Monkey, the ninth of the twelve zodiacs). It was used for storing medicine.

Preserved in Guangdong Chinese Medicine Museum

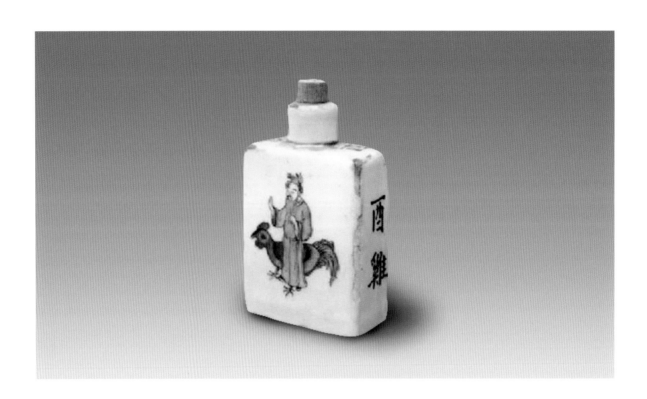

十二生肖方形瓷药瓶（酉鸡）

清

瓷质

口外径 1.75 厘米，通高 6.65 厘米，瓶身长 4.32 厘米，瓶身宽 2.13 厘米，瓶身高 5.4 厘米，重 55 克

Rectangular Porcelain Medicine Bottle with Zodiac Design (Rooster)

Qing Dynasty

Porcelain

Mouth Outer Diameter 1.75 cm/ Height 6.65 cm/ Body Length 4.32 cm/ Body Width 2.13 cm/ Body Height 5.4 cm/ Weight 55 g

一套十二件，上绘有生肖酉鸡像，书有"酉鸡"
二字。用于盛药。

广东中医药博物馆藏

This medicine bottle is one piece of a medicine bottle set, which has twelve pieces. It is rectangular and is adorned with an image of a rooster and on the side of its body are inscribed two Chinese characters "You Ji" (Rooster, the tenth of the twelve zodiacs). It was used for storing medicine.

Preserved in Guangdong Chinese Medicine Museum

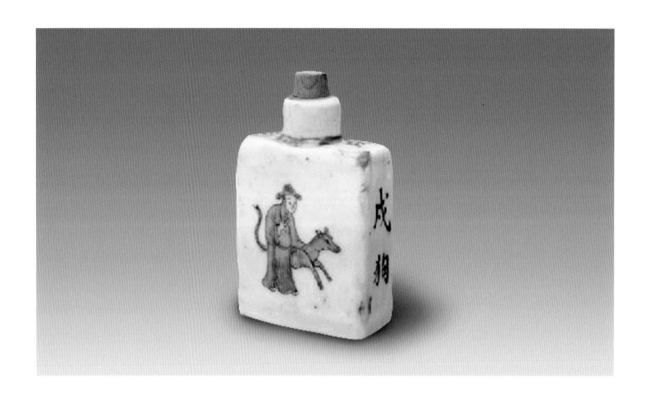

十二生肖方形瓷药瓶（戌狗）

清

瓷质

口外径 1.76 厘米，通高 6.39 厘米，瓶身长 4.38 厘米，瓶身宽 2 厘米，瓶身高 5.14 厘米，重 55 克

Rectangular Porcelain Medicine Bottle with Zodiac Design (Dog)

Qing Dynasty

Porcelain

Mouth Outer Diameter 1.76 cm/ Height 6.39 cm/ Body Length 4.38 cm/ Body Width 2 cm/ Body Height 5.14 cm/ Weight 55 g

一套十二件，上绘有生肖戌狗像，书有"戌狗"
二字。用于盛药。

广东中医药博物馆藏

This medicine bottle is one piece of a medicine bottle set, which has twelve pieces. It is rectangular and is adorned with an image of a dog and on the side of its body are inscribed two Chinese characters "Xu Gou" (Dog, the eleventh of the twelve zodiacs). It was used for storing medicine.

Preserved in Guangdong Chinese Medicine Museum

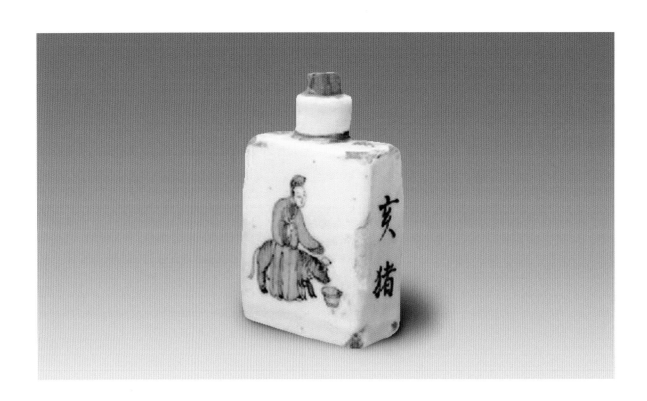

十二生肖方形瓷药瓶（亥猪）

清

瓷质

口外径 1.76 厘米，通高 6.39 厘米，瓶身长 4.38 厘米，瓶身宽 2 厘米，瓶身高 5.14 厘米，重 55 克

Rectangular Porcelain Medicine Bottle with Zodiac Design (Pig)

Qing Dynasty

Porcelain

Mouth Outer Diameter 1.76 cm/ Height 6.39 cm/ Body Length 4.38 cm/ Body Width 2 cm/ Body Height 5.14 cm/ Weight 55 g

一套十二件，上绘有生肖亥猪像，书有"亥猪"二字。用于盛药。

广东中医药博物馆藏

This medicine bottle is one piece of a medicine bottle set, which has twelve pieces. It is rectangular and is adorned with an image of a pig and on the side of its body are inscribed two Chinese characters "Hai Zhu" (Pig, the last of the twelve zodiacs). It was used for storing medicine.

Preserved in Guangdong Chinese Medicine Museum

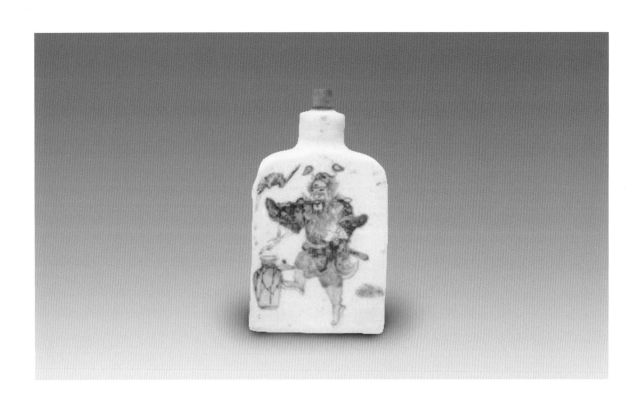

粉彩人物方形药瓶

清

瓷质

口外径 1.95 厘米，通高 7.86 厘米，瓶身长 5.12 厘米，瓶身宽 1.98 厘米，瓶身高 6.5 厘米，重 87 克

Rectangular Medicine Bottle with Famille Rose Decoration

Qing Dynasty

Porcelain

Mouth Outer Diameter 1.95 cm/ Height 7.86 cm/ Body Length 5.12 cm/ Body Width 1.98 cm/ Body Height 6.5 cm/ Weight 87 g

长方形，削肩，细直颈，平底，瓶身彩绘人
物像。用于装药。

广东中医药博物馆藏

This rectangular bottle has a sloping shoulder, a thin
and straight neck, and a flat bottom. The body is
adorned with a painted portraiture design. It was used
as a medicine container.

Preserved in Guangdong Chinese Medicine Museum

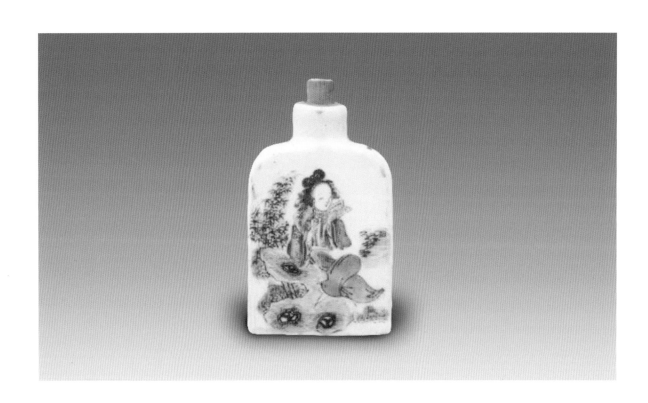

粉彩人物方形药瓶

清

瓷质

口外径 1.95 厘米，通高 7.82 厘米，瓶身长 5.12 厘米，瓶身宽 2 厘米，瓶身高 6.5 厘米，重 92 克

Rectangular Medicine Bottle with Famille Rose Decoration

Qing Dynasty

Porcelain

Mouth Outer Diameter 1.95 cm/ Height 7.82 cm/ Body Length 5.12 cm/ Body Width 2 cm/ Body Height 6.5 cm/ Weight 92 g

长方形，削肩，细直颈，平底，瓶身彩绘人
物像。用于装药。

广东中医药博物馆藏

This rectangular bottle has a sloping shoulder, a thin
and straight neck，and a flat bottom. The body is
adorned with a painted portraiture design. It was used
as a medicine container.

Preserved in Guangdong Chinese Medicine Museum

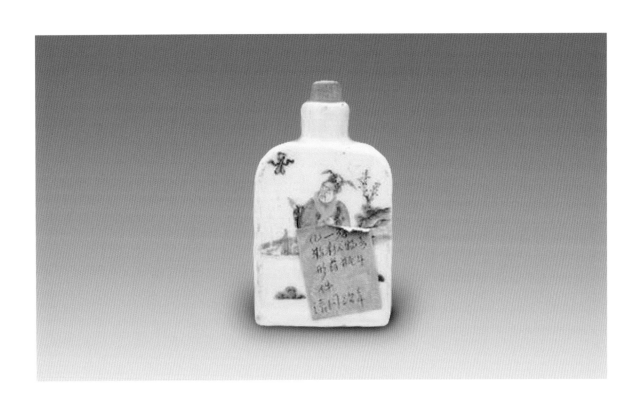

粉彩人物方形药瓶

清

瓷质

口外径 1.94 厘米，通高 7.97 厘米，瓶身长 5.06 厘米，瓶身宽 1.92 厘米，瓶身高 6.56 厘米，重 82 克

Rectangular Medicine Bottle with Famille Rose Decoration

Qing Dynasty

Porcelain

Mouth Outer Diameter 1.94 cm/ Height 7.97 cm/ Body Length 5.06 cm/ Body Width 1.92 cm/ Body Height 6.56 cm/ Weight 82 g

长方形，削肩，细直颈，平底，瓶身彩绘人
物像。用于装药。

广东中医药博物馆藏

This rectangular bottle has a sloping shoulder, a thin
and straight neck, and a flat bottom. The body is
adorned with a painted portraiture design. It was used
as a medicine container.

Preserved in Guangdong Chinese Medicine Museum

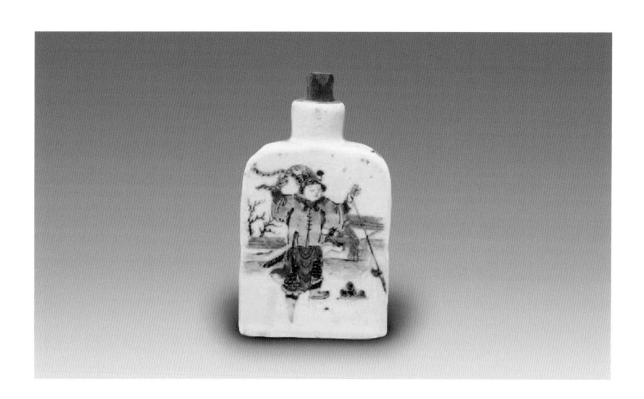

粉彩人物方形药瓶

清

瓷质

口外径 1.93 厘米，通高 7.76 厘米，瓶身长 5.15 厘米，瓶身宽 1.98 厘米，瓶身高 6.48 厘米，重 90 克

Rectangular Medicine Bottle with Famille Rose Decoration

Qing Dynasty

Porcelain

Mouth Outer Diameter 1.93 cm/ Height 7.76 cm/ Body Length 5.15 cm/ Body Width 1.98 cm/ Body Height 6.48 cm/ Weight 90 g

长方形，削肩，细直颈，平底，瓶身彩绘人
物像。用于装药。

广东中医药博物馆藏

This rectangular bottle has a sloping shoulder, a thin
and straight neck, and a flat bottom. The body is
adorned with a painted portraiture design. It was used
as a medicine container.

Preserved in Guangdong Chinese Medicine Museum

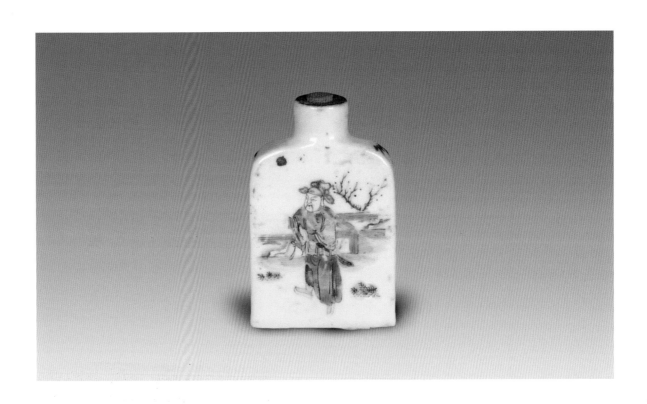

粉彩药瓶

清

瓷质

口外径 1.9 厘米，口内径 0.8 厘米，宽 5.2 厘米，高 7.8 厘米，厚 2.1 厘米

Medicine Bottle with Famille Rose Decoration

Qing Dynasty

Porcelain

Mouth Outer Diameter 1.9 cm/ Mouth Inner Diameter 0.8 cm/ Width 5.2 cm/ Height 7.8 cm/ Thickness 2.1 cm

方扁形，乳白釉，瓶身饰粉彩武官武士图案，
绘画精细，底部"大清同治年制"款识。盛
药器具。保存基本完好。1955 年入藏。

中华医学会 / 上海中医药大学医史博物馆藏

This oblate square bottle is coated with opaline glaze.
The body shows an exquisitely painted image of a
military officer in famille rose colour. The bottom
bears an inscription of "Da Qing Tong Zhi Nian
Zhi" (Made during the Reign of Tongzhi in the Qing
Dynasty). It was used as a medicine container. The
bottle was collected in the year 1955 and remains intact.
Preserved in Chinese Medical Association/ Museum
of Chinese Medicine, Shanghai University of
Traditional Chinese Medicine

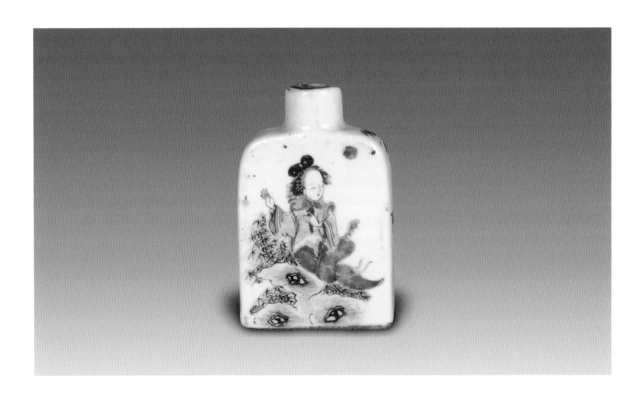

粉彩药瓶

清

瓷质

口外径 1.9 厘米，口内径 0.8 厘米，宽 5.25 厘米，高 7.9 厘米，厚 2.1 厘米

Medicine Bottle with Famille Rose Decoration

Qing Dynasty

Porcelain

Mouth Outer Diameter 1.9 cm/ Mouth Inner Diameter 0.8 cm/ Width 5.25 cm/ Height 7.9 cm/ Thickness 2.1cm

方扁形，乳白釉，瓶身饰粉彩贵妇图案，绘画精细，底部"大清同治年制"款识。盛药器具。保存基本完好。1955 年入藏。

中华医学会 / 上海中医药大学医史博物馆藏

This oblate square bottle is coated with opaline glaze. The body shows an exquisitely painted image of a lady in famille rose colour. The bottom bears an inscription of "Da Qing Tong Zhi Nian Zhi" (Made during the Reign of Tongzhi in the Qing Dynasty). It was used as a medicine container. The bottle was collected in the year 1955 and remains intact.
Preserved in Chinese Medical Association/ Museum of Chinese Medicine, Shanghai University of Traditional Chinese Medicine

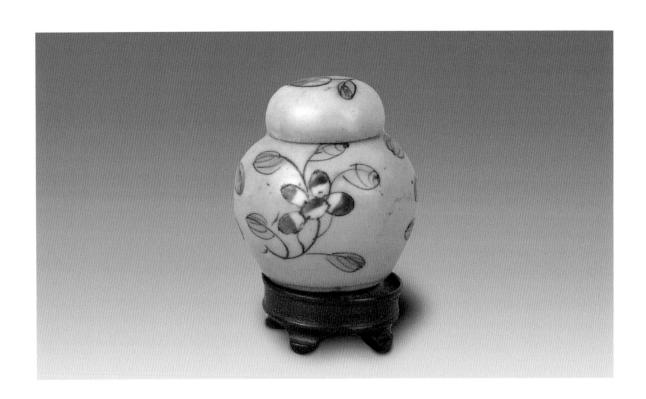

药瓶

清

瓷质

口径 1.7 厘米，腹径 3.7 厘米，通高 3.9 厘米

Medicine Bottle

Qing Dynasty

Porcelain

Mouth Diameter 1.7 cm/ Belly Diameter 3.7 cm/ Height 3.9 cm

圆瓶形，配扣盖，直口，平底，通身施绿釉，

彩绘花卉，小巧玲珑，工艺较好。盛药器具。

保存基本完好。1955 年入藏。

中华医学会 / 上海中医药大学医史博物馆藏

It is small and exquisite with a snap lid, a

straight mouth, and a flat bottom, showing good

craftsmanship. This green-glazed round bottle is

adorned with designs of famille rose flowers. It was

used as a medicine container, and was collected in

the year 1955. The bottle remains intact.

Preserved in Chinese Medical Association/ Museum

of Chinese Medicine, Shanghai University of Traditional

Chinese Medicine

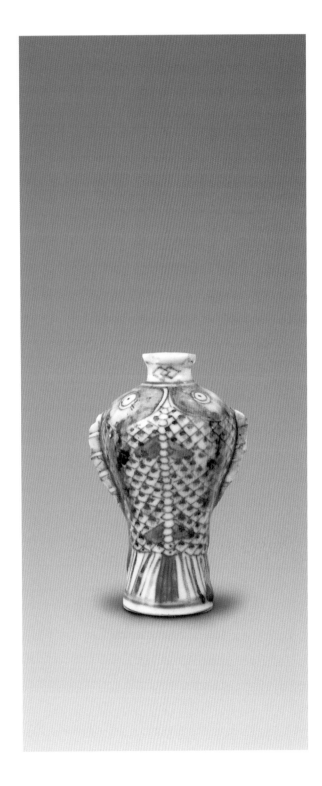

双鱼药瓶

清

瓷质

口径 1.8 厘米，底径 3.1 厘米，宽 5.2 厘米，通高 8.1 厘米

圆瓶形，五彩双鱼纹瓷瓶，直口，平底，双鱼鳍装饰耳，造型别致美观。盛药器具。保存基本完好。1955 年入藏。

中华医学会/上海中医药大学医史博物馆藏

Medicine Bottle with Double Fish Design

Qing Dynasty

Porcelain

Mouth Diameter 1.8 cm/ Bottom Diameter 3.1 cm/ Width 5.2 cm/ Height 8.1 cm

This round porcelain bottle is adorned with polychrome double fish patterns. The bottle, featuring a straight mouth, a flat bottom and two fin-shaped ears, is unique in appearance. The bottle which served as a medicine container is kept intact. It was collected in the year 1955. Preserved in Chinese Medical Association/ Museum of Chinese Medicine, Shanghai University of Traditional Chinese Medicine

药瓶

清

瓷质

口径 1.5 厘米，边长 2.9 厘米，通高 7.8 厘米

方瓶形，表面饰彩绘云龙纹，直口，平底，造

型美观，工艺较好。盛药器具。保存基本完好。

1954 年入藏。

中华医学会／上海中医药大学医史博物馆藏

Medicine Bottle

Qing Dynasty

Porcelain

Mouth Diameter 1.5 cm/ Side Length 2.9 cm/ Height 7.8 cm

This square bottle is adorned with designs of a dragon among clouds in famille rose colour. The gracefully shaped bottle with a straight mouth and a flat bottom shows good craftsmanship. The bottle which served as a medicine container is kept intact. The bottle was collected in the year 1954.

Preserved in Chinese Medical Association/ Museum of Chinese Medicine, Shanghai University of Traditional Chinese Medicine

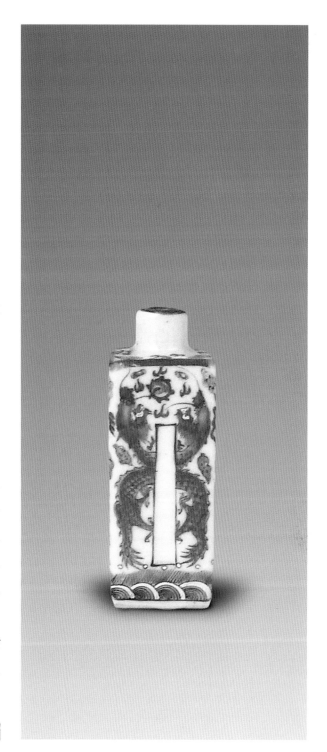

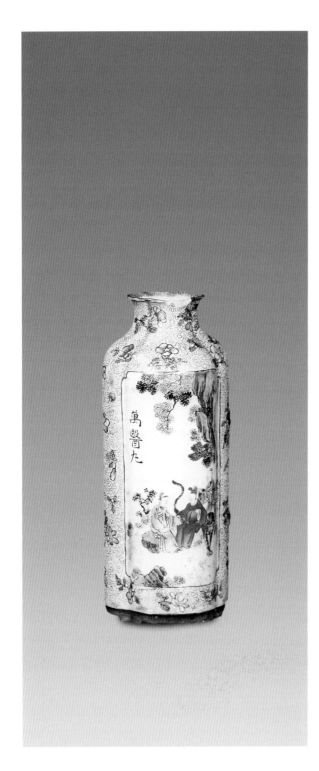

"万医丸" 药瓶

清

瓷质

口径 4.5 厘米，底径 5 厘米，高 13 厘米

圆柱形，敞口，束颈，溜肩，直腹，平底，卷足，表面饰粉彩，上有楷书 "万医丸" 三字。口沿有残。

上海中医药博物馆藏

Medicine Bottle with Chinese Label of "Wan Yi Wan"

Qing Dynasty

Porcelain

Mouth Diameter 4.5 cm/ Bottom Diameter 5 cm/ Height 13 cm

This cylindrical bottle has a flared mouth, a contracted neck, a sloping shoulder, a straight belly, a flat bottom, and a ring foot. It's painted with famille rose decoration. The bottle bears three Chinese characters in regular script "Wan Yi Wan" (the name of the drug). The mouth rim is cracked.

Preserved in Shanghai Museum of Traditional Chinese Medicine

瓷药瓶

清

瓷质

口外径 1.6 厘米，口内径 1.05 厘米，直径 3.7 厘米，

通高 8.15 厘米

圆瓶，瓶身绘有人物青花图案，无盖，制作工艺

一般，表面粗糙，瓶底无款识。盛药器具。保存

基本完好。1958 年入藏。

中华医学会 / 上海中医药大学医史博物馆藏

Porcelain Medicine Bottle

Qing Dynasty

Porcelain

Mouth Outer Diameter 1.6 cm/ Mouth Inner Diameter

1.05 cm/ Diameter 3.7 cm/ Height 8.15 cm

The blue-and-white bottle which has no lid is adorned

with portraiture designs. This round bottle shows a rough

surface with average quality workmanship. The bottom

of the bottle bears no reign mark or other inscription. The

bottle which served as a medicine container is kept intact.

The bottle was collected in the year 1958.

Preserved in Chinese Medical Association/ Museum of

Chinese Medicine, Shanghai University of Traditional

Chinese Medicine

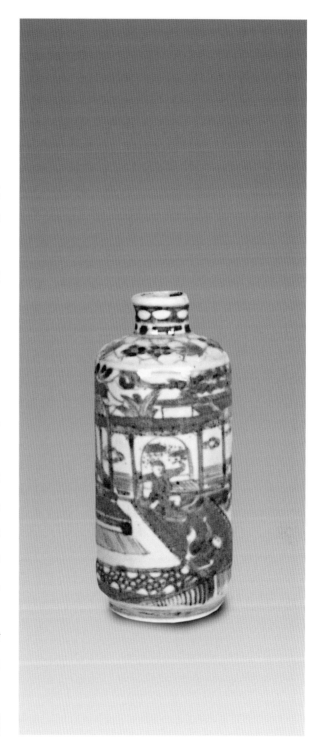

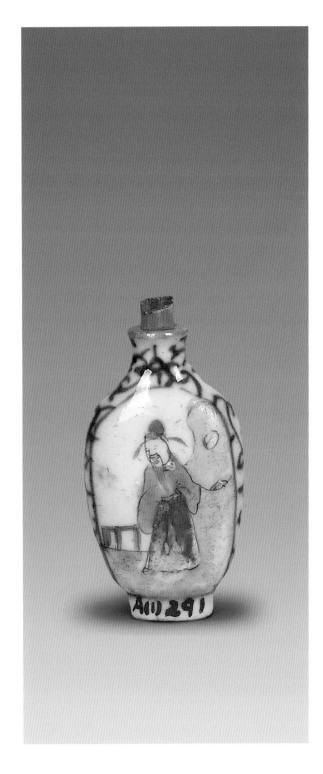

青花粉彩药瓶

清

瓷质

口外径 1.6 厘米，口内径 0.75 厘米，宽 4.1 厘米，

高 7.35 厘米，厚 1.9 厘米

Blue-and-white Medicine Bottle with Famille Rose Decoration

Qing Dynasty

Porcelain

Mouth Outer Diameter 1.6 cm/ Mouth Inner Diameter

0.75 cm/ Width 4.1 cm / Height 7.35 cm/ Thickness 1.9 cm

扁瓶状，瓶身彩绘人物，两侧青花缠枝纹，

平底，工艺一般，表面不光滑。盛药器具。

保存基本完好。1955 年入藏。

中华医学会 / 上海中医药大学医史博物馆藏

This oblate flat-bottomed bottle is adorned with a

painted portraiture on the front surface and blue

interlocking branches of flowers on the side surfaces.

The bottle shows a rough surface with average

quality workmanship. The bottle which served as a

medicine container is kept in good condition. The

bottle was collected in the year 1955.

Preserved in Chinese Medical Association/ Museum

of Chinese Medicine, Shanghai University of

Traditional Chinese Medicine

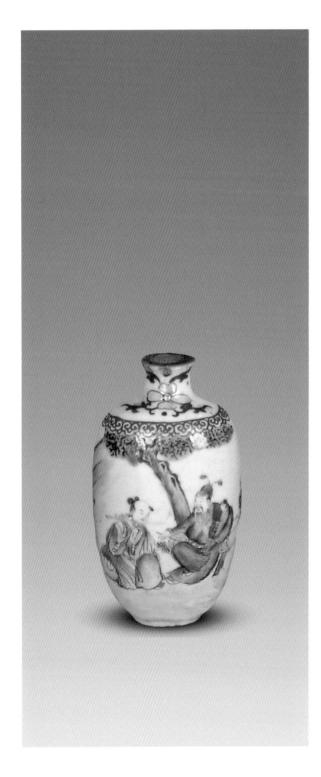

粉彩瓷药瓶

清

瓷质

口外径 1.6 厘米，口内径 0.8 厘米，宽 4.4 厘米，

高 7.65 厘米，厚 3.4 厘米

Porcelain Medicine Bottle with Famille Rose Decoration

Qing Dynasty

Porcelain

Mouth Outer Diameter 1.6 cm/ Mouth Inner Diameter 0.8 cm/

Width 4.4 cm/ Height 7.65 cm/ Thickness 3.4 cm

扁瓶状，表面饰粉彩人物故事图案，底有图案款识，画工精细。盛药器具。保存基本完好。1956 年入藏。

　中华医学会 / 上海中医药大学医史博物馆藏

This oblate bottle is adorned with famille rose decoration of narrative scenes. Exquisite designs and inscriptions are also found at the bottom of the bottle. The bottle which served as a medicine container is kept in good condition. The bottle was collected in the year 1956.

Preserved in Chinese Medical Association/ Museum of Chinese Medicine, Shanghai University of Traditional Chinese Medicine

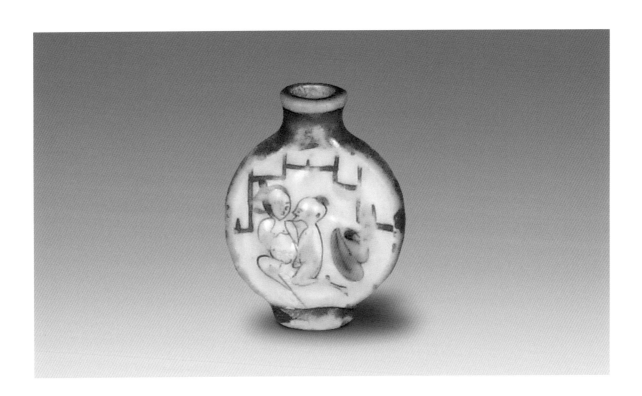

粉彩药瓶

清

瓷质

口外径 1.5 厘米，口内径 0.75 厘米，宽 3.85 厘米，高 4.95 厘米，厚 1.45 厘米

Medicine Bottle with Famille Rose Decoration

Qing Dynasty

Porcelain

Mouth Outer Diameter 1.5 cm/ Mouth Inner Diameter 0.75 cm/ Width 3.85 cm / Height 4.95 cm/ Thickness 1.45 cm

扁圆瓶，表面绘粉彩春宫图，底部无款识，

工艺一般。盛药器具。保存基本完好。1955 年

入藏。

中华医学会 / 上海中医药大学医史博物馆藏

This oblate bottle, which is adorned with famille rose

decoration of erotic paintings, shows average quality

workmanship. The bottom of the bottle bears no reign

mark or other inscription. The bottle which served as

a medicine container was kept in good condition. The

object was collected in the year 1955.

Preserved in Chinese Medical Association/ Museum

of Chinese Medicine, Shanghai University of

Traditional Chinese Medicine

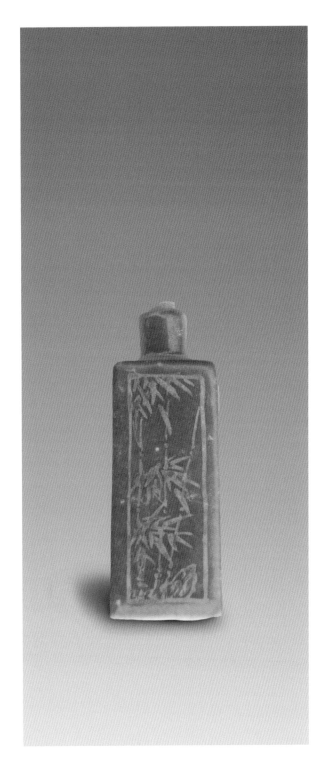

小药瓶

清

瓷质

口外径 1.3 厘米，宽 2.8 厘米，通高 7.5 厘米，重 54 克

方形，直口，平沿，折肩，平底，瓶身绘竹叶纹。用于装药。

广东中医药博物馆藏

Small Medicine Bottle

Qing Dynasty

Porcelain

Mouth Outer Diameter 1.3 cm/ Width 2.8 cm/ Height 7.5 cm/ Weight 54 g

This square medicine bottle has a straight mouth, a flat mouth rim, an angular shoulder, and a flat bottom. It is painted with patters bamboo leaves.It was used as a medicine container.

Preserved in Guangdong Chinese Medicine Museum

豇豆红圆柱形药瓶

清

瓷质

口外径 1.5 厘米，腹径 5.1 厘米，底径 4.4 厘米，

通高 12.15 厘米，重 172 克

圆柱形，直口，平沿，细长颈，溜肩，腹渐收至

底，平底，圈足，外施豇豆红釉。用于装药。

广东中医药博物馆藏

Cylindrical Medicine Bottle in Cowpea Red

Qing Dynasty

Porcelain

Mouth Outer Diameter 1.5 cm/ Belly Diameter 5.1 cm/

Bottom Diameter 4.4 cm/ Height 12.15 cm/ Weight 172 g

This cylindrical medicine bottle has a straight mouth, a

flat mouth rim, a long and slim neck, a sloping shoulder,

a flat bottom, and a ring foot. Its belly narrows down to

the bottom.It is coated with cowpea red glaze. It was used

as a medicine container.

Preserved in Guangdong Chinese Medicine Museum

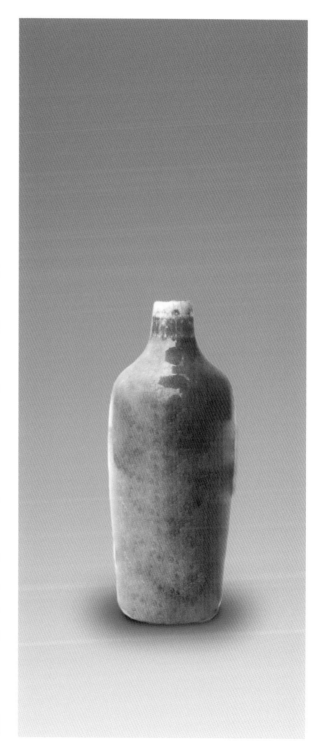

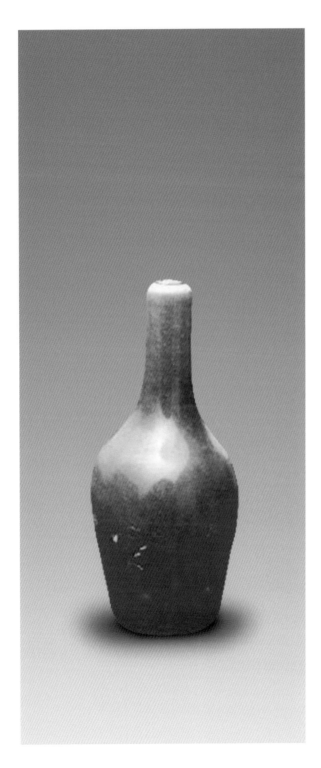

祭药长颈圆形药瓶

清

瓷质

口外径1.26厘米，腹径3.58厘米，底径2.74厘米，

通高7.65厘米，瓶颈长2.22厘米，重43克

细直颈，鼓腹，其下收敛，平底。用于装药。

广东中医药博物馆藏

Altar Red Round Medicine Bottle with Elongated Neck

Qing Dynasty

Porcelain

Mouth Outer Diameter 1.26 cm/ Belly Diameter 3.58 cm/ Bottom Diameter 2.74 cm/ Height 7.65cm/ Neck Length 2.22 cm/ Weight 43 g

This bottle has a slim and straight neck, a drum-like belly that narrows down to the flat bottom. It was used as a medicine container.

Preserved in Guangdong Chinese Medicine Museum

祭红圆形小药瓶

清

瓷质

口外径 1.48 厘米，腹径 3.63 厘米，底径 2.21 厘米，

通高 7.42 厘米，重 45 克

口微敞，短颈，丰肩，肩以下渐收，圈足。用于装药。

广东中医药博物馆藏

Small Altar Red Round Medicine Bottle

Qing Dynasty

Porcelain

Mouth Outer Diameter 1.48 cm/ Belly Diameter 3.63 cm/

Bottom Diameter 2.21 cm/ Height 7.42 cm/ Weight 45 g

This bottle has a slightly flared mouth, a short bottleneck, and an abundant shoulder that narrows down to the ring foot. It was used as a medicine container.

Preserved in Guangdong Chinese Medicine Museum

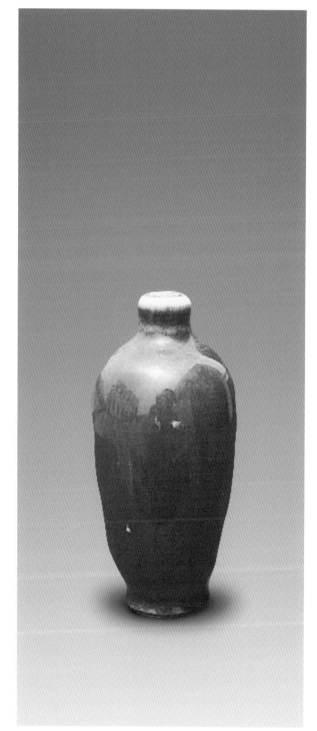

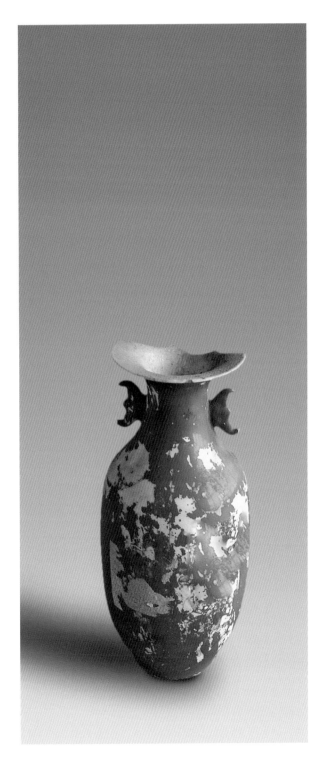

药瓶

清

瓷质

口径 7.5 厘米，底径 6 厘米，高 21 厘米

敞口，束颈，溜肩，平底，圈足，颈部有蝙蝠形对耳，外壁被人为漆了层红漆。口部残。由民间征集。

成都中医药大学中医药传统文化博物馆藏

Medicine Bottle

Qing Dynasty

Porcelain

Mouth Diameter 7.5 cm/ Bottom Diameter 6 cm/ Height 21 cm

This medicine bottle has a flared and broken mouth, a contracted neck, a sloping shoulder, a flat bottom, and a ring foot. A pair of batwing-shaped ears are stuck on the bottle's neck symmetrically. It is painted with red lacquer. The object was collected from a private owner.

Preserved in Museum of Traditional Chinese Medicine Culture, Chengdu University of Traditional Chinese Medicine

药瓶

清

瓷质

口径 9 厘米，高 4.5 厘米

敞口，束颈，鼓肩，直腹，圈足，颈部有两个蝙蝠形对耳，后人在器身表面涂了层红漆。由民间征集。

成都中医药大学中医药传统文化博物馆藏

Medicine Bottle

Qing Dynasty

Porcelain

Mouth Diameter 9 cm/ Height 4.5 cm

This medicine bottle has a flared mouth, a contracted neck, a drum-like shoulder, a straight belly, and a ring foot. There are two batwing-shaped ears stuck on the bottle's neck. The outer wall was coated later with red lacquer. It was collected from a private owner.

Preserved in Museum of Traditional Chinese Medicine Culture, Chengdu University of Traditional Chinese Medicine

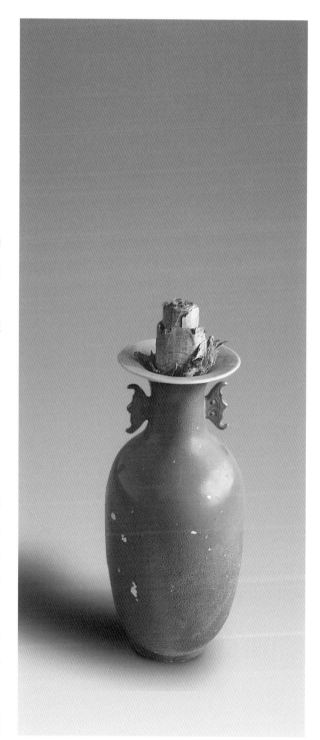

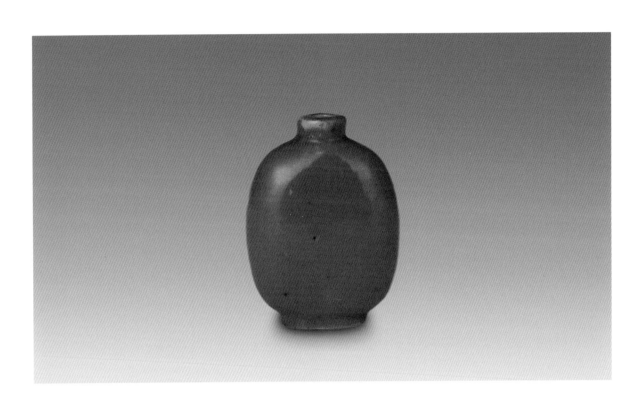

药瓶

清

瓷质

口径 1.4 厘米，宽 4.2 厘米，通高 5.7 厘米，厚 2.2 厘米

Medicine Bottle

Qing Dynasty

Porcelain

Mouth Diameter 1.4 cm/ Width 4.2 cm/ Height 5.7 cm/ Thickness 2.2 cm

扁瓶状，通身施棕黄釉，直口，平底，圈足，小巧玲珑，造型美观。盛药器具。保存基本完好。1954 年入藏。

中华医学会 / 上海中医药大学医史博物馆藏

This brown-glazed oblate bottle has a straight mouth, a flat bottom, and a ring foot. This exquisitely designed small bottle was used as a medicine container. The bottle was collected in the year 1954 and remains intact.
Preserved in Chinese Medical Association/ Museum of Chinese Medicine, Shanghai University of Traditional Chinese Medicine

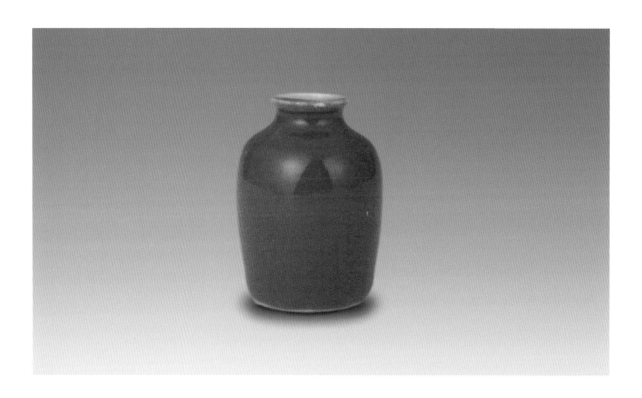

药瓶

清

瓷质

口径 1.8 厘米，腹径 4.8 厘米，通高 6.2 厘米

Medicine Bottle

Qing Dynasty

Porcelain

Mouth Diameter 1.8 cm/ Belly Diameter 4.8 cm/ Height 6.2 cm

圆瓶形，褐色釉，口沿施青灰釉，平底，翻沿，朴实大方，底有"大清康熙年制"款识。盛药器具。口有残。1955 年入藏。

中华医学会 / 上海中医药大学医史博物馆藏

This brown-glazed round bottle has a blue ash glazed mouth rim which is folded outward and a flat bottom, bearing an inscription of "Da Qing Kang Xi Nian Zhi" (Made during the Reign of Kangxi in the Qing Dynasty). This simple but elegant bottle was used as a medicine container. Its mouth is damaged. It was collected in the year 1955.

Preserved in Chinese Medical Association/ Museum of Chinese Medicine, Shanghai University of Traditional Chinese Medicine

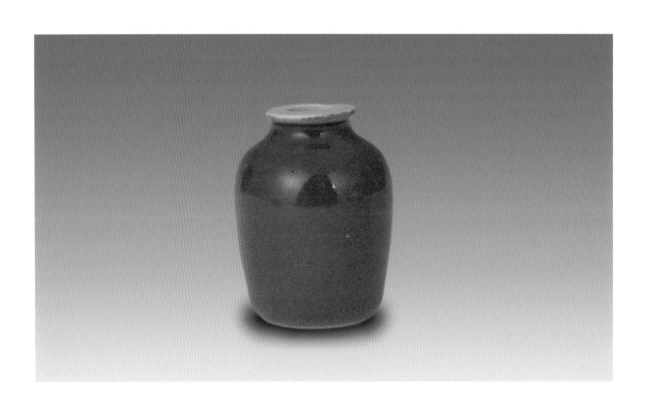

药瓶

清

瓷质

口径 2.6 厘米，腹径 4.8 厘米，通高 6.5 厘米

Medicine Bottle

Qing Dynasty

Porcelain

Mouth Diameter 2.6 cm/ Belly Diameter 4.8 cm/ Height 6.5 cm

圆瓶形，褐色釉，口沿施青灰釉，平底，翻沿，朴实大方，底有"大清康熙年制"款识。盛药器具。口有残。1955年入藏。

中华医学会 / 上海中医药大学医史博物馆藏

This brown-glazed round bottle has a blue ash glazed mouth rim which is folded outward and a flat bottom, bearing an inscription of "Da Qing Kang Xi Nian Zhi" (Made during the Reign of Kangxi in the Qing Dynasty). This simple but elegant bottle was used as a medicine container. Its mouth is damaged. It was collected in the year 1955.

Preserved in Chinese Medical Association/ Museum of Chinese Medicine, Shanghai University of Traditional Chinese Medicine

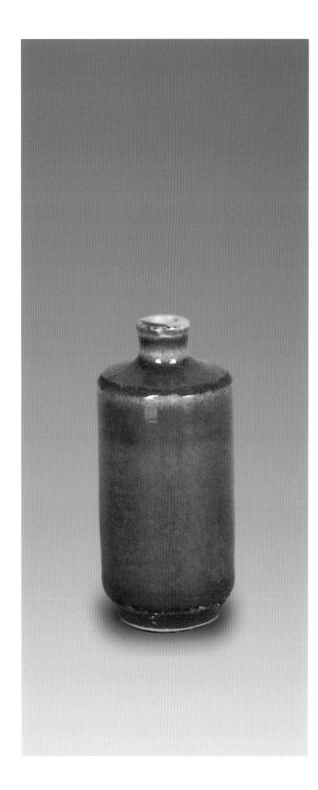

瓷药瓶

清

瓷质

口外径 1.3 厘米，口内径 0.6 厘米，直径 3.25 厘米，
高 7.05 厘米

Porcelain Medicine Bottle

Qing Dynasty

Porcelain

Mouth Outer Diameter 1.3 cm/ Mouth Inner Diameter 0.6 cm/

Diameter 3.25 cm/ Height 7.05 cm

圆柱形，通身施猪肝色釉，圈足，平底无款

识，工艺较好。盛药器具。保存基本完好。

1955 年入藏。

中华医学会 / 上海中医药大学医史博物馆藏

This cylindrical medicine bottle is coated with liver-

coloured glaze. The bottom of the ring foot bears no

reign mark or other inscription. The bottle with good

workmanship was used as a medicine container. It

was collected in the year 1955 and remains intact.

Preserved in Chinese Medical Association/ Museum

of Chinese Medicine, Shanghai University of

Traditional Chinese Medicine

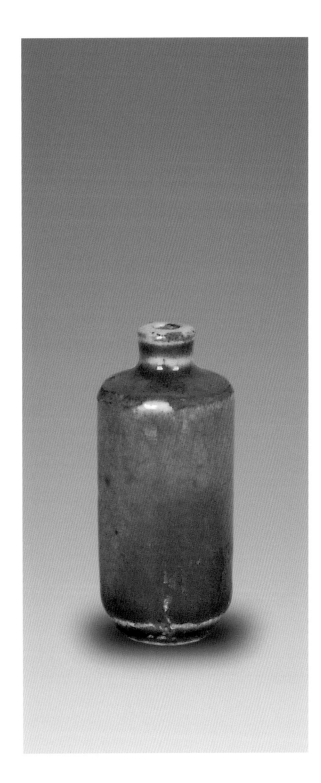

瓷药瓶

清

瓷质

口外径 1.45 厘米，口内径 0.6 厘米，直径 3.3 厘米，
高 7.45 厘米

Porcelain Medicine Bottle

Qing Dynasty

Porcelain

Mouth Outer Diameter 1.45 cm/ Mouth Inner Diameter 0.6 cm/

Diameter 3.3 cm/ Height 7.45 cm

圆柱形，通身施猪肝色釉，圈足，平底无款识，工艺较好。盛药器具。保存基本完好。1955 年入藏。

中华医学会 / 上海中医药大学医史博物馆藏

This cylindrical medicine bottle is coated with liver-coloured glaze. The bottom of the ring foot bears no reign mark or other inscription. The bottle with good workmanship was used as a medicine container. It was collected in the year 1955 and remains intact.

Preserved in Chinese Medical Association/ Museum of Chinese Medicine, Shanghai University of Traditional Chinese Medicine

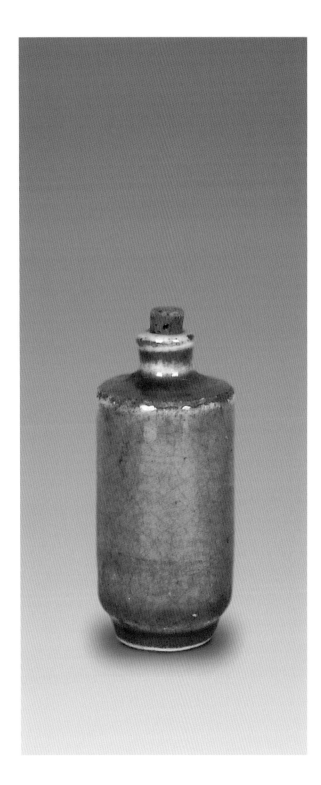

瓷药瓶

清

瓷质

口外径 1.5 厘米，口内径 0.7 厘米，直径 3.4 厘米，
高 7.5 厘米

Porcelain Medicine Bottle

Qing Dynasty

Porcelain

Mouth Outer Diameter 1.5 cm/ Mouth Inner Diameter 0.7 cm/

Diameter 3.4 cm/ Height 7.5 cm

圆柱形，通身施猪肝色釉，圈足，平底无款
识，工艺较好。盛药器具。保存基本完好。
1955 年入藏。

中华医学会 / 上海中医药大学医史博物馆藏

This cylindrical medicine bottle is coated with liver-
coloured glaze. The bottom of the ring foot bears no
reign mark or other inscription. The bottle with good
workmanship was used as a medicine container. It
was collected in the year 1955 and remains intact.
Preserved in Chinese Medical Association/ Museum
of Chinese Medicine, Shanghai University of
Traditional Chinese Medicine

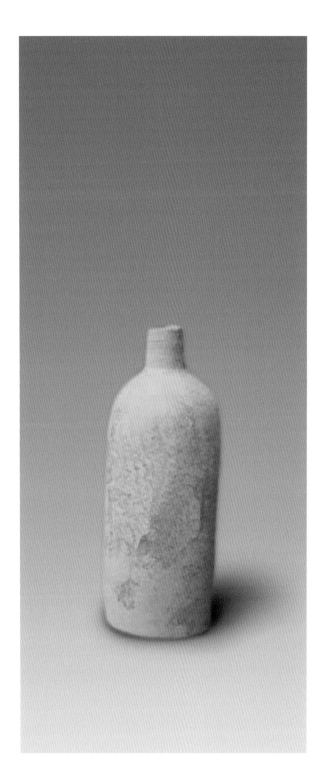

小药瓶

清

瓷质

口外径 1 厘米，腹径 2.9 厘米，通高 7.3 厘米，

重 38 克

Small Medicine Bottle

Qing Dynasty

Porcelain

Mouth Outer Diameter 1 cm/ Belly Diameter 2.9 cm/

Height 7.3 cm/ Weight 38 g

圆柱形，敛口，直颈，溜肩，直腹，平底，圈足，通体施黄釉。用于装药。

广东中医药博物馆藏

This cylindrical bottle has a contracted mouth, a straight neck, a sloping shoulder, a straight belly, a flat bottom, and a ring foot. It is entirely coated with yellow glaze, and was used as a medicine container.

Preserved in Guangdong Chinese Medicine Museum

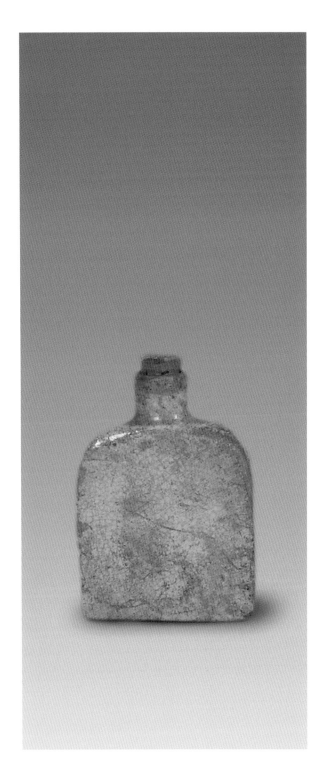

瓷药瓶

清

瓷质

口外径 1.3 厘米，口内径 0.7 厘米，宽 3.8 厘米，
高 5.5 厘米，厚 1.5 厘米

Porcelain Medicine Bottle

Qing Dynasty

Porcelain

Mouth Outer Diameter 1.3 cm/ Mouth Inner Diameter 0.7 cm/

Width 3.8 cm / Height 5.5 cm/ Thickness 1.5 cm

扁方形，通身施黄釉，小开片，直口，平
底，底无款识，工艺粗糙。保存基本完好。
1955 年入藏。

中华医学会 / 上海中医药大学医史博物馆藏

This oblate square bottle is fully coated with crackled
yellow glaze. The bottle with a straight mouth and
a flat bottom without inscription. It is rough in
workmanship. It was collected in the year 1955, and
remains intact.

Preserved in Chinese Medical Association/ Museum
of Chinese Medicine, Shanghai University of Traditional
Chinese Medicine

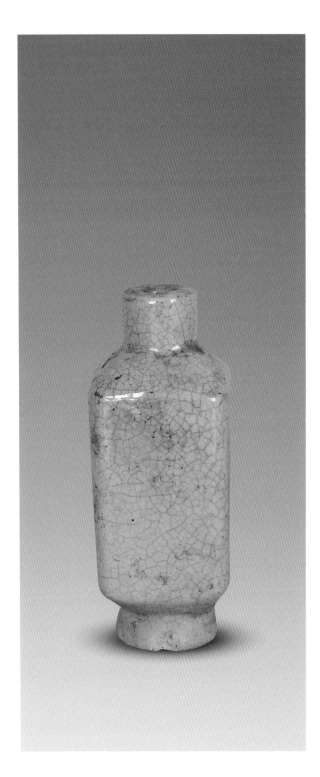

瓷药瓶

清

瓷质

口外径 1.9 厘米，口内径 0.6 厘米，宽 3.6 厘米，
高 8.85 厘米

Porcelain Medicine Bottle

Qing Dynasty

Porcelain

Mouth Outer Diameter 1.9 cm/ Mouth Inner Diameter 0.6 cm/

Width 3.6 cm/ Height 8.85 cm

方瓶形，通身施黄色釉，小开片，直口，圈足，平底无款，工艺一般。盛药器具。保存基本完好。1955 年入藏。

中华医学会 / 上海中医药大学医史博物馆藏

This square bottle, fully coated with crackled yellow glaze, features a straight mouth, a ring foot and a flat bottom without inscription. The bottle with average quality workmanship was used as a medicine container. It was collected in the year 1955 and remains intact.

Preserved in Chinese Medical Association/ Museum of Chinese Medicine, Shanghai University of Traditional Chinese Medicine

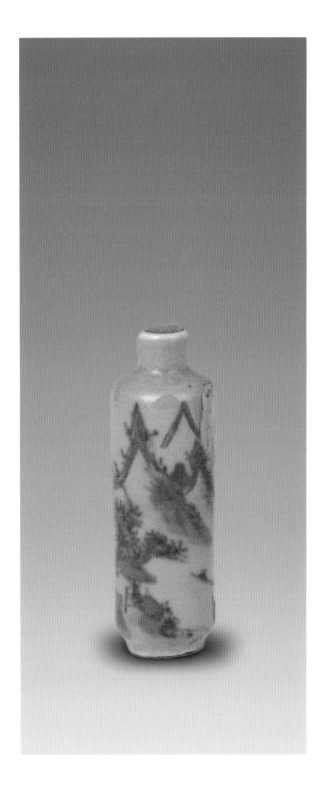

药瓶

清

瓷质

口径 1.3 厘米，腹径 2.7 厘米，通高 7.7 厘米

Medicine Bottle

Qing Dynasty

Porcelain

Mouth Diameter 1.3 cm/ Belly Diameter 2.7 cm/

Height 7.7 cm

圆柱形，表面绘黄釉彩绘山水图，直口，平
底，圈足，小巧玲珑，造型美观。盛药器具。
保存基本完好。1955 年入藏。

中华医学会 / 上海中医药大学医史博物馆藏

Adorned with painted landscape designs, this yellow-
glazed cylindrical bottle features a straight mouth,
a flat bottom and a ring foot. The tiny and exquisite
object with pretty shape was used as a medicine
container. It was collected in the year 1955 and
remains intact.

Preserved in Chinese Medical Association/ Museum of
Chinese Medicine, Shanghai University of Traditional
Chinese Medicine

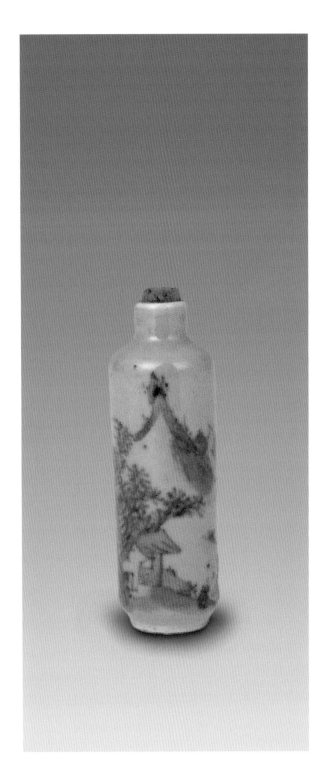

药瓶

清

瓷质

口径 1.3 厘米，腹径 2.6 厘米，通高 7.6 厘米

Medicine Bottle

Qing Dynasty

Porcelain

Mouth Diameter 1.3 cm/ Belly Diameter 2.6 cm/ Height

7.6 cm

圆柱形，表面绘黄釉彩绘山水图，直口，平底，圈足，小巧玲珑，造型美观。盛药器具。保存基本完好。1955 年入藏。

中华医学会 / 上海中医药大学医史博物馆藏

Adorned with painted landscape designs, this yellow-glazed cylindrical medicine bottle features a straight mouth, a flat bottom and a ring foot. The tiny and exquisite object with pretty shape was used as a medicine container. It was collected in the year 1955 and remains intact.

Preserved in Chinese Medical Association/ Museum of Chinese Medicine, Shanghai University of Traditional Chinese Medicine

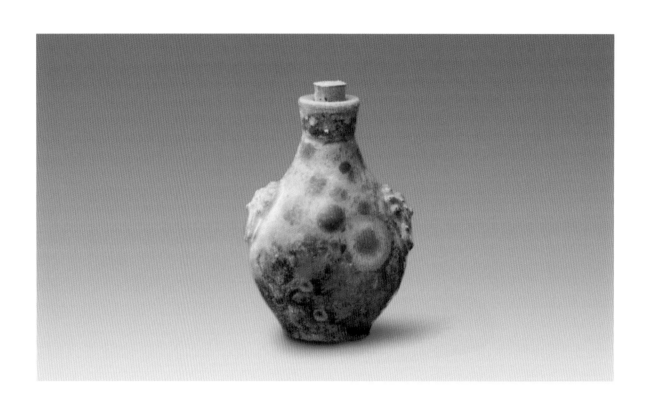

小药瓶

清

瓷质

瓶颈直径 1.2 厘米，瓶腹宽 3.6 厘米，瓶腹厚 2.6 厘米，通高 5.15 厘米，重 20 克

扁圆形，直口，平沿，竖颈，溜肩，对耳，鼓腹，平底，圈足。用于装药。

广东中医药博物馆藏

Small Medicine Bottle

Qing Dynasty

Porcelain

Bottleneck Diameter 1.2 cm/ Belly Width 3.6 cm/ Belly Thickness 2.6 cm/ Height 5.15 cm/ Weight 20 g

This oblate round bottle was used as a medicine container, which has a straight mouth, a flat mouth rim, a straight neck, a sloping shoulder, a pair of ears, a drum-like belly, a flat bottom, and a ring foot.

Preserved in Guangdong Chinese Medicine Museum

绿瓷玉米瓶

清

瓷质

口径 0.5 厘米，底径 1.6 厘米，通高 7 厘米，重 50 克

玉米状，通身施绿釉，直口，圈足。贮药器具。完整无损。

陕西医史博物馆藏

Green Corn-shaped Porcelain Bottle

Qing Dynasty

Porcelain

Mouth Diameter 0.5 cm/ Bottom Diameter 1.6 cm/ Height 7 cm/ Weight 50 g

This corn-shaped bottle with a straight mouth and a ring foot is fully coated with green glaze. It was used as a medicine container and remains intact.

Preserved in Shaanxi Museum of Medical History

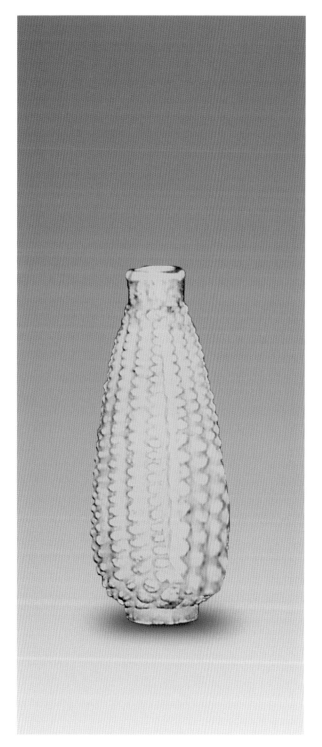

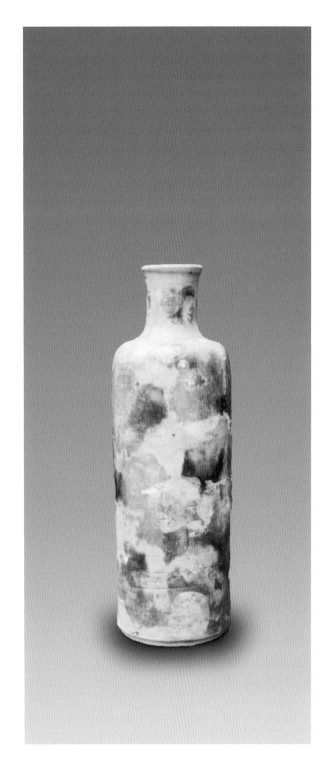

黄绿银色釉瓷瓶

清

瓷质

口外径 2.46 厘米，底径 4.66 厘米，通高 14.27 厘米，瓶身高 11.43 厘米，瓶深 12.4 厘米，重 140 克

Green Yellow and Silver Glazed Porcelain Bottle

Qing Dynasty

Porcelain

Mouth Outer Diameter 2.46 cm/ Bottom Diameter 4.66 cm/ Height 14.27 cm/ Body Height 11.43 cm/ Depth 12.4 cm/ Weight 140 g

圆柱形，口微敞，平沿，直长颈，溜肩，直
腹，平底，圈足，外施黄绿银色釉，底无釉。
装药用。

广东中医药博物馆藏

This cylindrical bottle has a slightly-flared mouth,
a flat mouth rim, a long and straight neck, a sloping
shoulder, a straight belly, a flat bottom, and a ring
foot,the exterior of which is glazed in silver. The
bottom is left unglazed. It was used as a medicine
container.

Preserved in Guangdong Chinese Medicine Museum

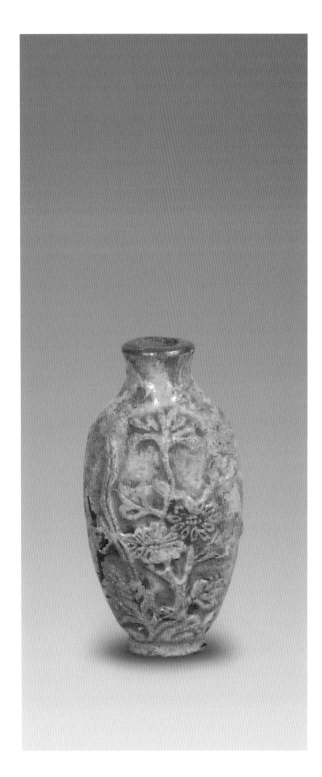

瓷药瓶

清

瓷质

口外径 1.7 厘米，口内径 0.85 厘米，宽 3.6 厘米，高 6.9 厘米，厚 2.55 厘米

Porcelain Medicine Bottle

Qing Dynasty

Porcelain

Mouth Outer Diameter 1.7 cm/ Mouth Inner Diameter 0.85 cm/

Width 3.6 cm/ Height 6.9 cm/ Thickness 2.55 cm

扁瓶状，通身施黄绿釉，绘浮雕花草图案，平口，平底，底无款识，工艺一般。盛药器具。保存基本完好。1955 年入藏。

中华医学会 / 上海中医药大学医史博物馆藏

Adorned with relief carving of flower and grass designs, this yellow and green glazed oblate bottle has a flat mouth and a flat bottom with no inscription. The bottle with average quality workmanship was used as a medicine container. It was collected in the year 1955 and remains intact.

Preserved in Chinese Medical Association/ Museum of Chinese Medicine, Shanghai University of Traditional Chinese Medicine

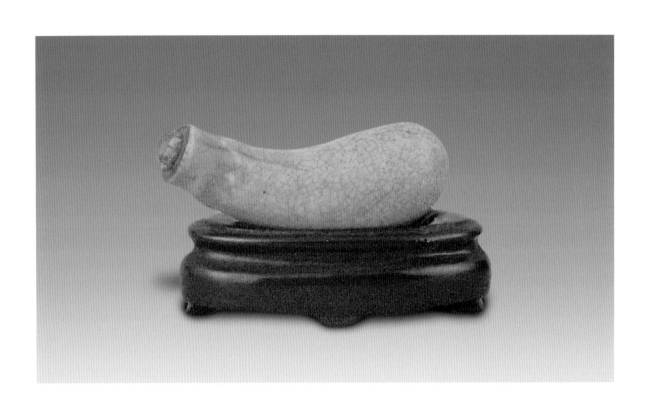

瓷药瓶

清

瓷质

长 3.8 厘米，宽 1.5 厘米

茄形，施黄绿釉，小开片，一端有嘴并配木塞，
造型小巧别致，工艺较好。保存基本完好。
1954 年入藏。

中华医学会 / 上海中医药大学医史博物馆藏

Porcelain Medicine Bottle

Qing Dynasty

Porcelain

Length 3.8 cm/ Width 1.5 cm

This eggplant-shaped bottle is fully coated with small crackle glaze in yellow and green. There is a spout and a wooden plug at one end. The tiny and exquisite bottle shows good workmanship. It was collected in the year 1954 and remains intact.

Preserved in Chinese Medical Association/ Museum of Chinese Medicine, Shanghai University of Traditional Chinese Medicine

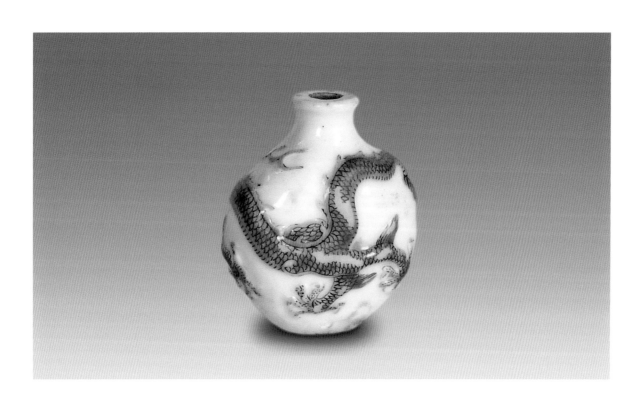

瓷药瓶

清

瓷质

口外径 1.6 厘米，口内径 0.7 厘米，宽 4.65 厘米，

通高 5.58 厘米，厚 2.9 厘米

扁瓶状，上有突起之绿釉祥龙图案。盛药器具。

保存基本完好，上口有残。1955 年入藏。

中华医学会 / 上海中医药大学医史博物馆藏

Porcelain Medicine Bottle

Qing Dynasty

Porcelain

Mouth Outer Diameter 1.6 cm/ Mouth Inner Diameter 0.7 cm/

Width 4.65 cm/ Height 5.58 cm/ Thickness 2.9 cm

This oblate bottle is adorned with raised auspicious patterns

of a dragon covered with green glaze. The bottle was used as

a medicine container, and is kept in good condition except a

cracked mouth. It was collected in the year 1955.

Preserved in Chinese Medical Association/ Museum of

Chinese Medicine, Shanghai University of Traditional

Chinese Medicine

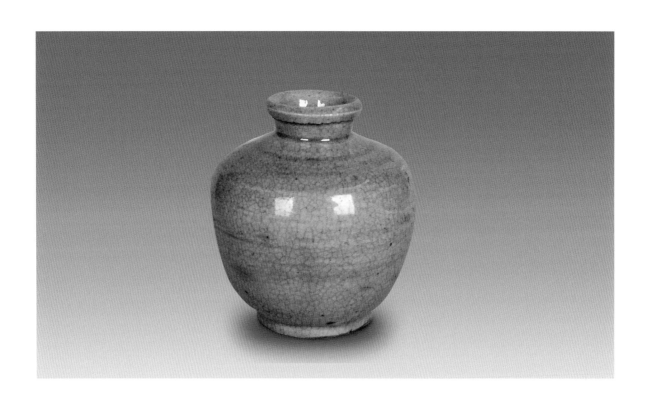

瓷药瓶

清

瓷质

口外径 4.85 厘米，口内径 3.1 厘米，腹径 15 厘米，底径 5.9 厘米，高 11.3 厘米

Porcelain Medicine Bottle

Qing Dynasty

Porcelain

Mouth Outer Diameter 4.85 cm/ Mouth Inner Diameter 3.1 cm/ Belly Diameter 15 cm/ Bottom Diameter 5.9 cm/ Height 11.3 cm

圆形，施黄绿釉，小开片，有旋纹，圈足，平底，无款识，工艺精良。盛药器具。保存基本完好。1958 年入藏。

中华医学会 / 上海中医药大学医史博物馆藏

This round bottle is fully coated with yellow and green crackle glaze. Adorned with whorl designs, the bottle has a ring foot and a flat bottom with no inscription. The bottle with exquisite workmanship was used as a medicine container. It was collected in the year 1958 and remains intact.

Preserved in Chinese Medical Association/ Museum of Chinese Medicine, Shanghai University of Traditional Chinese Medicine

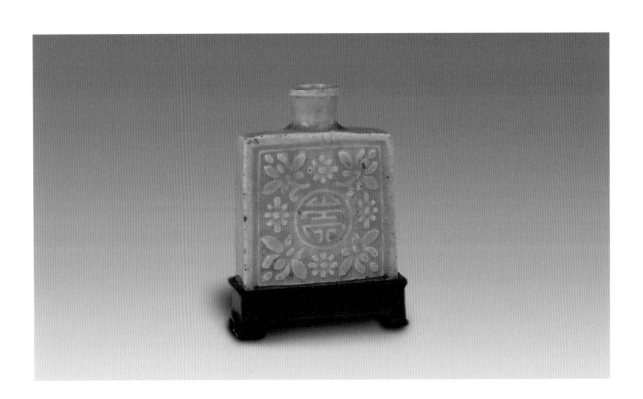

瓷药瓶

清

瓷质

口径 2 厘米，宽 6.2 厘米，通高 7.8 厘米，厚 2.4 厘米

Porcelain Medicine Bottle

Qing Dynasty

Porcelain

Mouth Diameter 2 cm/ Width 6.2 cm/ Height 7.8 cm/ Thickness 2.4 cm

方瓶形，施青绿釉，浮雕"寿"字、花卉等图案，直口，平底，圈足，小巧玲珑，工艺精良。盛药器具。保存基本完好。1954 年入藏。

中华医学会 / 上海中医药大学医史博物馆藏

This blue-and-green square bottle is decorated with a Chinese character "Shou" (longevity) cut in relief as well as some patterns of flowers and plants. This tiny bottle, featuring a straight mouth, a flat bottom and a ring foot, shows exquisite workmanship. It was used as a medicine container, and is still in good condition. It was collected in the year 1954.

Preserved in Chinese Medical Association/ Museum of Chinese Medicine, Shanghai University of Traditional Chinese Medicine

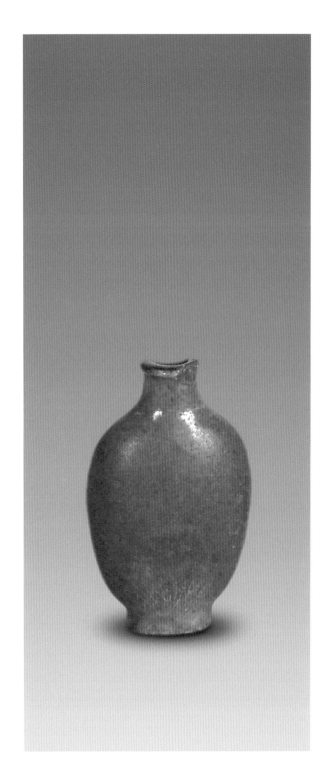

瓷药瓶

清

瓷质

口外径 1.4 厘米，口内径 0.7 厘米，宽 3.6 厘米，

通高 5.9 厘米，厚 1.88 厘米

扁瓶状，通身施绿釉。盛药器具。保存基本完好，

上口有残。1955 年入藏。

中华医学会 / 上海中医药大学医史博物馆藏

Porcelain Medicine Bottle

Qing Dynasty

Porcelain

Mouth Outer Diameter 1.4 cm/ Mouth Inner Diameter 0.7 cm/

Width 3.6 cm/ Height 5.9 cm/ Thickness 1.88 cm

This green-glazed oblate bottle was used as a medicine

container, which is kept intact except the cracked mouth.

It was collected in the year 1955.

Preserved in Chinese Medical Association/ Museum of

Chinese Medicine, Shanghai University of Traditional

Chinese Medicine

小药瓶

清

瓷质

口外径 1.5 厘米，通高 5.1 厘米，腹宽 3.5 厘米，腹厚 2.2 厘米，重 17 克

扁圆形，敞口，平沿，直颈，溜肩，鼓腹，平底，圈足，腹身雕青蝉一只，伏于器身，形象生动，纹理清晰。用于装药。

广东中医药博物馆藏

Small Medicine Bottle

Qing Dynasty

Porcelain

Mouth Outer Diameter 1.5 cm/ Height 5.1 cm/Belly Width 3.5 cm/ Belly Thickness 2.2 cm/ Weight 17 g

This oblate bottle has a flared mouth, a flat mouth rim, a straight neck, a sloping shoulder, a drum-like belly, a flat bottom, and a ring foot. The belly was engraved a cicada, which is very lively and clear in lines and veins. It was used as a medicine container.

Preserved in Guangdong Chinese Medicine Museum

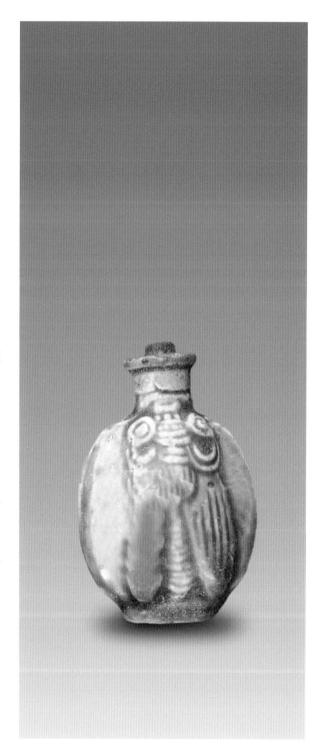

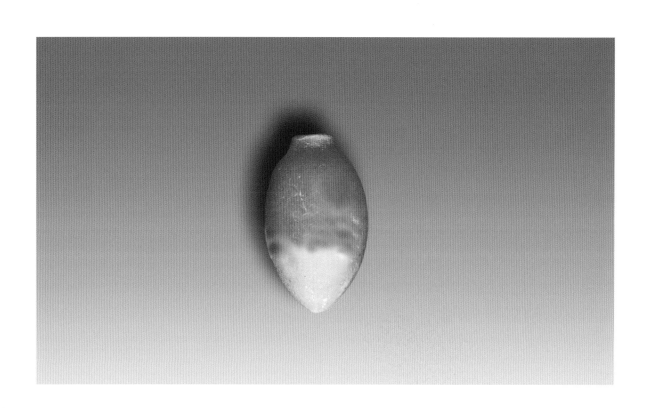

小药瓶

清

瓷质

口外径 0.75 厘米，腹径 1.7 厘米，通高 3 厘米，
重 6 克

蛋形，直口，平沿，溜肩，鼓腹，尖底，器身施
绿釉。用于装药。

广东中医药博物馆藏

Small Medicine Bottle

Qing Dynasty

Porcelain

Mouth Outer Diameter 0.75 cm/ Belly Diameter 1.7 cm/
Height 3 cm/ Weight 6 g

This egg-shaped bottle has a straight mouth, a flat mouth
rim, a sloping shoulder, a drum-like belly, an ogival
bottom. Its body is glazed in green. This bottle was used
for storing medicine.

Preserved in Guangdong Chinese Medicine Museum

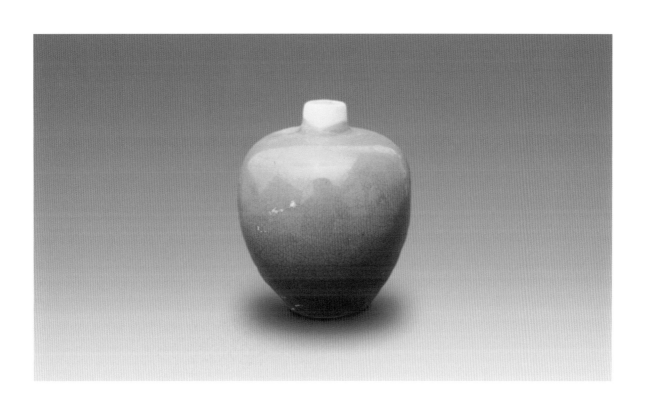

古翠绿小药瓶

清

瓷质

口外径 1.63 厘米，腹径 6.27 厘米，底径 3.02 厘米，

通高 7.61 厘米，腹深 6.9 厘米，重 94 克

直口，平沿，平肩，鼓腹，腹渐收至底，平底，

圈足。装药用。

广东中医药博物馆藏

Jade-green Small Medicine Bottle

Qing Dynasty

Porcelain

Mouth Outer Diameter 1.63 cm/ Belly Diameter 6.27 cm/

Bottom Diameter 3.02 cm/ Height 7.61 cm/ Belly Depth

6.9 cm/ Weight 94 g

This bottle has a straight mouth, a flat mouth rim, a flat

shoulder, a drum-like belly, which contracted slowly on

the lower part, a flat bottom, and a ring foot. The bottle

served as a medicine container.

Preserved in Guangdong Chinese Medicine Museum

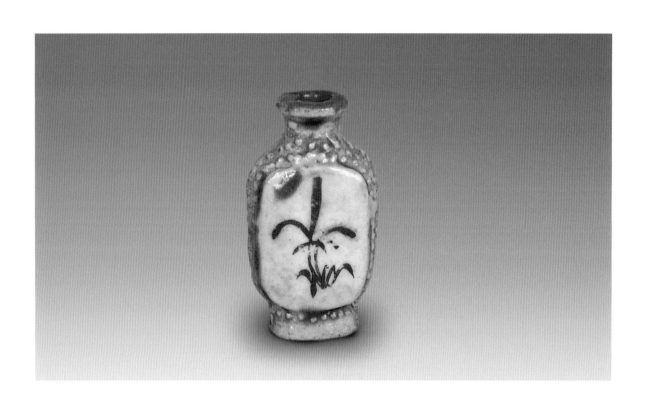

瓷药瓶

清

瓷质

口外径 1.6 厘米，口内径 0.7 厘米，宽 2.95 厘米，
高 5.3 厘米，厚 0.85 厘米

扁瓶状，施绿釉和乳白釉，器表绘有褐色植物图
案，工艺粗糙，施釉不匀。盛药器具。口沿有残。
1955 年入藏。

中华医学会 / 上海中医药大学医史博物馆藏

Porcelain Medicine Bottle

Qing Dynasty

Porcelain

Mouth Outer Diameter 1.6 cm/ Mouth Inner Diameter
0.7 cm/ Width 2.95 cm/ Height 5.3 cm/ Thickness 0.85 cm

The bottle is oblate in shape and is coated with green
glaze and opal glaze. On its body are painted brown
floral patterns. Due to rough craftsmanship, the glaze
is unevenly enameled. The bottle was used for storing
medicine and its mouth rim was damaged. It was
collected in 1955.

Preserved in Chinese Medical Association/ Museum of
Chinese Medicine, Shanghai University of Traditional
Chinese Medicine

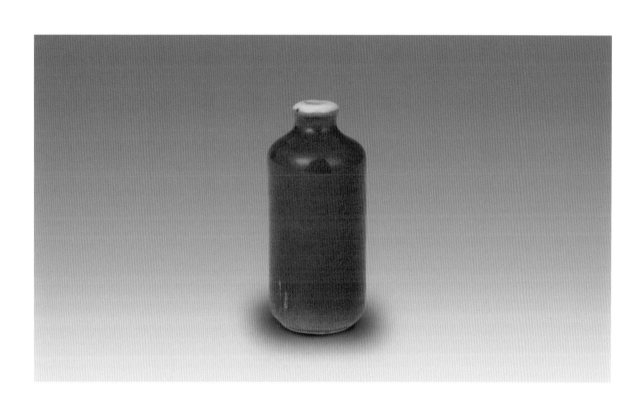

药瓶

清

瓷质

口径 1.6 厘米，腹径 3.3 厘米，通高 7.6 厘米

圆瓶形，蓝色釉，表面润泽光亮，直口，平底，

小巧玲珑，工艺较好。盛药器具。保存基本完好。

1955 年入藏。

中华医学会 / 上海中医药大学医史博物馆藏

Medicine Bottle

Qing Dynasty

Porcelain

Mouth Diameter 1.6 cm/ Belly Diameter 3.3 cm/ Height 7.6 cm

This round bottle is coated with lustrous blue glaze. It is small and exquisite with a straight mouth and a flat bottom. The bottle was used for storing medicine and is basically well-preserved. It was collected in 1955.

Preserved in Chinese Medical Association/ Museum of Chinese Medicine, Shanghai University of Traditional Chinese Medicine

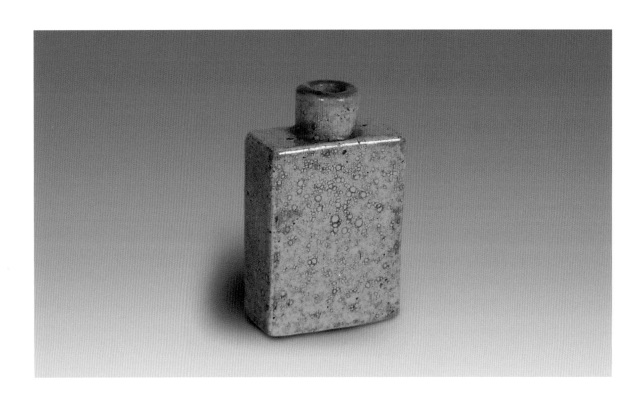

瓷药瓶

清

瓷质

口外径 1.55 厘米，口内径 0.7 厘米，宽 3.55 厘米，通高 5.7 厘米，厚 1.75 厘米

Porcelain Medicine Bottle

Qing Dynasty

Porcelain

Mouth Outer Diameter 1.55 cm/ Mouth Inner Diameter 0.7 cm/ Width 3.55 cm/ Height 5.7 cm/ Thickness 1.75 cm

扁方形，通身施蓝灰釉，瓶口为棕黄釉，瓶底无款识。盛药器具。有残。 1955 年入藏。

中华医学会 / 上海中医药大学医史博物馆藏

This bottle is cuboid in shape and is coated entirely with bluish-grey glaze, except its mouth rim, which is enameled with brownish-yellow glaze. There is no inscription on its bottom. It was for storing medicine and is slightly damaged. It was collected in 1955. Preserved in Chinese Medical Association/ Museum of Chinese Medicine, Shanghai University of Traditional Chinese Medicine

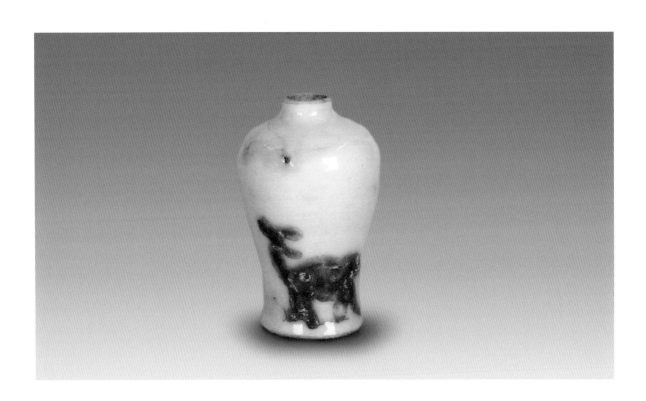

瓷药瓶

清

瓷质

口外径 1.4 厘米，口内径 1.05 厘米，直径 3.95 厘米，通高 6.3 厘米

Porcelain Medicine Bottle

Qing Dynasty

Porcelain

Mouth Outer Diameter 1.4 cm/ Mouth Inner Diameter 1.05 cm/ Diameter 3.95 cm/ Height 6.3 cm

圆形，通身施青灰釉，瓶身饰赭色动物图案，无盖，表面光滑，瓶底无款识，制作工艺一般。盛药器具。保存基本完好。1957 年入藏。

中华医学会 / 上海中医药大学医史博物馆藏

This round bottle, with average craftsmanship, was used for storing medicine. Its whole body is coated with smooth celadon-gray glaze. It has no inscription on the bottom and no lid on the top with a reddish brown animal motif on the body. The basically well-preserved bottle was collected in 1957.

Preserved in Chinese Medical Association/ Museum of Chinese Medicine, Shanghai University of Traditional Chinese Medicine

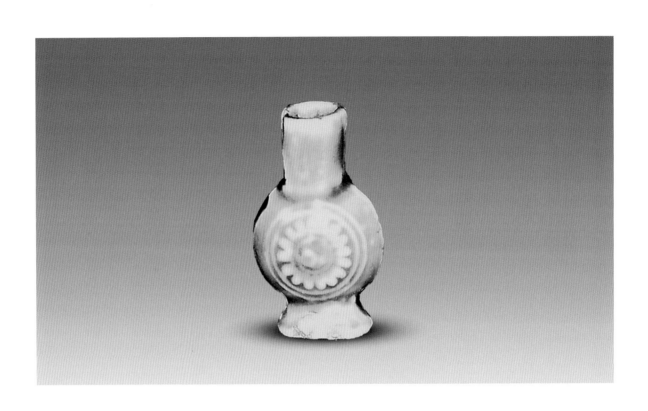

瓷药瓶

清

瓷质

口径 1 厘米，底径 1.5 厘米，高 4.2 厘米，重
12 克

直口，圆腹，平底，腹中有葵花太极纹。医药器
具。口、底略残。2001 年 9 月入藏，陕西省西
安市古玩市场征集。

陕西医史博物馆藏

Porcelain Medicine Bottle

Qing Dynasty

Porcelain

Mouth Diameter 1 cm/ Bottom Diameter 1.5 cm/ Height
4.2 cm/ Weight 12 g

The bottle has a straight mouth, a rounded belly, and a flat
bottom. The centre of its belly is decorated with sunflower
and Taiji patterns. It served as a medicine utensil. Both
its mouth and bottom are slightly damaged. The bottle
was collected from the Antique Market in Xi'an, Shaanxi
Province, in September 2001.

Preserved in Shaanxi Museum of Medical History

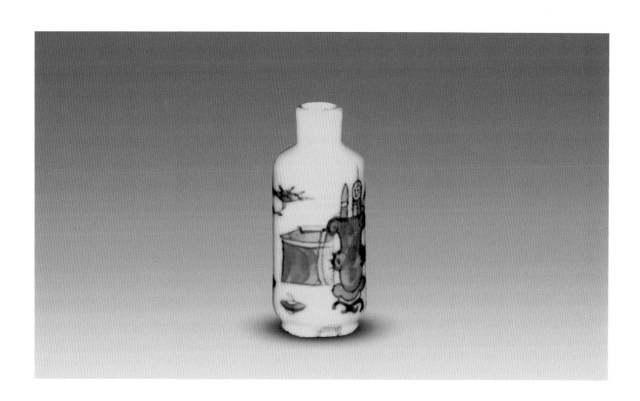

青花小药瓶

清

瓷质

口径 1.2 厘米，底径 1.9 厘米，高 5.5 厘米，重 34 克

直圆口，平肩，直腹，圈足，腹饰有青花花瓶图案。医药器具。保存完整。2001 年 9 月入藏，陕西省西安市古玩市场征集。

陕西医史博物馆藏

Small Medicine Bottle with Blue-and-white Design

Qing Dynasty

Porcelain

Mouth Diameter 1.2 cm/ Bottom Diameter 1.9 cm/ Height 5.5 cm/ Weight 34 g

The bottle has a straight and round mouth, a flat shoulder, a straight belly, and a ring foot. Its belly is decorated with blue-and-white vase patterns. It served as a medicine utensil and remains intact. The bottle was collected from the Antique Market in Xi'an, Shaanxi Province, in September 2001.

Preserved in Shaanxi Museum of Medical History

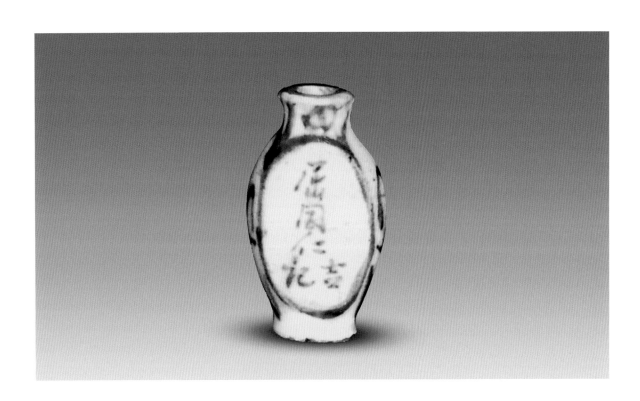

青花小药瓶

清

瓷质

口径 1.4 厘米，底径 1.1 厘米 ×1.7 厘米，高 5.1 厘米，重 16 克

Small Medicine Bottle with Blue-and-white Design

Qing Dynasty

Porcelain

Mouth Diameter 1.4 cm/ Bottom Diameter 1.1 cm ×1.7 cm/ Height 5.1 cm/ Weight 16 g

平口沿，扁腹，椭圆圈足，腹两侧饰青花缠枝纹，腹一面有"屈同仁吉记"，一面有"痧气丹"。医药器具。保存完整。2001 年 9 月入藏，陕西省西安市古玩市场征集。

陕西医史博物馆藏

The bottle has a flat mouth rim, an oblate belly and an oval-shaped ring foot. Blue-and-white interlocking patterns can be seen on both flanks of its belly. On one side of its belly is written the name of the pharmacy "Qu Tong Ren Ji Ji", while on the other side the name of the drug "Sha Qi Dan". The bottle served as a medicine utensil and remains intact. It was collected from the Antique Market in Xi'an, Shaanxi Province, in September 2001.

Preserved in Shaanxi Museum of Medical History

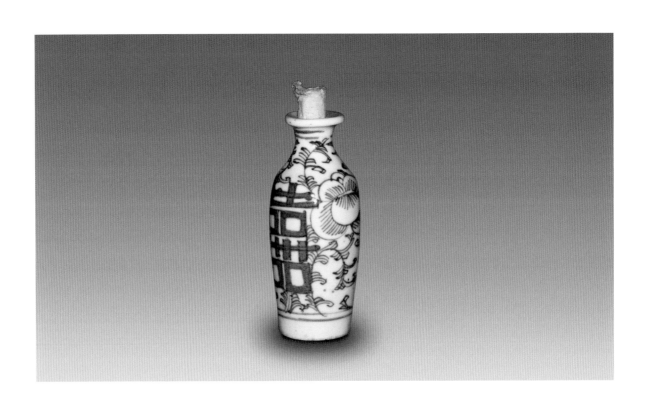

青花药瓶

清

瓷质

口径 3 厘米，底径 3.6 厘米，高 11.2 厘米，重 150 克

Medicine Bottle with Blue-and-white Design

Qing Dynasty

Porcelain

Mouth Diameter 3 cm/ Bottom Diameter 3.6 cm/ Height 11.2 cm/ Weight 150 g

小喇叭口，圆唇，溜肩，直斜腹，圈足，瓶身有朱砂面标签，青花"喜"字缠枝花卉图案。医药器具。保存完整。2001 年 9 月入藏，陕西省西安市鼓楼文物市场征集。

陕西医史博物馆藏

The bottle has a small trumpet mouth, a round lip, a sloping shoulder, a straight and oblique belly, and a ring foot. Its belly is painted with cinnabar pigment, which serves as a label. Its belly is embellished with blue-and-white interlocking floral patterns together with Chinese character "Xi" (happiness). It served as a medicine utensil and is still in good shape. The bottle was collected from the Drum Tower Market of Culture Relics in Xi'an, Shaanxi Province, in September 2001.

Preserved in Shaanxi Museum of Medical History

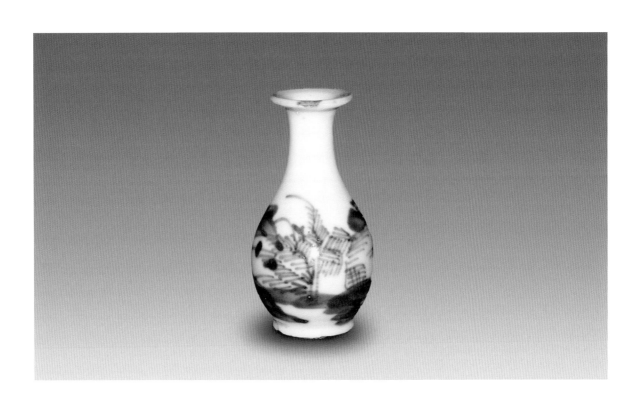

青花小药瓶

清

瓷质

口径 2.8 厘米，底径 2.8 厘米，高 7.8 厘米

小喇叭口，长颈，圆腹，圈足，腹饰青花花卉。
医药器具。口沿略残。陕西省西安市古玩市场征集。

陕西医史博物馆藏

Small Medicine Bottle with Blue-and-white Floral Design

Qing Dynasty

Porcelain

Mouth Diameter 2.8 cm/ Bottom Diameter 2.8 cm/ Height 7.8 cm

The bottle has a small trumpet mouth, a long neck, a rounded belly, and a ring foot. Its belly is decorated with blue-and-white floral patterns. It served as a medicine utensil and its mouth rim is slightly damaged. The bottle was collected from the Antique Market in Xi'an, Shaanxi Province.

Preserved in Shaanxi Museum of Medical History

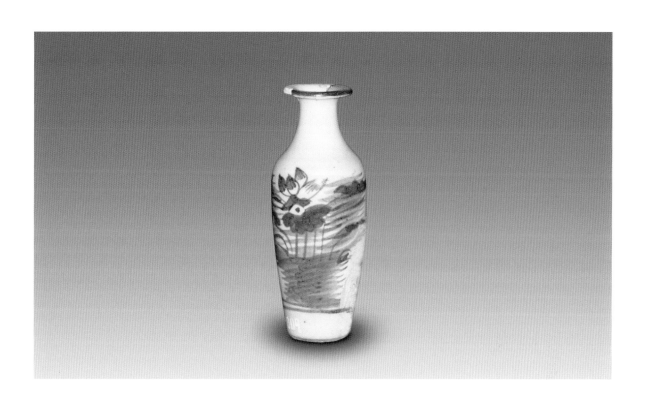

青花瓷药瓶

清

瓷质

口径 3.5 厘米，底径 3.8 厘米，通高 13 厘米，重 150 克

喇叭口，折肩，斜腹，平底，圈足，腹饰水纹图案。贮药器具。口沿有修补。

陕西医史博物馆藏

Blue-and-white Porcelain Medicine Bottle

Qing Dynasty

Porcelain

Mouth Diameter 3.5 cm/ Bottom Diameter 3.8 cm/ Height 13 cm/ Weight 150 g

The bottle has a trumpet mouth, an angular shoulder, an oblique belly, a flat bottom, and a ring foot. Water patterns decorate the body. It is a medicine container. The mouth rim has been repaired.

Preserved in Shaanxi Museum of Medical History

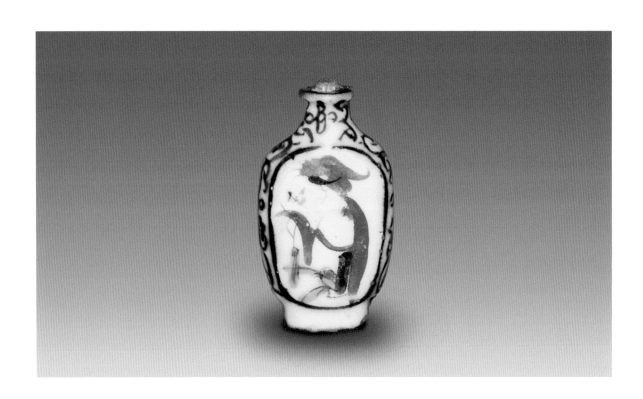

青花人物图案瓷药瓶

清

瓷质

口径 1.6 厘米，底径 1.5 厘米 ×2.5 厘米，高 6.8 厘米，重 40 克

Porcelain Medicine Bottle with Blue-and-white Figure Pattern

Qing Dynasty

Porcelain

Mouth Diameter 1.6 cm/ Bottom Diameter 1.5 cm×2.5 cm/ Height 6.8 cm/ Weight 40 g

平口沿，扁腹，椭圆圈足，腹两侧有青花缠枝纹，腹两面有彩色人物图案，一面贴有"金疮散"药签。医药器具。口沿残。2001 年 9 月入藏，陕西省西安市古玩市场征集。

陕西医史博物馆藏

The bottle has a flat mouth rim, an oblate belly, and an oval-shaped ring foot. On the two sides are blue-and-white patterns of interlocking branches, while on the two faces of it are coloured figure patterns. A medicine label"Jin Chuang San"can be seen on one face of the bottle. It was used as a medicine container, whose mouth rim was broken. It was collected from the Antique Market in Xi'an, Shaanxi Province, in September 2001.

Preserved in Shaanxi Museum of Medical History

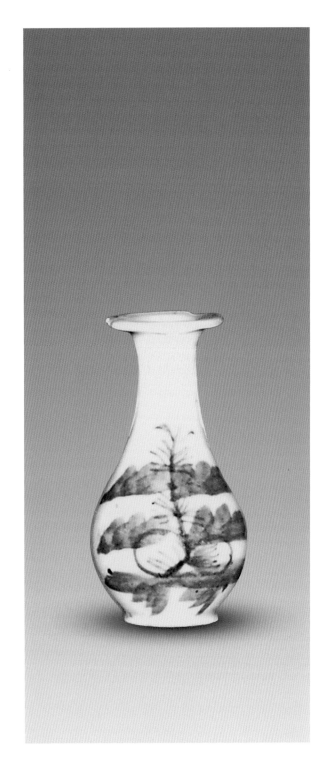

青花瓷药瓶

清

瓷质

口径 3 厘米，底径 2.5 厘米，通高 7.5 厘米，重 500 克

喇叭口，长颈，鼓腹，圈足，腹饰青瓷蓝花。贮药器具。口沿小残。

陕西医史博物馆藏

Blue-and-white Porcelain Medicine Bottle

Qing Dynasty

Porcelain

Mouth Diameter 3 cm/ Bottom Diameter 2.5 cm/ Height 7.5 cm/ Weight 500 g

The bottle has a trumpet mouth, a long neck, a drum-like belly, and a ring foot. Its belly is decorated with blue flower patterns. It was used for storing medicine and its mouth rim is slightly damaged.

Preserved in Shaanxi Museum of Medical History

青花瓷药瓶

清

瓷质

口径 2.3 厘米，底径 2.5 厘米，通高 8.5 厘米，
重 500 克

喇叭口，细颈，鼓腹，圈足，腹饰青瓷菊花图。
贮药器具。口沿小残。

陕西医史博物馆藏

Blue-and-white Porcelain Medicine Bottle

Qing Dynasty

Porcelain

Mouth Diameter 2.3 cm/ Bottom Diameter 2.5 cm/
Height 8.5 cm/ Weight 500 g

The bottle has a trumpet mouth, a narrow neck, a drum-like
belly, and a ring foot. A blue-and-white chrysanthemum
pattern is painted on its belly. It was used for storing
medicine and its mouth rim is slightly damaged.

Preserved in Shaanxi Museum of Medical History

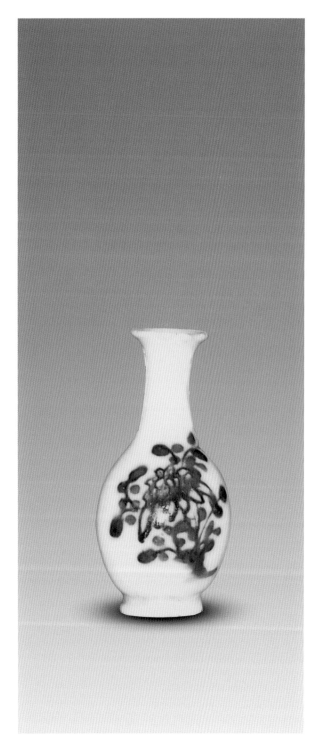

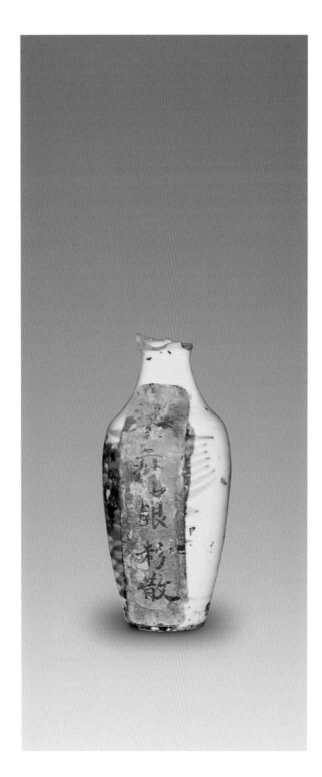

青花瓷药瓶

清

瓷质

口径 3 厘米，底径 3.5 厘米，通高 12 厘米，重
150 克

喇叭口，圆腹，圈足，腹饰兰花，药签名为"疝
银粉散"。贮药器具。口沿有残。陕西省汉中市
公兴大药店征集。

陕西医史博物馆藏

Blue-and-white Porcelain Medicine Bottle

Qing Dynasty

Porcelain

Mouth Diameter 3 cm/ Bottom Diameter 3.5 cm/ Height
12 cm/ Weight 150 g

The bottle has a trumpet mouth, a rounded belly, and a
ring foot. Blue-and-white orchid patterns are painted on
its belly upon which is pasted the name of the medicine
"Shan Yin Fen San". The bottle was used for storing
medicine and its mouth rim is damaged. It was collected from
Gongxing Pharmacy, Hanzhong City, Shaanxi Province.

Preserved in Shaanxi Museum of Medical History

瓷药瓶

清

瓷质

口径 4.5 厘米，底径 4.5 厘米，通高 17 厘米，
重 250 克

喇叭口，直斜腹，圈足，腹饰几何图形。贮药器
具。口沿有残。陕西省华阴市征集。

陕西医史博物馆藏

Porcelain Medicine Bottle

Qing Dynasty

Porcelain

Mouth Diameter 4.5 cm/ Bottom Diameter 4.5 cm/
Height 17 cm/ Weight 250 g

The bottle has a trumpet mouth, a straight and oblique
belly, and a ring foot. Its belly is decorated with
geometrical patterns. The bottle was used for storing
medicine and its mouth rim is damaged. It was collected
from Huayin City, Shaanxi Province.

Preserved in Shaanxi Museum of Medical History

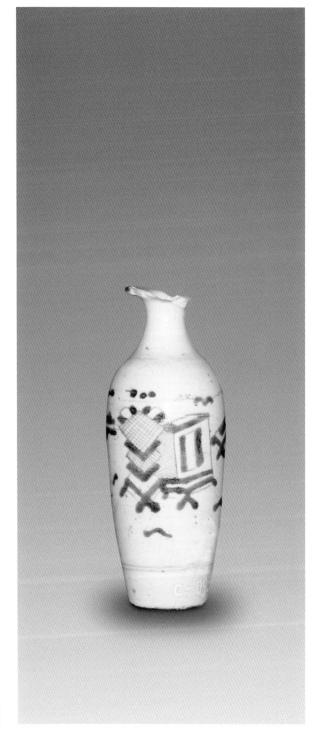

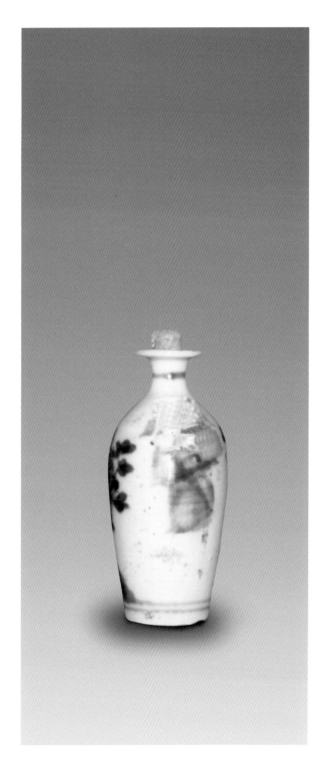

青花瓷小药瓶

清

瓷质

口径 3.5 厘米，底径 4.3 厘米，通高 14 厘米，重 300 克

喇叭口，溜肩，圆腹，圈足，腹饰小兰花。贮药器具。口沿有残。陕西省周至县广育堂遗物。

陕西医史博物馆藏

Small Blue-and-white Porcelain Medicine Bottle

Qing Dynasty

Porcelain

Mouth Diameter 3.5 cm/ Bottom Diameter 4.3 cm/ Height 14 cm/ Weight 300 g

The bottle has a trumpet mouth, a sloping shoulder, a rounded belly, and a ring foot. Small orchid patterns are painted on its belly. The bottle was used for storing medicine and its mouth rim is damaged. It was the relic of Guang Yu Tang in Zhouzhi County, Shaanxi Province. Preserved in Shaanxi Museum of Medical History

瓷药瓶

清

瓷质

口径 3 厘米，底径 3.5 厘米，通高 12 厘米，重 150 克

喇叭口，圆肩，斜腹，圈足，腹饰荷花图，底有 "诤花□先生石羔用"。贮药器具。完整无损。

陕西医史博物馆藏

Porcelain Medicine Bottle

Qing Dynasty

Porcelain

Mouth Diameter 3 cm/ Bottom Diameter 3.5 cm/ Height 12 cm/ Weight 150 g

The bottle has a trumpet mouth, a rounded shoulder, an oblique belly, and a ring foot. Lotus patterns are painted on its belly. There is an inscription on its bottom. The bottle was used for storing medicine and remains intact.

Preserved in Shaanxi Museum of Medical History

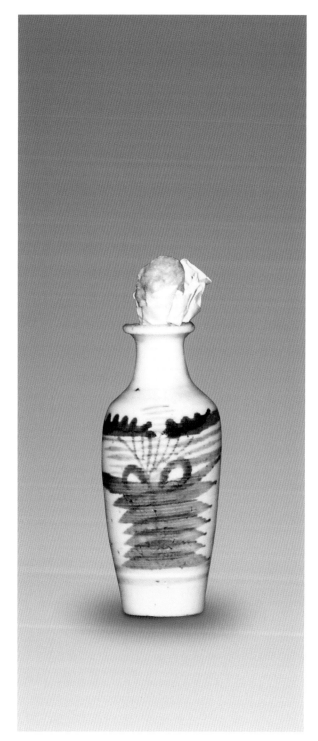

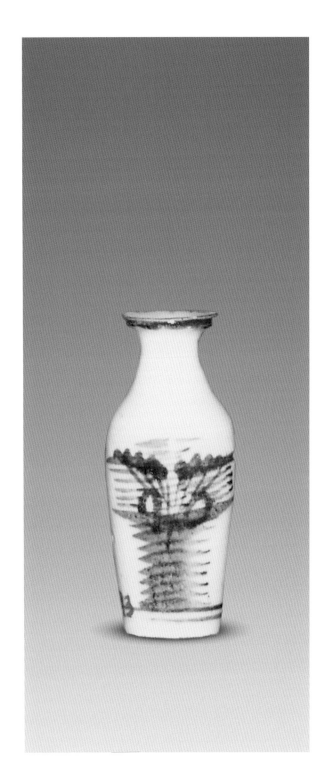

瓷药瓶

清

瓷质

口径 3.2 厘米，底径 3.2 厘米，通高 10.5 厘米，重 150 克

喇叭口，圆肩，斜腹，圈足，腹饰青瓷荷花图。贮药器具。底有残。陕西省汉中市公兴大药店征集。

陕西医史博物馆藏

Porcelain Medicine Bottle

Qing Dynasty

Porcelain

Mouth Diameter 3.2 cm/ Bottom Diameter 3.2 cm/ Height 10.5 cm/ Weight 150 g

The bottle has a trumpet mouth, a rounded shoulder, an oblique belly, and a ring foot. On its belly are painted blue-and-white lotus patterns. It was used for storing medicine and its bottom is damaged. The bottle was collected from Gongxing Pharmacy, Hanzhong City, Shaanxi Province.

Preserved in Shaanxi Museum of Medical History

瓷药瓶

清

瓷质

口径 2.8 厘米，底径 3 厘米，通高 10 厘米，重
100 克

喇叭口，折肩，斜腹，圈足，腹饰水纹图。医药
器具。完整无损。

陕西医史博物馆藏

Porcelain Medicine Bottle

Qing Dynasty

Porcelain

Mouth Diameter 2.8 cm/ Bottom Diameter 3 cm/ Height
10 cm/ Weight 100 g

The bottle has a trumpet mouth, an angular shoulder, an
oblique belly, and a ring foot. On its belly are painted
ripple patterns. The bottle served as a medicine utensil
and remains intact.

Preserved in Shaanxi Museum of Medical History

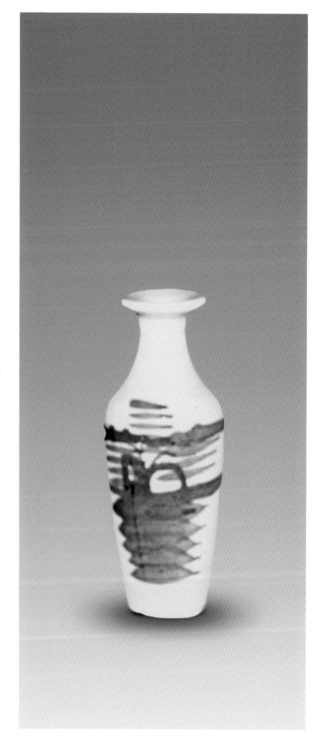

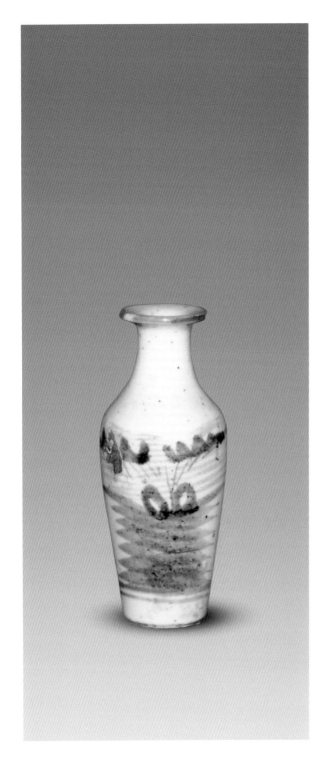

瓷药瓶

清

瓷质

口径 3.4 厘米，底径 3.2 厘米，通高 3.1 厘米，重 150 克

喇叭口，折肩，斜腹，圈足，腹饰荷花图。医药器具。完整无损。

陕西医史博物馆藏

Porcelain Medicine Bottle

Qing Dynasty

Porcelain

Mouth Diameter 3.4 cm/ Bottom Diameter 3.2 cm/ Height 3.1 cm/ Weight 150 g

The bottle has a trumpet mouth, an angular shoulder, an oblique belly, and a ring foot. Its belly is decorated with lotus patterns. The bottle served as a medicine utensil and remains intact.

Preserved in Shaanxi Museum of Medical History

瓷药瓶

清

瓷质

口径 3.8 厘米，底径 3.8 厘米，通高 11.6 厘米，重 150 克

喇叭口，折肩，斜腹，圈足，腹饰兰花图，标签名为"万应痧"。医药器具。口沿有残。

陕西医史博物馆藏

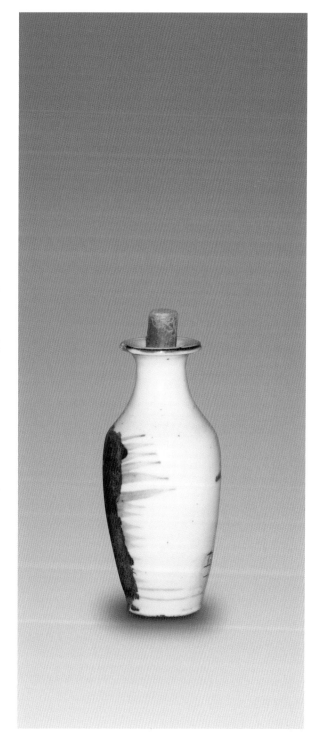

Porcelain Medicine Bottle

Qing Dynasty

Porcelain

Mouth Diameter 3.8 cm/ Bottom Diameter 3.8 cm/ Height 11.6 cm/ Weight 150 g

The bottle has a trumpet mouth, an angular shoulder, an oblique belly, and a ring foot. Its belly is decorated with orchid patterns, together with a label of the name of the medicine "Wan Ying Sha". The bottle served as a medicine utensil and its mouth rim is damaged.

Preserved in Shaanxi Museum of Medical History

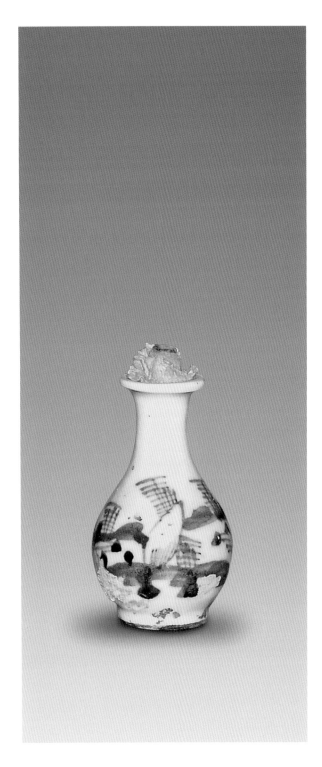

瓷药瓶

清

瓷质

口径 2.6 厘米，底径 2.9 厘米，通高 7.8 厘米，重 50 克

喇叭口，长颈，圆腹，圈足，标签名"梅花点舌丹"。贮药器具。完整无损。

陕西医史博物馆藏

Porcelain Medicine Bottle

Qing Dynasty

Porcelain

Mouth Diameter 2.6 cm/ Bottom Diameter 2.9 cm/ Height 7.8 cm/ Weight 50 g

The bottle has a trumpet mouth, a long neck, a rounded belly, and a ring foot. On its belly is inscribed the name of the medicine "Mei Hua Dian She Dan". The bottle was used for storing medicine and remains intact.

Preserved in Shaanxi Museum of Medical History

青花瓷药瓶

清

瓷质

口径 0.9 厘米，底径 2.9 厘米，通高 7.4 厘米，
重 50 克

小圆口，直腹，圈足，腹上饰小狗戏球图，底有
"康熙年制"字样。医药器具。完整无损。

陕西医史博物馆藏

Blue-and-white Porcelain Medicine Bottle

Qing Dynasty

Porcelain

Mouth Diameter 0.9 cm/ Bottom Diameter 2.9 cm/
Height 7.4 cm/ Weight 50 g

The bottle has a small and round mouth, a straight belly,
and a ring foot. On its belly is painted a motif of a dog
playing with a ball and on its bottom are inscribed four
Chinese characters "Kang Xi Nian Zhi" (Made during the
Reign of Kangxi). The bottle served as a medicine utensil
and remains intact.

Preserved in Shaanxi Museum of Medical History

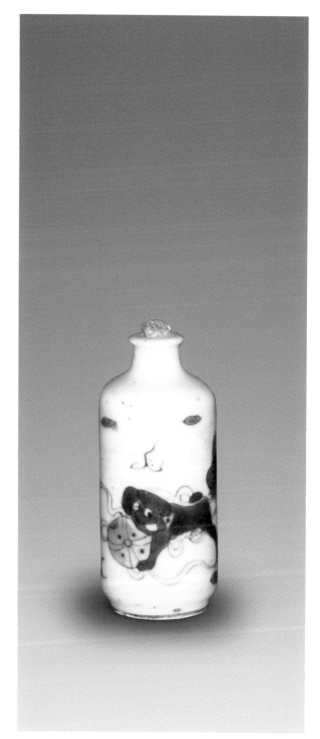

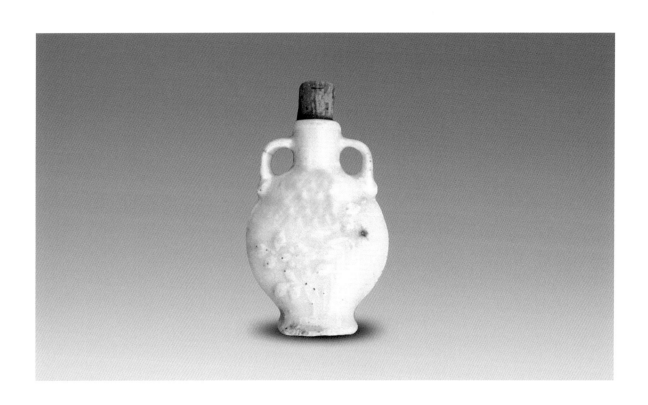

仿影青小药壶

清

瓷质

口径 1.6 厘米，腹径 2.7 厘米，腹厚 2 厘米，通高 6.3 厘米，重 45 克

仿影青，平口，直颈，扁腹，平底，底呈长方形，腹部刻有花纹，肩部有双系。

广东中医药博物馆藏

Small Medicine Pot, Imitation of Misty Blue Porcelain

Qing Dynasty

Porcelain

Mouth Diameter 1.6 cm/ Belly Diameter 2.7 cm/ Belly Thickness 2 cm/ Height 6.3 cm/ Weight 45 g

The pot has a flat mouth, a straight neck, an oblate belly, and a rectangular bottom. It is coated with fake misty blue glaze. There are two rings on its shoulder with floral patterns on its belly.

Preserved in Guangdong Chinese Medicine Museum

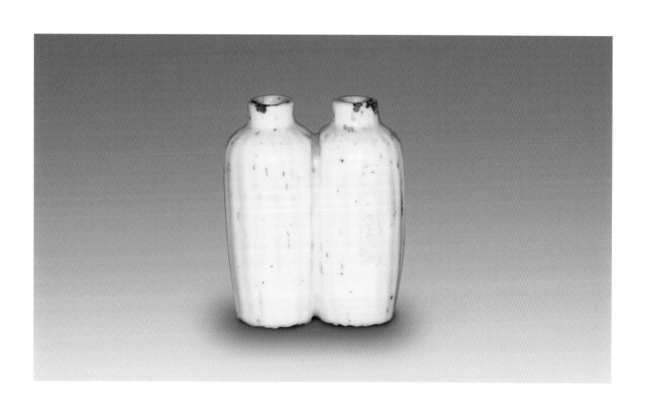

双连瓷瓶

清

瓷质

口径 1.2 厘米，底径 2.2 厘米，通高 6.2 厘米，

重 90 克

直口，圆肩，直腹，圈足，两瓶相连腹上有一条

直纹。医药器具。完整无损。

陕西医史博物馆藏

Two Conjoined Porcelain Bottles

Qing Dynasty

Porcelain

Mouth Diameter 1.2 cm/ Bottom Diameter 2.2 cm/

Height 6.2 cm/ Weight 90 g

The bottles have straight mouths, rounded shoulders,

straight bellies, and ring feet. A straight line can be seen

on the belly where the twin bottles are conjoined together.

The bottles served as medicine utensils and remain intact.

Preserved in Shaanxi Museum of Medical History

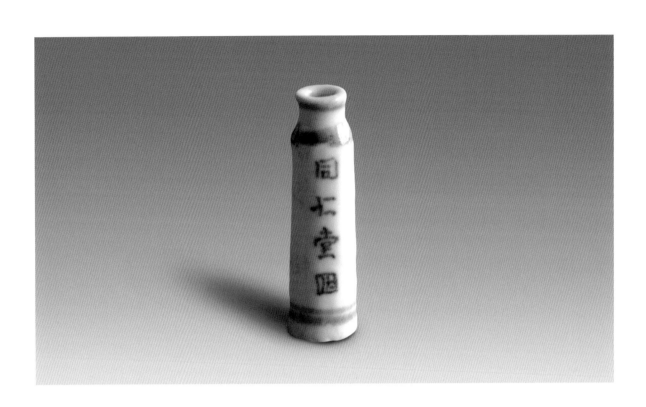

药瓶

清

瓷质

口径 1.5 厘米，高 5.5 厘米

圆柱状，平底，腹部有"同仁堂"铭和印章图案。

由民间征集。

成都中医药大学中医药传统文化博物馆藏

Medicine Bottle

Qing Dynasty

Porcelain

Mouth Diameter 1.5 cm/ Height 5.5 cm

This cylindrical bottle was collected from a private owner. The inscription and the seal of "Tong Ren Tang" can be seen respectively on its belly and flat bottom.

Preserved in Museum of Traditional Chinese Medicine Culture, Chengdu University of Traditional Chinese Medicine

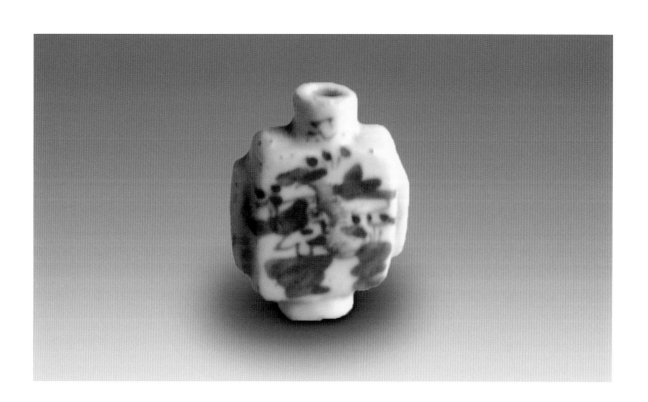

青花小药瓶

清

瓷质

高 5.5 厘米

器身扁平，口为圈柱状，圈足，器身上有青花山水纹饰。由民间征集。

　　　成都中医药大学中医药传统文化博物馆藏

Small Blue-and-white Medicine Bottle

Qing Dynasty

Porcelain

Height 5.5 cm

This flat bottle has a cylindrical mouth and a ring foot. Blue-and-white landscape patterns are painted on its body. The bottle was collected from a private owner.

Preserved in Museum of Traditional Chinese Medicine Culture, Chengdu University of Traditional Chinese Medicine

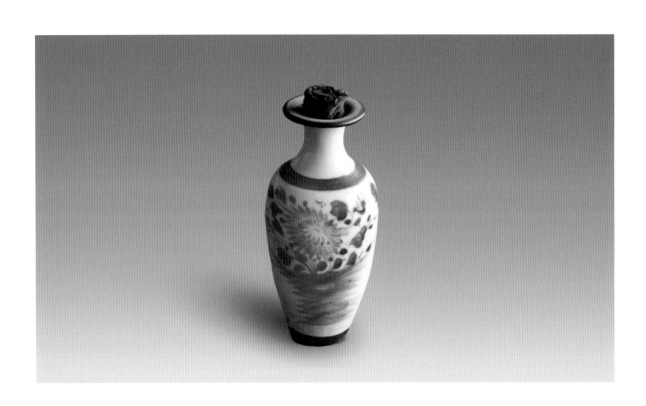

青花药瓶

清

瓷质

口径 6 厘米，高 17 厘米

束颈，鼓肩，直斜腹，浅圈足，腹部有青花草叶纹饰。由民间征集。

成都中医药大学中医药传统文化博物馆藏

Blue-and-white Medicine Bottle

Qing Dynasty

Porcelain

Mouth Diameter 6 cm/ Height 17 cm

The bottle has a contracted neck, a drum-like shoulder, a straight and oblique belly, and a shallow ring foot. Its belly is decorated with blue-and-white patterns of grass and leaves. It was collected from a private owner.

Preserved in Museum of Traditional Chinese Medicine Culture, Chengdu University of Traditional Chinese Medicine

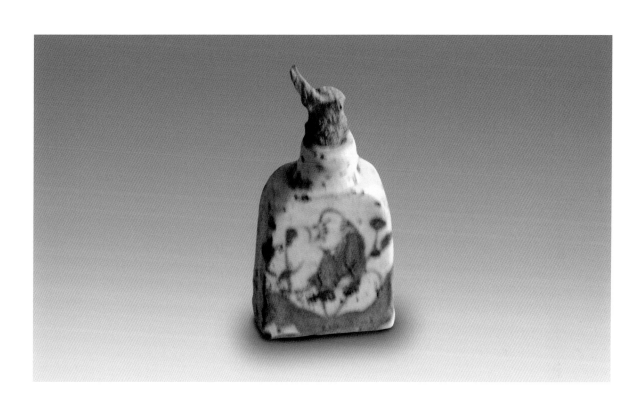

药瓶

清

瓷质

高 6.5 厘米

瓶身扁平，圆柱形口，平底，腹部饰青花枝叶纹
和动物纹。由民间征集。

　　　　成都中医药大学中医药传统文化博物馆藏

Medicine Bottle

Qing Dynasty

Porcelain

Height 6.5cm

This oblate bottle has a cylindrical mouth and a flat
bottom. Its belly is embellished with blue-and-white
flower and leaf patterns and an animal pattern. It was
collected from a private owner.

Preserved in Museum of Traditional Chinese Medicine
Culture, Chengdu University of Traditional Chinese
Medicine

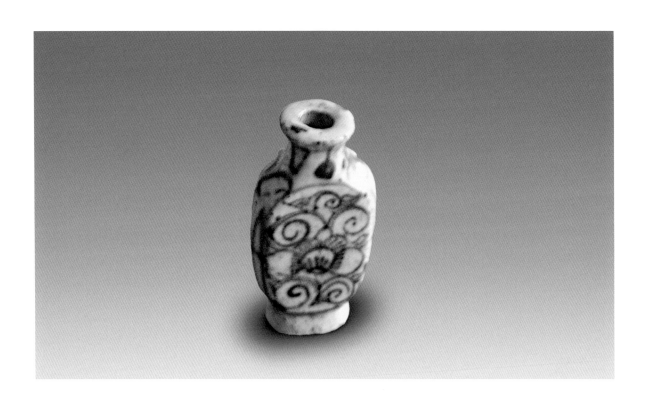

药瓶

清

瓷质

高 5 厘米

平口，瓶近似于鱼形，圈足，表面饰青花纹。用
于盛放粉状药物或小型药物颗粒。

成都中医药大学中医药传统文化博物馆藏

Medicine Bottle

Qing Dynasty

Porcelain

Height 5 cm

The bottle resembles a fish in shape and has a flat mouth
and a ring foot. It is decorated with blue-and-white floral
patterns. It was used for storing powdery medicine or
small granular medicine.

Preserved in Museum of Traditional Chinese Medicine
Culture, Chengdu University of Traditional Chinese
Medicine

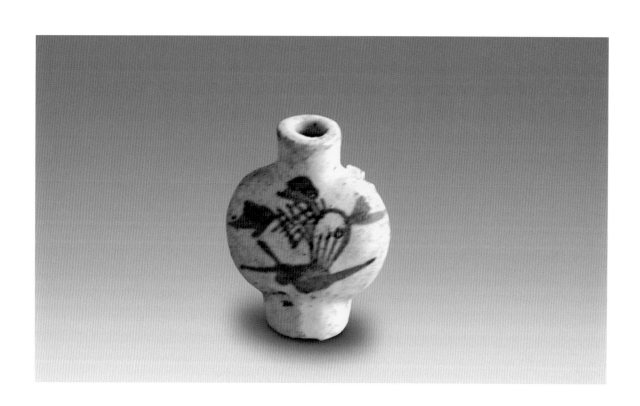

药瓶

清

瓷质

高 5 厘米

圆柱形口，瓶身较扁，鼓腹，圈足。

　　　成都中医药大学中医药传统文化博物馆藏

Medicine Bottle

Qing Dynasty

Porcelain

Height 5 cm

This oblate bottle has a cylindrical mouth, a drum-like belly, and a ring foot.

Preserved in Museum of Traditional Chinese Medicine Culture, Chengdu University of Traditional Chinese Medicine

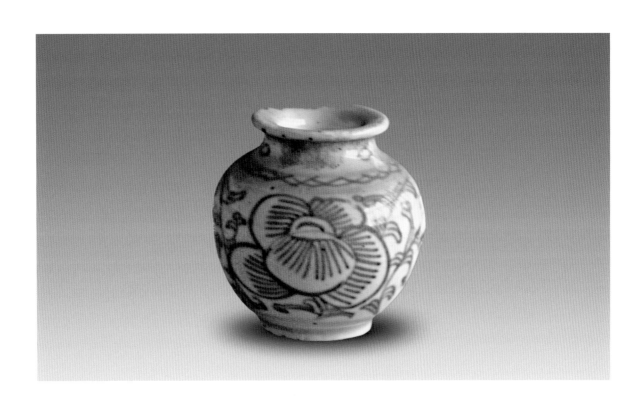

小药瓶

清

瓷质

口径 3.5 厘米，高 5 厘米

圆口，束颈，腹微鼓，浅圈足，腹部有青花纹饰。
口部残。由民间征集。

　　　　　成都中医药大学中医药传统文化博物馆藏

Small Medicine Bottle

Qing Dynasty

Porcelain

Mouth Diameter 3.5 cm/ Height 5 cm

The bottle has a round mouth, a contracted neck, a
slightly swollen belly, and a shallow ring foot. On its
belly are painted blue-and-white floral patterns. The
bottle was collected from a private owner and its mouth
rim is damaged.

Preserved in Museum of Traditional Chinese Medicine
Culture, Chengdu University of Traditional Chinese
Medicine

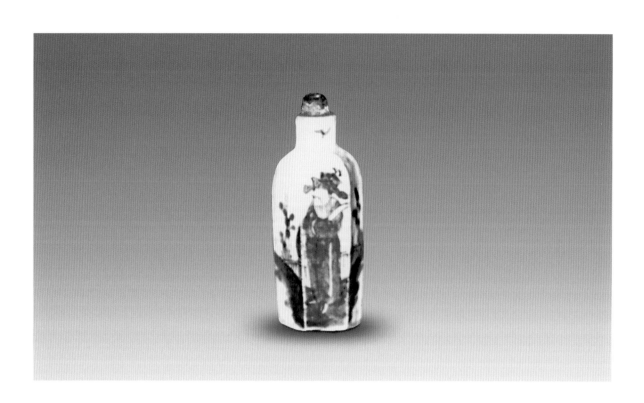

六棱瓷药瓶

清

瓷质

口径 1.6 厘米，底径 2.4 厘米，通高 7.5 厘米，
重 50 克

直口，腹为六棱，圈足，腹上有一人物图案。贮
药器具。完整无损。

陕西医史博物馆藏

Porcelain Medicine Bottle with Six Ribs

Qing Dynasty

Porcelain

Mouth Diameter 1.6 cm/ Bottom Diameter 2.4 cm/
Height 7.5 cm/ Weight 50 g

The bottle has a straight mouth, a six-ribbed belly, and
a ring foot. On its belly is painted a figurine motif. The
bottle was used for storing medicine and remains intact.

Preserved in Shaanxi Museum of Medical History

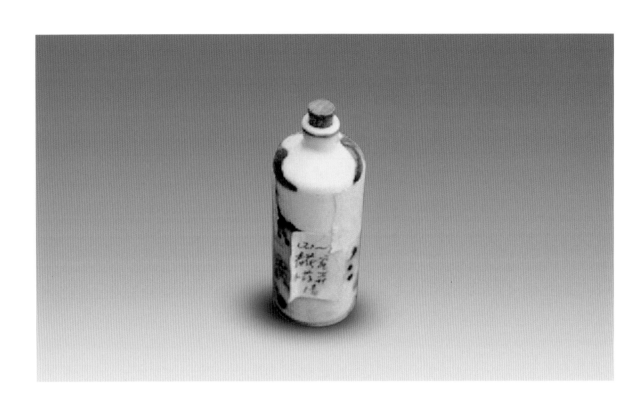

小药瓶

清

瓷质

口径 1.1 厘米，底径 2.9 厘米，通高 7.3 厘米，腹深 2.9 厘米，重 41 克

青花，直口，平底，腹部呈圆柱形。盛药用。

广东中医药博物馆藏

Small Medicine Bottle

Qing Dynasty

Porcelain

Mouth Diameter 1.1 cm/ Bottom Diameter 2.9 cm/ Height 7.3 cm/ Belly Depth 2.9 cm/ Weight 41 g

The blue-and-white bottle has a straight mouth, a flat bottom and a cylindrical belly. It was used for storing medicine.

Preserved in Guangdong Chinese Medicine Museum

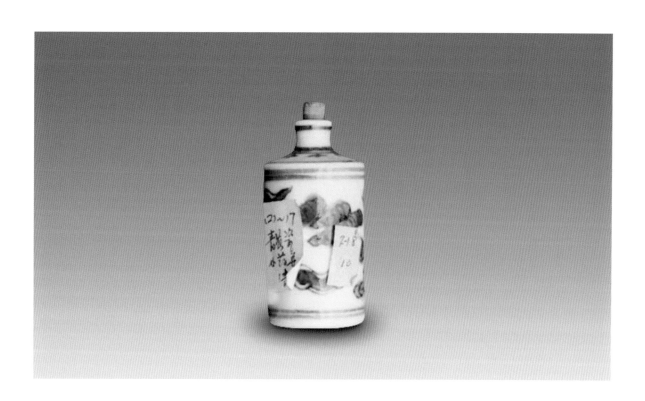

小药瓶

清

瓷质

口径 1.3 厘米，腹径 3.1 厘米，底径 3.1 厘米，

通高 6.2 厘米，重 41 克

青花，平口，口沿外侈，束颈，腹部呈圆柱形，

小圈足。用于装细碎药物。

广东中医药博物馆藏

Small Medicine Bottle

Qing Dynasty

Porcelain

Mouth Diameter 1.3 cm/ Belly Diameter 3.1 cm/ Bottom

Diameter 3.1 cm/ Height 6.2 cm/ Weight 41 g

This blue-and-white glazed bottle has a flat mouth, a

flared mouth rim, a contracted neck, a cylindrical belly,

and a small ring foot. It was used for storing ground

medicine.

Preserved in Guangdong Chinese Medicine Museum

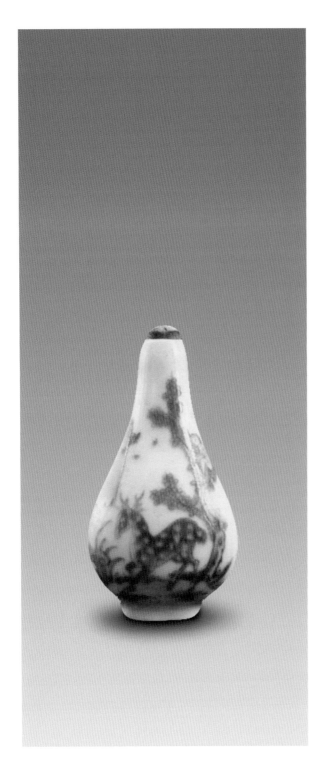

小药瓶

清

瓷质

瓶颈宽 1.3 厘米，瓶颈厚 1.2 厘米，瓶腹宽 3.5 厘米，

瓶腹厚 2.3 厘米，通高 6.15 厘米，重 17 克

Small Medicine Bottle

Qing Dynasty

Porcelain

Bottleneck Width 1.3 cm/ Bottleneck Thickness 1.2 cm/

Belly Width 3.5 cm/ Belly Thickness 2.3 cm/ Height

6.15 cm/ Weight 17 g

水滴形，敛口，溜肩，鼓腹，平底，圈足，表面绘梅花鹿等图案。用于装药。

广东中医药博物馆藏

The bottle is in the shape of a water drop, a flat bottom, a ring foot, and was used for storing medicine.This bottle has a contracted mouth,a sloping shoulder, a drum-like belly, on which are painted patterns of sika deer.

Preserved in Guangdong Chinese Medicine Museum

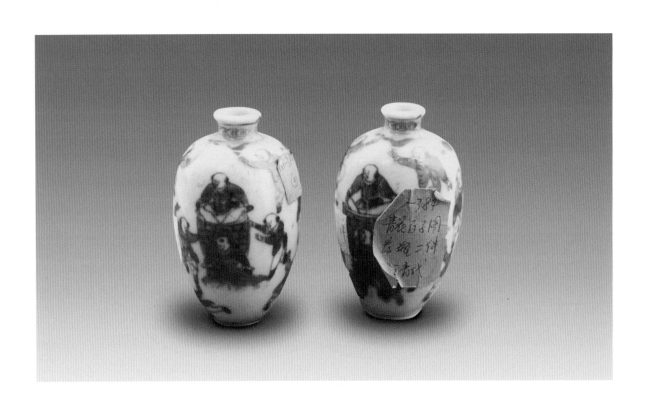

青花百子图药瓶

清

瓷质

左：口径 2.1 厘米，腹径 4.3 厘米，底径 2 厘米，通高 7.1 厘米，重 51 克

右：口径 1.55 厘米，腹径 4.35 厘米，底径 2.15 厘米，通高 7.2 厘米，重 53 克

Two Blue-and-white Small Medicine Bottles with a Hundred Children Motif

Qing Dynasty

Porcelain

Left: Mouth Diameter 2.1 cm/ Belly Diameter4.3 cm/ Bottom Diameter 2 cm/ Height 7.1 cm/ Weight 51 g

Right: Mouth Diameter 1.55 cm/ Belly Diameter 4.35 cm/ Bottom Diameter 2.15 cm/ Height 7.2 cm/ Weight 53 g

共两件。圆形，敞口，平沿，束颈，溜肩，鼓腹，腹部渐收至底，平底，圈足，上绘百子图案。用于装药。

广东中医药博物馆藏

These two bottles are round in shape and each has a flared mouth, a flat mouth rim, a contracted neck,a sloping shoulder, a drum-like belly, which narrows down to the flat bottom,and a ring foot. They are decorated with motifs of a hundred children on their bellies. They were used for storing medicine.

Preserved in Guangdong Chinese Medicine Museum

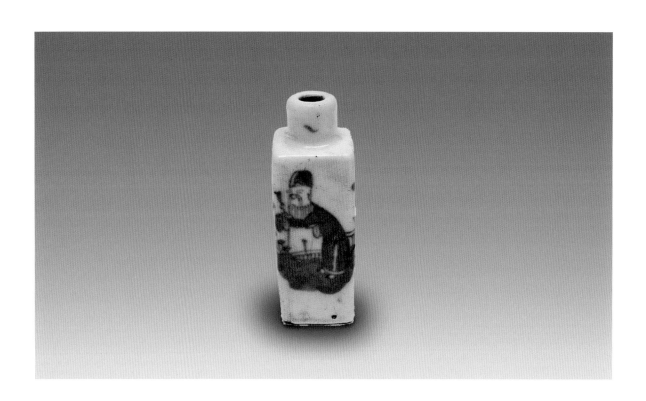

药瓶

清

瓷质

高 8.5 厘米

上圆下方形，寓意天圆地方，腹饰青花人物纹。由民间征集。

成都中医药大学中医药传统文化博物馆藏

Medicine Bottle

Qing Dynasty

Porcelain

Height 8.5 cm

The bottle has a round mouth and a square body, embodying the round heaven and the square earth. A blue-and-white figurine motif is painted on its belly. The bottle was collected from a private owner.

Preserved in Museum of Traditional Chinese Medicine Culture, Chengdu University of Traditional Chinese Medicine

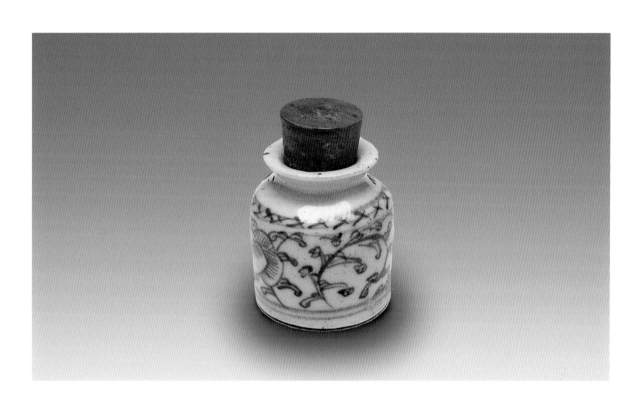

药瓶

清

瓷质

口径 3.8 厘米，底径 4.7 厘米，高 5 厘米

平口，圆唇，束颈，腹微敞，平底，腹饰青花缠
枝纹。由民间征集。

成都中医药大学中医药传统文化博物馆藏

Medicine Bottle

Qing Dynasty

Porcelain

Mouth Diameter 3.8 cm/ Bottom Diameter 4.7 cm/
Height 5 cm

The bottle has a flat mouth, a round lip, a contracted
neck, a slightly flared belly, and a flat bottom. Its belly
is decorated with blue-and-white interlocking floral
patterns. The bottle was collected from a private owner.

Preserved in Museum of Traditional Chinese Medicine
Culture, Chengdu University of Traditional Chinese
Medicine

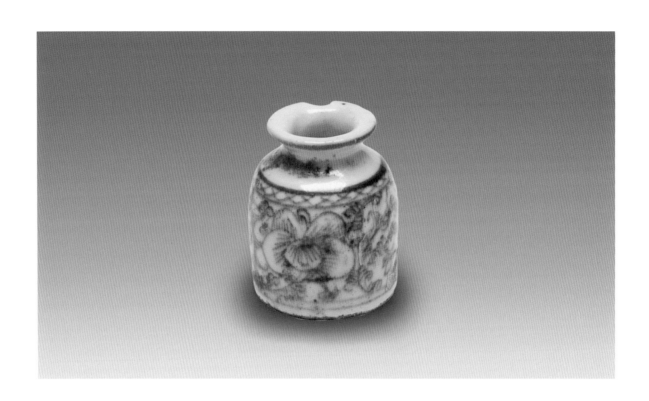

瓷药瓶

清

瓷质

口径 3.8 厘米，底径 4.7 厘米，高 5 厘米

平口，圆唇，束颈，腹微敞，平底，腹饰青花缠枝纹。盛装较小型药物的用具。

成都中医药大学中医药传统文化博物馆藏

Porcelain Medicine Bottle

Qing Dynasty

Porcelain

Mouth Diameter 3.8 cm/ Bottom Diameter 4.7 cm/ Height 5 cm

The bottle has a flat mouth, a round lip, a contracted neck, a slightly flared belly, and a flat bottom. Its belly is decorated with blue-and-white interlocking floral patterns. The bottle was used for storing small-sized medicine.

Preserved in Museum of Traditional Chinese Medicine Culture, Chengdu University of Traditional Chinese Medicine

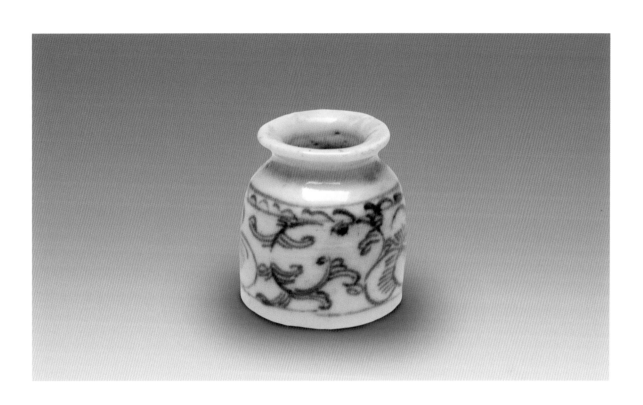

药瓶

清

瓷质

口径 3.8 厘米，底径 4.7 厘米，高 5 厘米

平口，圆唇，束颈，腹微敞，平底，腹饰青花缠枝纹。盛装较小型药物的用具。保存完好。

成都中医药大学中医药传统文化博物馆藏

Medicine Bottle

Qing Dynasty

Porcelain

Mouth Diameter 3.8 cm/ Bottom Diameter 4.7 cm/ Height 5 cm

The bottle has a flat mouth, a round lip, a contracted neck, a slightly flared belly, and a flat bottom. Its belly is decorated with blue-and-white interlocking floral patterns. The bottle was used for storing small-sized medicine and is well-preserved.

Preserved in Museum of Traditional Chinese Medicine Culture, Chengdu University of Traditional Chinese Medicine

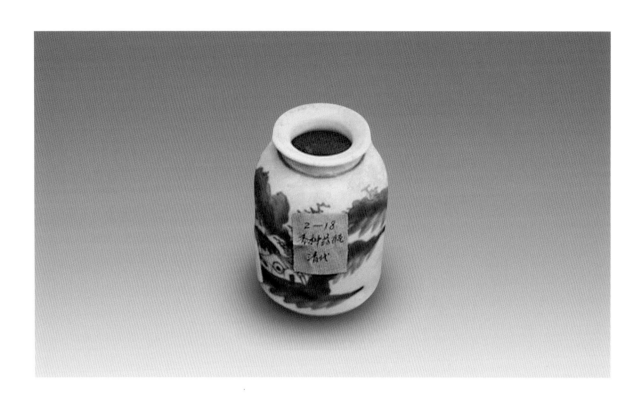

小药瓶

清

瓷质

口径 4.5 厘米，腹径 6.8 厘米，底径 6.9 厘米，通高 8.8 厘米，腹深 8.3 厘米，重 141 克

青花，盘口，束颈，溜肩，腹部近似圆柱形，上稍窄，小圈足。用于装细碎药物。

广东中医药博物馆藏

Small Medicine Bottle

Qing Dynasty

Porcelain

Mouth Diameter 4.5 cm/ Belly Diameter 6.8 cm/ Bottom Diameter 6.9 cm/ Height 8.8 cm/ Belly Depth 8.3 cm/ Weight 141 g

This bottle is coated with blue-and-white glaze and its belly is cylinder in shape, despite its slightly smaller upper part. It has a dish-shaped mouth, a contracted neck, a sloping shoulder, and a small ring foot. It was used for storing ground medicine.

Preserved in Guangdong Chinese Medicine Museum

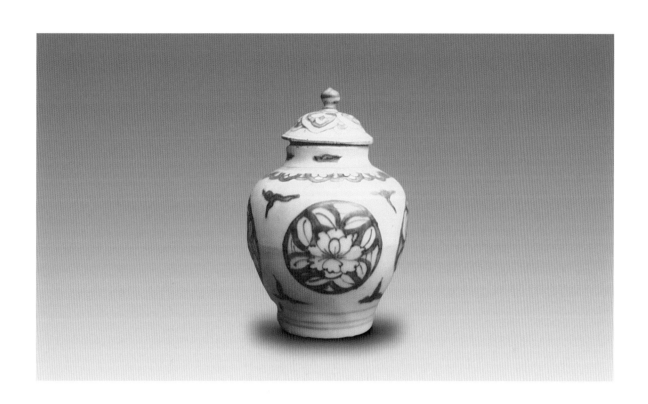

瓷釉裹红仙佛药瓶

清

瓷质

口径 4.85 厘米，腹径 9.4 厘米，底径 5.65 厘米，
带盖高 13.4 厘米，腹深 9.4 厘米，重 255 克

直口，溜肩，鼓腹，平底，圈足，宝塔形盖，表
面绘芍药花和蝙蝠纹。用于装药。

广东中医药博物馆藏

Porcelain Medicine Bottle with Buddha Motif

Qing Dynasty

Porcelain

Mouth Diameter 4.85 cm/ Belly Diameter 9.4 cm/ Bottom
Diameter 5.65 cm/ Height (with the lid) 13.4 cm/ Belly
Depth 9.4 cm/ Weight 255 g

This bottle has a straight mouth, a sloping shoulder, a drum-
like belly, a flat bottom, and a ring foot. Its lid is in the shape
of a pagoda. On its body are painted patterns of bat and
peony blossom. The bottle served as a medicine container.

Preserved in Guangdong Chinese Medicine Museum

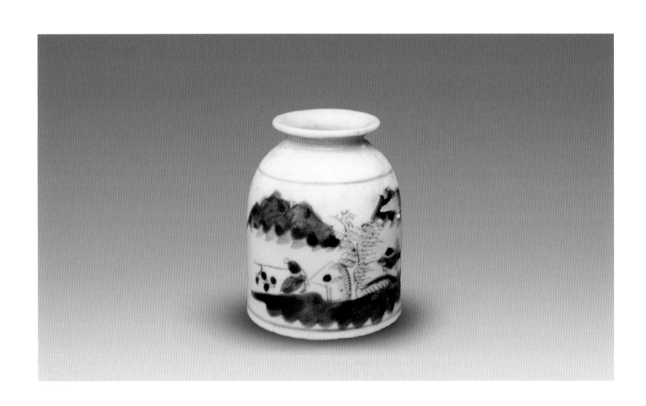

青花药瓶

清

瓷质

口径 4.46 厘米，底径 7.19 厘米，高 8.64 厘米，
腹深 7.8 厘米，重 150 克

敞口，束颈，溜肩，直腹，平底，圈足，腹饰青
花山水画。装药用。

广东中医药博物馆藏

Blue-and-white Medicine Bottle

Qing Dynasty

Porcelain

Mouth Diameter 4.46 cm/ Bottom Diameter 7.19 cm/
Height 8.64 cm/ Belly Depth 7.8 cm/ Weight 150 g

The bottle has a flared mouth, a contracted neck, a sloping
shoulder, a straight belly, a flat bottom, and a ring foot. Its
belly is decorated with blue-and-white landscape patterns.
It was used for storing medicine.

Preserved in Guangdong Chinese Medicine Museum

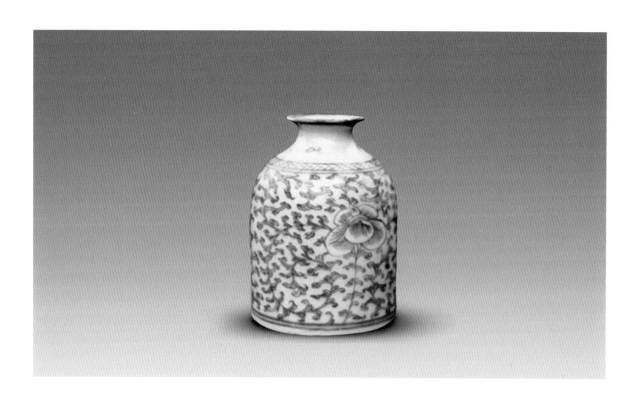

青花药瓶

清

瓷质

口径 4.3 厘米，底径 8.26 厘米，通高 11.11 厘米，

腹深 9.7 厘米，重 252 克

盘口，溜肩，平底。盛药用。

广东中医药博物馆藏

Blue-and-white Medicine Bottle

Qing Dynasty

Porcelain

Mouth Diameter 4.3 cm/ Bottom Diameter 8.26 cm/

Height 11.11 cm/ Belly Depth 9.7 cm/ Weight 252 g

The bottle has a dish-shaped mouth, a sloping shoulder,

and a flat bottom. It was used for storing medicine.

Preserved in Guangdong Chinese Medicine Museum

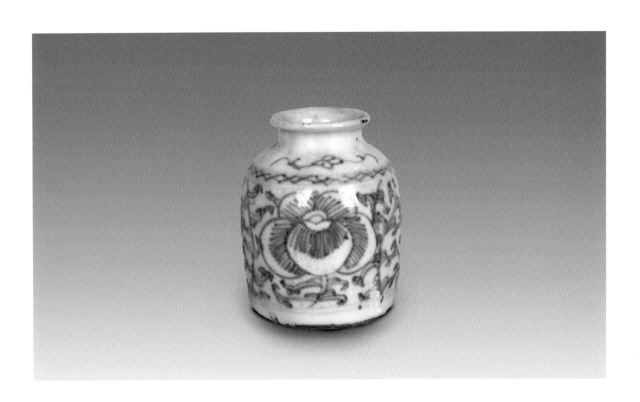

青花药瓶

清

瓷质

口外径 4.05 厘米，口内径 2.55 厘米，直径 6.55 厘米，高 7.7 厘米

Blue-and-white Medicine Bottle

Qing Dynasty

Porcelain

Mouth Outer Diameter 4.05 cm/ Mouth Inner Diameter 2.55 cm/ Diameter 6.55 cm/ Height 7.7 cm

圆形，翻沿，平底，浅圈足，表面饰青花花
卉缠枝纹，上釉不匀，工艺粗糙。盛药器具。
保存基本完好。1955 年入藏。

中华医学会 / 上海中医药大学医史博物馆藏

This round bottle has an everted mouth rim, a flat
bottom, and a shallow ring foot. On its surface are
carved blue-and-white interlocking floral designs. It
is glazed unevenly with coarse craftsmanship. The
bottle was used for storing medicine and is basically
well-preserved. It was collected in 1955.
Preserved in Chinese Medical Association/ Museum
of Chinese Medicine, Shanghai University of
Traditional Chinese Medicine

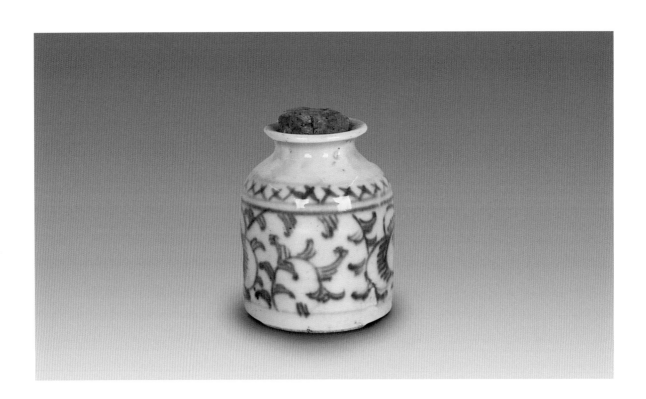

青花药瓶

清

瓷质

口外径 4.3 厘米，口内径 2.45 厘米，直径 6.35 厘米，高 7.55 厘米

Blue-and-white Medicine Bottle

Qing Dynasty

Porcelain

Mouth Outer Diameter 4.3 cm/ Mouth Inner Diameter 2.45 cm/ Diameter 6.35 cm/ Height 7.55 cm

圆形，翻沿，平底，浅圈足，表面饰青花花
卉缠枝纹，上釉不匀，工艺粗糙。盛药器具。
口沿与圈足有残。1955 年入藏。

中华医学会 / 上海中医药大学医史博物馆藏

This round bottle has an everted mouth rim, a flat
bottom, and a shallow ring foot. On its surface are
carved blue-and-white interlocking floral designs. It
is glazed unevenly with coarse craftsmanship. The
bottle was used for storing medicine and its mouth
rim and bottom were damaged to different degrees. It
was collected in 1955.

Preserved in Chinese Medical Association/ Museum
of Chinese Medicine, Shanghai University of
Traditional Chinese Medicine

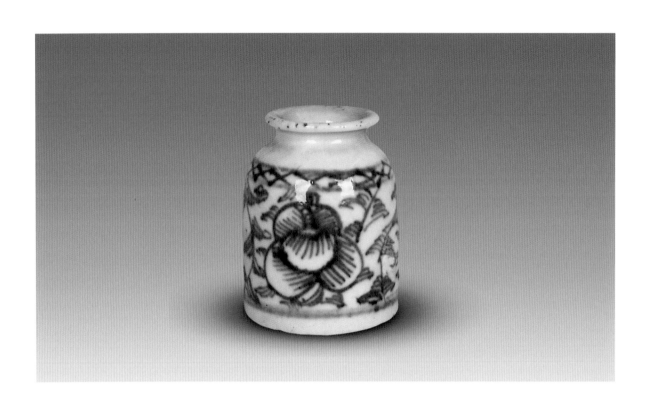

青花药瓶

清

瓷质

口外径 4.2 厘米，口内径 2.3 厘米，直径 5.8 厘米，高 7.2 厘米

Blue-and-white Medicine Bottle

Qing Dynasty

Porcelain

Mouth Outer Diameter 4.2 cm/ Mouth Inner Diameter 2.3 cm/ Diameter 5.8 cm/ Height 7.2 cm

圆形，翻沿，平底，浅圈足，表面饰青花花
卉缠枝纹，上釉不匀，工艺粗糙。盛药器具。
口沿有残。1955 年入藏。

中华医学会 / 上海中医药大学医史博物馆藏

This round bottle has an everted mouth rim, a flat
bottom, and a shallow ring foot. On its surface are
carved blue-and-white interlocking floral designs. It
is glazed unevenly with coarse craftsmanship. The
bottle was used for storing medicine and its mouth
rim is damaged. It was collected in 1955.
Preserved in Chinese Medical Association/ Museum
of Chinese Medicine, Shanghai University of
Traditional Chinese Medicine

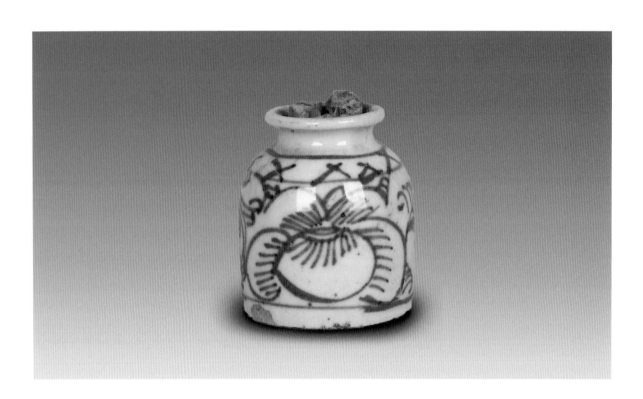

青花药瓶

清

瓷质

口外径 3.65 厘米，口内径 2 厘米，直径 5.4 厘米，高 6.1 厘米

Blue-and-white Medicine Bottle

Qing Dynasty

Porcelain

Mouth Outer Diameter 3.65 cm/ Mouth Inner Diameter 2 cm/ Diameter 5.4 cm/ Height 6.1 cm

圆形，翻沿，平底，浅圈足，表面饰青花花

卉缠枝纹，上釉不匀，工艺粗糙。盛药器具。

保存基本完好。1955 年入藏。

中华医学会 / 上海中医药大学医史博物馆藏

This round medicine bottle has an everted mouth rim,

a flat bottom, and a shallow ring foot. On its surface

are carved blue-and-white interlocking floral designs.

It is glazed unevenly with rough workmanship. The

bottle was used for storing medicine. It is kept intact

and was collected in 1955.

Preserved in Chinese Medical Association/ Museum

of Chinese Medicine, Shanghai University of

Traditional Chinese Medicine

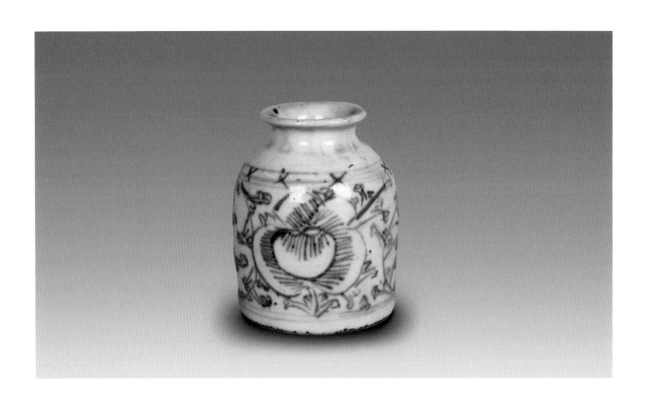

青花药瓶

清

瓷质

口外径 4.2 厘米，口内径 2.45 厘米，直径 6.4 厘米，高 7.95 厘米

Blue-and-white Medicine Bottle

Qing Dynasty

Porcelain

Mouth Outer Diameter 4.2 cm/ Mouth Inner Diameter 2.45 cm/ Diameter 6.4 cm/ Height 7.95 cm

圆形，翻沿，平底，浅圈足，表面饰青花花
卉缠枝纹，上釉不匀，工艺粗糙。盛药器具。
保存基本完好。1955 年入藏。

中华医学会 / 上海中医药大学医史博物馆藏

This round medicine bottle has an everted mouth rim,
a flat bottom, and a shallow ring foot. On its surface
are carved blue- and-white interlocking floral designs.
It is glazed unevenly with rough workmanship. The
bottle was used for storing medicine. It is kept intact
and was collected in 1955.

Preserved in Chinese Medical Association/ Museum
of Chinese Medicine, Shanghai University of
Traditional Chinese Medicine

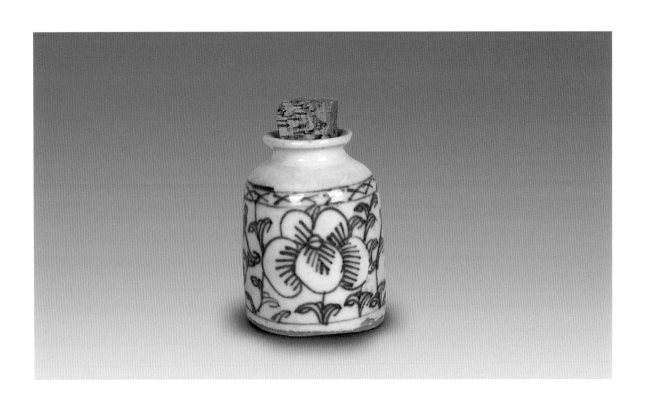

青花药瓶

清

瓷质

口外径 4.1 厘米，口内径 2.6 厘米，直径 6.8 厘米，高 8.55 厘米

Blue-and-white Medicine Bottle

Qing Dynasty

Porcelain

Mouth Outer Diameter 4.1 cm/ Mouth Inner Diameter 2.6 cm/ Diameter 6.8 cm/ Height 8.55 cm

圆形，翻沿，平底，浅圈足，表面饰青花花

卉缠枝纹，上釉不匀，工艺粗糙。盛药器具。

保存基本完好。1955 年入藏。

中华医学会／上海中医药大学医史博物馆藏

This round medicine bottle has an everted mouth rim,

a flat bottom, and a shallow ring foot. On its surface

are carved blue-and-white interlocking floral designs.

It is glazed unevenly with rough workmanship. The

bottle was used for storing medicine. It is kept intact

and was collected in 1955.

Preserved in Chinese Medical Association/ Museum

of Chinese Medicine, Shanghai University of

Traditional Chinese Medicine

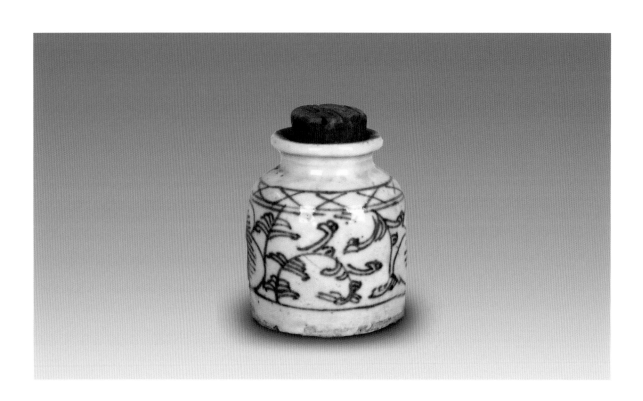

青花药瓶

清

瓷质

口外径 4.2 厘米，口内径 2.5 厘米，直径 6 厘米，高 6.9 厘米

Blue-and-white Medicine Bottle

Qing Dynasty

Porcelain

Mouth Outer Diameter 4.2 cm/ Mouth Inner Diameter 2.5 cm/ Diameter 6 cm/ Height 6.9 cm

圆形，翻沿，平底，浅圈足，表面饰青花花
卉缠枝纹，上釉不匀，工艺粗糙。盛药器具。
保存基本完好。1955 年入藏。

中华医学会 / 上海中医药大学医史博物馆藏

This round medicine bottle has an everted mouth rim,
a flat bottom, and a shallow ring foot. On its surface
are carved blue-and-white interlocking floral designs.
It is glazed unevenly with rough workmanship. The
bottle was used for storing medicine. It is kept intact
and was collected in 1955.

Preserved in Chinese Medical Association/ Museum
of Chinese Medicine, Shanghai University of
Traditional Chinese Medicine

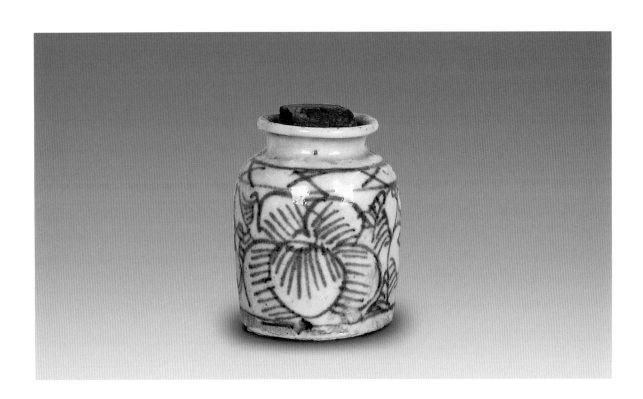

青花药瓶

清

瓷质

口外径 4 厘米，口内径 2.4 厘米，直径 5.5 厘米，高 6.6 厘米

Blue-and-white Medicine Bottle

Qing Dynasty

Porcelain

Mouth Outer Diameter 4 cm/ Mouth Inner Diameter 2.4 cm/ Diameter 5.5 cm/ Height 6.6 cm

圆形，翻沿，平底，浅圈足，表面饰青花花
卉缠枝纹，上釉不匀，工艺粗糙。盛药器具。
保存基本完好。1955 年入藏。

中华医学会 / 上海中医药大学医史博物馆藏

This round medicine bottle has an everted mouth rim,
a flat bottom, and a shallow ring foot. On its surface
are carved blue-and-white interlocking floral designs.
It is glazed unevenly with rough workmanship. The
bottle was used for storing medicine. It is kept intact
and was collected in 1955.

Preserved in Chinese Medical Association/ Museum
of Chinese Medicine, Shanghai University of
Traditional Chinese Medicine

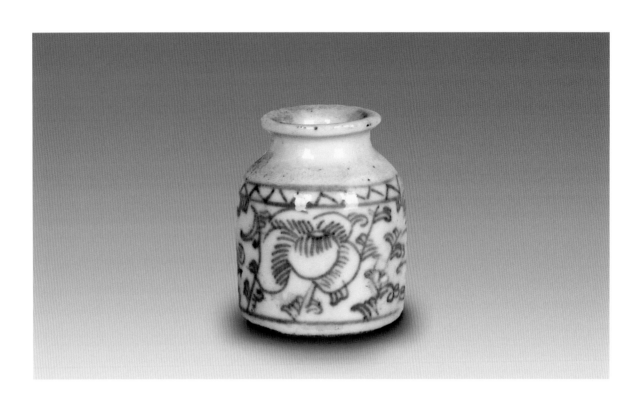

青花药瓶

清

瓷质

口外径 3.3 厘米，口内径 1.95 厘米，直径 4.7 厘米，高 5.55 厘米

Blue-and-white Medicine Bottle

Qing Dynasty

Porcelain

Mouth Outer Diameter 3.3 cm/ Mouth Inner Diameter 1.95 cm/ Diameter 4.7 cm/ Height 5.55 cm

圆形，翻沿，平底，浅圈足，表面饰青花花
卉缠枝纹，上釉不匀，工艺粗糙。盛药器具。
口有残。1955 年入藏。

中华医学会 / 上海中医药大学医史博物馆藏

This round medicine bottle has an everted mouth rim,
a flat bottom, and a shallow ring foot. On its surface
are carved blue-and-white interlocking floral designs.
It is glazed unevenly with rough workmanship. The
bottle was used for storing medicine and its mouth
was damaged. It was collected in 1955.
Preserved in Chinese Medical Association/ Museum
of Chinese Medicine, Shanghai University of
Traditional Chinese Medicine

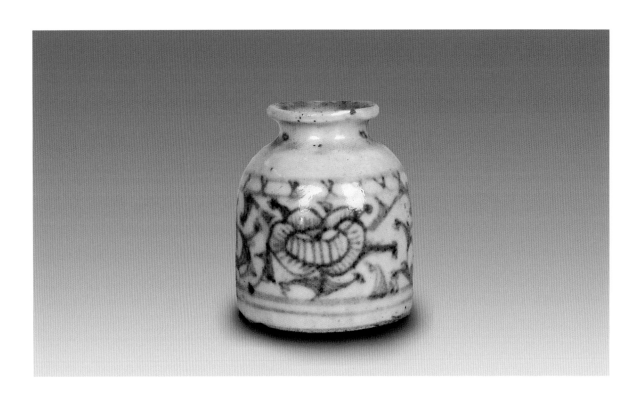

青花药瓶

清

瓷质

口外径 3.1 厘米，口内径 1.65 厘米，直径 5.1 厘米，高 5.75 厘米

Blue-and-white Medicine Bottle

Qing Dynasty

Porcelain

Mouth Outer Diameter 3.1 cm/ Mouth Inner Diameter 1.65 cm/ Diameter 5.1 cm/ Height 5.75 cm

圆形，翻沿，平底，浅圈足，表面饰青花花
卉缠枝纹，上釉不匀，工艺粗糙。盛药器具。
保存基本完好。1955 年入藏。

中华医学会 / 上海中医药大学医史博物馆藏

This round medicine bottle has an everted mouth rim,
a flat bottom, and a shallow ring foot. On its surface
are carved blue-and-white interlocking floral designs.
It is glazed unevenly with rough workmanship. The
bottle was used for storing medicine. It is kept intact
and was collected in 1955.

Preserved in Chinese Medical Association/ Museum
of Chinese Medicine, Shanghai University of
Traditional Chinese Medicine

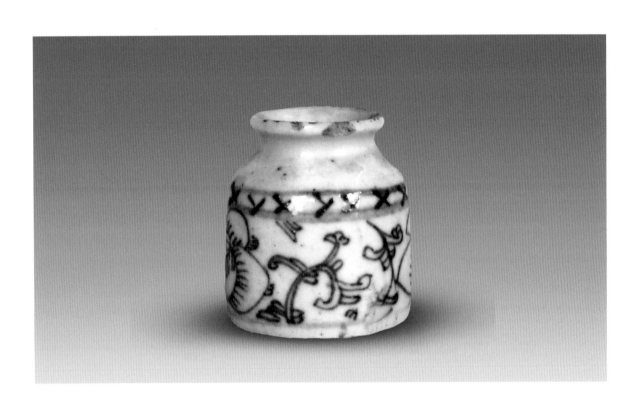

青花药瓶

清

瓷质

口外径 3.6 厘米，口内径 2.1 厘米，直径 4.9 厘米，高 5.25 厘米

Blue-and-white Medicine Bottle

Qing Dynasty

Porcelain

Mouth Outer Diameter 3.6 cm/ Mouth Inner Diameter 2.1 cm/ Diameter 4.9 cm/ Height 5.25 cm

圆形，翻沿，平底，浅圈足，表面饰青花花

卉缠枝纹，上釉不匀，工艺粗糙。盛药器具。

口有残。1955 年入藏。

中华医学会 / 上海中医药大学医史博物馆藏

This round medicine bottle has an everted mouth rim,

a flat bottom, and a shallow ring foot. On its surface

are carved blue-and-white interlocking floral designs.

It is glazed unevenly with rough workmanship. The

bottle was used for storing medicine and its mouth

was damaged. It was collected in 1955.

Preserved in Chinese Medical Association/ Museum

of Chinese Medicine, Shanghai University of

Traditional Chinese Medicine

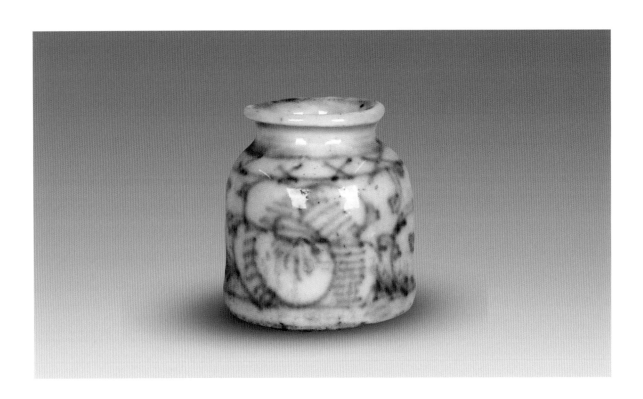

青花药瓶

清

瓷质

口外径 3.5 厘米，口内径 2.1 厘米，直径 4.6 厘米，高 4.8 厘米

Blue-and-white Medicine Bottle

Qing Dynasty

Porcelain

Mouth Outer Diameter 3.5 cm/ Mouth Inner Diameter 2.1 cm/ Diameter 4.6 cm/ Height 4.8 cm

圆形，翻沿，平底，浅圈足，表面饰青花花卉缠枝纹，上釉不匀，工艺粗糙。盛药器具。保存基本完好。1955 年入藏。

中华医学会 / 上海中医药大学医史博物馆藏

This round medicine bottle has an everted mouth rim, a flat bottom, and a shallow ring foot. On its surface are carved blue-and-white interlocking floral designs. It is glazed unevenly with rough workmanship. The bottle was used for storing medicine. It is kept intact and was collected in 1955.

Preserved in Chinese Medical Association/ Museum of Chinese Medicine, Shanghai University of Traditional Chinese Medicine

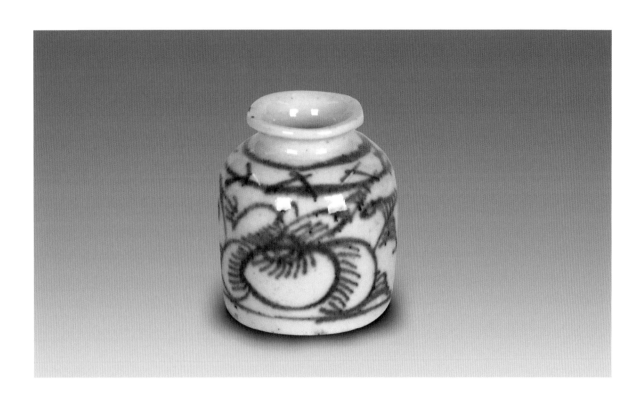

瓷药瓶

清

瓷质

口外径 3.6 厘米，口内径 2.05 厘米，直径 5.95 厘米，通高 6.1 厘米

Porcelain Medicine Bottle

Qing Dynasty

Porcelain

Mouth Outer Diameter 3.6 cm/ Mouth Inner Diameter 2.05 cm/ Diameter 5.95 cm/ Height 6.1 cm

圆形，敞口，外撇，折沿，束颈，溜肩，直腹，平底，圈足，表面绘青花萱草图，底面无款识，工艺一般。盛药器具。1958 年入藏。

中华医学会 / 上海中医药大学医史博物馆藏

This bottle has a flared mouth, an everted mouth rim, a contracted neck, a sloping shoulder, a straight belly, a flat bottom, and a ring foot. This round bottle was made with average workmanship. Blue-and-white daylily patterns are painted on it. There is no inscription on its bottom. It was used as a medicine container and was collected in 1958.

Preserved in Chinese Medical Association/ Museum of Chinese Medicine, Shanghai University of Traditional Chinese Medicine

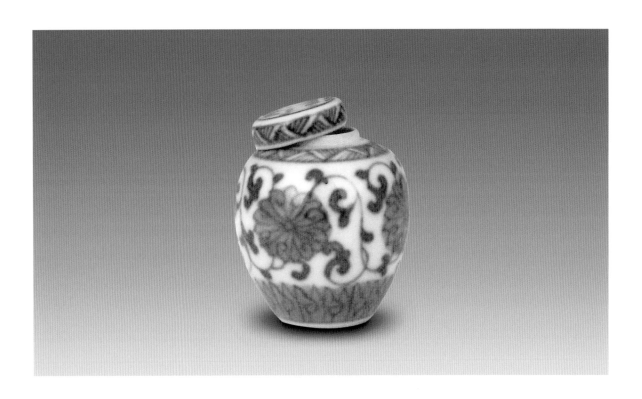

药瓶

清

瓷质

口径 2 厘米，腹径 4.9 厘米，通高 5.9 厘米

Medicine Bottle

Qing Dynasty

Porcelain

Mouth Diameter 2 cm/ Belly Diameter 4.9 cm/ Height 5.9 cm

青花瓷，配平扣盖，直口，平底，表面饰菊花缠枝纹，小巧玲珑，工艺精良。盛药器具。保存基本完好。1982 年入藏。

中华医学会 / 上海中医药大学医史博物馆藏

This medicine bottle is a blue-and-white porcelain bottle. It has a straight mouth, a flat bottom and a flat lid. Interlocking chrysanthemum branches are painted on its body. The small bottle looks beautiful with exquisite workmanship. It is kept intact and was collected in 1982.

Preserved in Chinese Medical Association/ Museum of Chinese Medicine, Shanghai University of Traditional Chinese Medicine

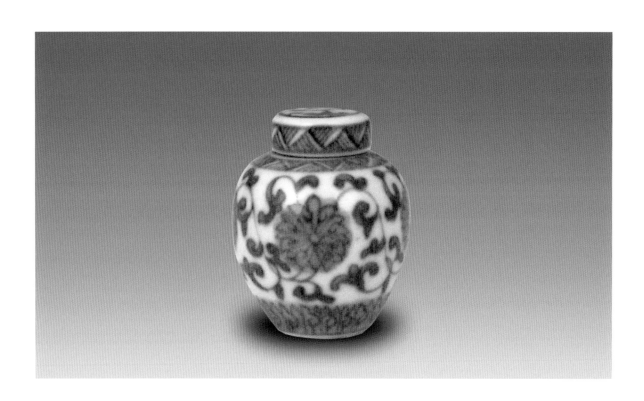

药瓶

清

瓷质

口径 2.2 厘米，腹径 5 厘米，通高 5.8 厘米

Medicine Bottle

Qing Dynasty

Porcelain

Mouth Diameter 2.2 cm/ Belly Diameter 5 cm/ Height 5.8 cm

青花瓷，配平扣盖，直口，平底，表面饰菊花缠枝纹，小巧玲珑，工艺精良。盛药器具。保存基本完好。1982 年入藏。

中华医学会 / 上海中医药大学医史博物馆藏

This medicine bottle is a blue-and-white porcelain bottle. It has a straight mouth, a flat bottom and a flat lid. Interlocking chrysanthemum branches are painted on its body. The small bottle looks beautiful with exquisite workmanship. It is kept intact and was collected in 1982.

Preserved in Chinese Medical Association/ Museum of Chinese Medicine, Shanghai University of Traditional Chinese Medicine

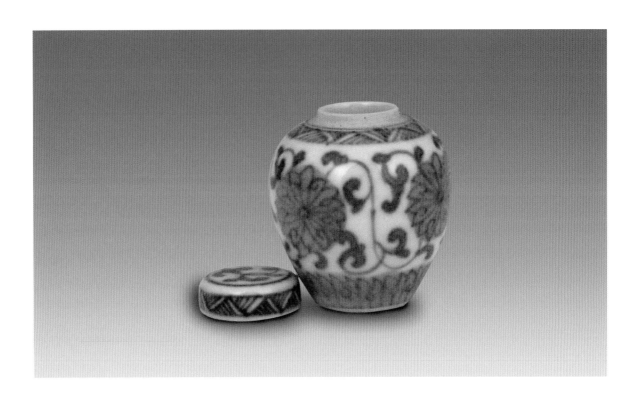

药瓶

清

瓷质

口径 2.1 厘米，腹径 4.8 厘米，通高 5.6 厘米

Medicine Bottle

Qing Dynasty

Porcelain

Mouth Diameter 2.1 cm/ Belly Diameter 4.8 cm/ Height 5.6 cm

青花瓷，配扣盖，直口，平底，表面饰菊花
缠枝纹，小巧玲珑，工艺精良。盛药器具。
保存基本完好。1982 年入藏。

中华医学会 / 上海中医药大学医史博物馆藏

This medicine bottle is a blue-and-white porcelain
bottle. It has a straight mouth, a flat bottom and a
flat lid. Interlocking chrysanthemum branches are
painted on its body. The small bottle looks beautiful
with exquisite workmanship. It is kept intact and was
collected in 1982.

Preserved in Chinese Medical Association/ Museum
of Chinese Medicine, Shanghai University of
Traditional Chinese Medicine

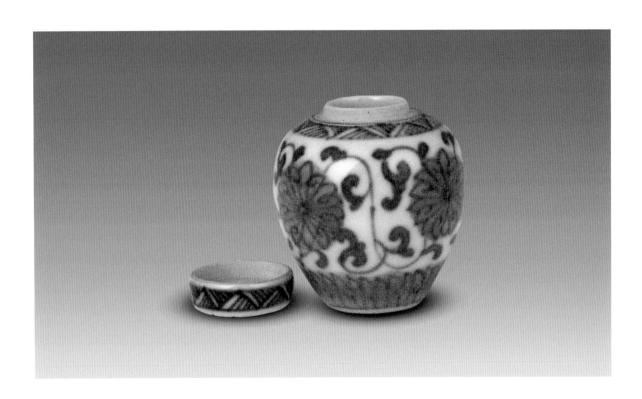

药瓶

清

瓷质

口径 2.2 厘米，腹径 5 厘米，通高 5.9 厘米

Medicine Bottle

Qing Dynasty

Porcelain

Mouth Diameter 2.2 cm/ Belly Diameter 5 cm/ Height 5.9 cm

青花瓷，配扣盖，直口，平底，表面饰菊花缠枝纹，小巧玲珑，工艺精良。盛药器具。保存基本完好。1982 年入藏。

中华医学会 / 上海中医药大学医史博物馆藏

This medicine bottle is a blue-and-white porcelain bottle. It has a straight mouth, a flat bottom and a flat lid. Interlocking chrysanthemum branches are painted on its body. The small bottle looks beautiful with exquisite workmanship. It is kept intact and was collected in 1982.

Preserved in Chinese Medical Association/ Museum of Chinese Medicine, Shanghai University of Traditional Chinese Medicine

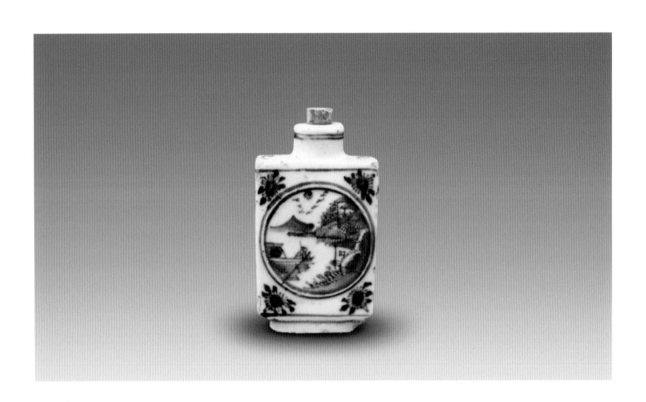

青花瓷药瓶

清

瓷质

口外径 1.48 厘米，通高 6.55 厘米，瓶身长 3.84 厘米，瓶身宽 1.58 厘米，瓶身高 5.06 厘米，重 40 克

长方形，细直颈，平肩，圈足。用于装药。

广东中医药博物馆藏

Blue-and-white Porcelain Medicine Bottle

Qing Dynasty

Porcelain

Mouth Outer Diameter 1.48 cm/ Height 6.55 cm/ Body Length 3.84 cm/ Body Width 1.58 cm/ Body Height 5.06 cm/ Weight 40 g

This rectangular bottle has a thin and straight neck, a flat shoulder, and a ring foot. It was used for storing medicine.

Preserved in Guangdong Chinese Medicine Museum

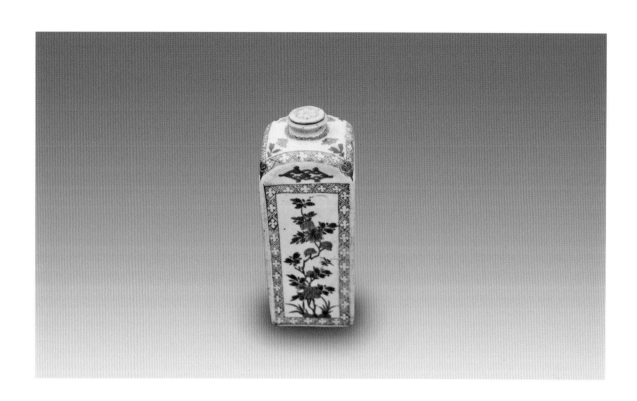

青花方形大药瓶

清

瓷质

口外径 3.85 厘米，腹宽 9 厘米，通高 21.6 厘米，
重 912 克

敞口，平沿，溜肩，平底，方形药瓶。用于储存药物。

广东中医药博物馆藏

Large Square Blue-and-white Medicine Bottle

Qing Dynasty

Porcelain

Mouth Outer Diameter 3.85 cm/ Belly Width 9 cm/
Height 21.6 cm/ Weight 912 g

This bottle has a flared mouth, a flat mouth rim, a sloping
shoulder, and a flat bottom.This square bottle is used for
storing medicine.

Preserved in Guangdong Chinese Medicine Museum

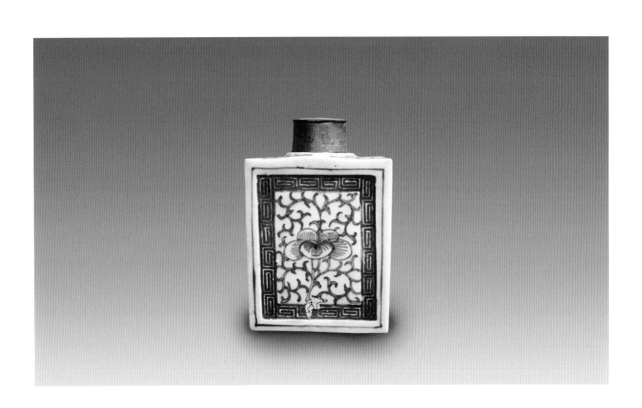

青花方形药瓶

清

瓷质

口外径3.6厘米，通高11.9厘米，瓶身长9.3厘米，瓶身宽4.8厘米，瓶身高11厘米，重376克

长方形，细圆颈，平口，平底，青花。用于装药。

广东中医药博物馆藏

Rectangular Blue-and-white Medicine Bottle

Qing Dynasty

Porcelain

Mouth Outer Diameter 3.6 cm/ Height 11.9 cm/ Body Length 9.3 cm/ Body Width 4.8 cm/ Body Height 11 cm/ Weight 376 g

This rectangular blue-and-white bottle has a thin round neck, a flat mouth, and a flat bottom. It was used as a medicine container.

Preserved in Guangdong Chinese Medicine Museum

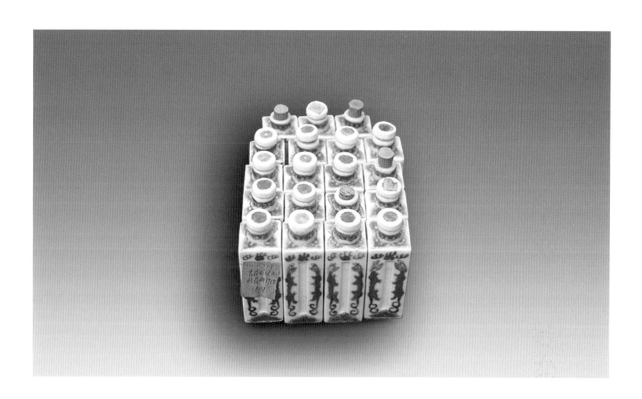

青花方形龙纹小药瓶

清

瓷质

通高8.8厘米，瓶身长2.7厘米，瓶身宽2.7厘米，瓶身高7.2厘米，单个重60克

共19件。直口，平沿，瓶身绘青花龙纹，方形小药瓶。用于装药。

广东中医药博物馆藏

Small Cubic Porcelain Medicine Bottles with Dragon Design

Qing Dynasty

Porcelain

Height 8.8 cm/ Body Length 2.7 cm/ Body Width 2.7 cm/ Body Height 7.2 cm/ Weight (a single bottle) 60 g

There are nineteen square medicine bottle. Their mouths are upright,while their mouth rims are flat.Blue-and-white dragon patterns are painted on their bodies. These square medicine bottles are used for storing medicine.

Preserved in Guangdong Chinese Medicine Museum

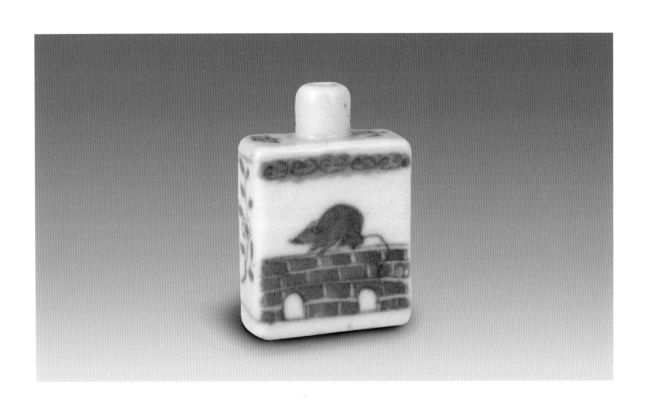

生肖药瓶（子鼠）

清

瓷质

口径 1.4 厘米，宽 4.1 厘米，通高 5.9 厘米，厚 1.9 厘米

Medicine Bottle with Chinese Zodiac Design （Zi Shu）

Qing Dynasty

Porcelain

Mouth Diameter 1.4 cm/ Width 4.1 cm/ Height 5.9 cm/ Thickness 1.9 cm

方瓶形青花瓷瓶，直口，平底，浅圈足。该套药瓶瓶肩分别书有"子鼠""丑牛"等标记，该藏为子鼠瓶，工艺精良，美观大方。盛药器具。保存基本完好。1957 年入藏。

中华医学会 / 上海中医药大学医史博物馆藏

This cuboid bottle, beautiful and elegant, belongs to blue-and-white porcelain with delicate workmanship. It has a straight mouth, a flat bottom, and a shallow ring foot. On the shoulder of this set of bottle is inscribed the name of the lunar year such as "Zi Shu" (Rat, the first of the twelve zodiac signs), "Chou Niu" (Ox, the second of the twelve zodiac signs) and so on. This is a "Zi Shu" bottle and was used as a medicine container. It is kept basically intact and was collected in 1957.

Preserved in Chinese Medical Association/ Museum of Chinese Medicine, Shanghai University of Traditional Chinese Medicine

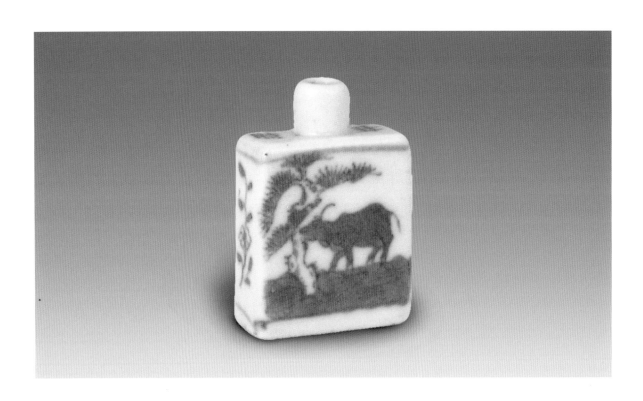

生肖药瓶（丑牛）

清

瓷质

口径 1.4 厘米，宽 4.1 厘米，通高 5.9 厘米，厚 1.9 厘米

Medicine Bottle with Chinese Zodiac Design (Chou Niu)

Qing Dynasty

Porcelain

Mouth Diameter 1.4 cm/ Width 4.1 cm/ Height 5.9 cm/ Thickness 1.9 cm

方瓶形青花瓷瓶，直口，平底，浅圈足。该
套药瓶瓶肩分别书有"子鼠""丑牛"等标记，
该藏为丑牛瓶，工艺精良，美观大方。盛药
器具。保存基本完好。1957 年入藏。

中华医学会 / 上海中医药大学医史博物馆藏

This cuboid bottle, beautiful and elegant, belongs to
blue-and-white porcelain with delicate workmanship.
It has a straight mouth, a flat bottom, and a shallow
ring foot. On the shoulder of this set of bottle is
inscribed the name of the lunar year such as "Zi
Shu" (Rat, the first of the twelve zodiac signs), "Chou
Niu" (Ox, the second of the twelve zodiac signs) and
so on. This is a "Chou Niu" bottle and was used as a
medicine container. It is kept basically intact and was
collected in 1957.

Preserved in Chinese Medical Association/ Museum
of Chinese Medicine, Shanghai University of
Traditional Chinese Medicine

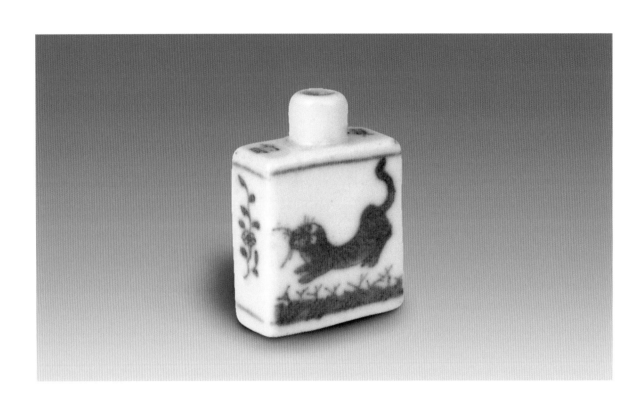

生肖药瓶（寅虎）

清

瓷质

口径 1.4 厘米，宽 4.1 厘米，通高 5.9 厘米，厚 1.9 厘米

Medicine Bottle with Chinese Zodiac Design （Yin Hu）

Qing Dynasty

Porcelain

Mouth Diameter 1.4 cm/ Width 4.1 cm/ Height 5.9 cm/ Thickness 1.9 cm

方瓶形青花瓷瓶，直口，平底，浅圈足。该套药瓶瓶肩分别书有"子鼠""丑牛"等标记，该藏为"寅虎瓶"，工艺精良，美观大方。盛药器具。保存基本完好。 1957 年入藏。

中华医学会 / 上海中医药大学医史博物馆藏

This cuboid bottle, beautiful and elegant, belongs to blue-and-white porcelain with delicate workmanship. It has a straight mouth, a flat bottom, and a shallow ring foot. On the shoulder of this set of bottle is inscribed the name of the lunar year such as "Zi Shu" (Rat, the first of the twelve zodiac signs), "Chou Niu" (Ox, the second of the twelve zodiac signs) and so on. This is a "Yin Hu" (Tiger, the third of the twelve zodiac signs) bottle and was used as a medicine container. It is kept basically intact and was collected in 1957.

Preserved in Chinese Medical Association/ Museum of Chinese Medicine, Shanghai University of Traditional Chinese Medicine

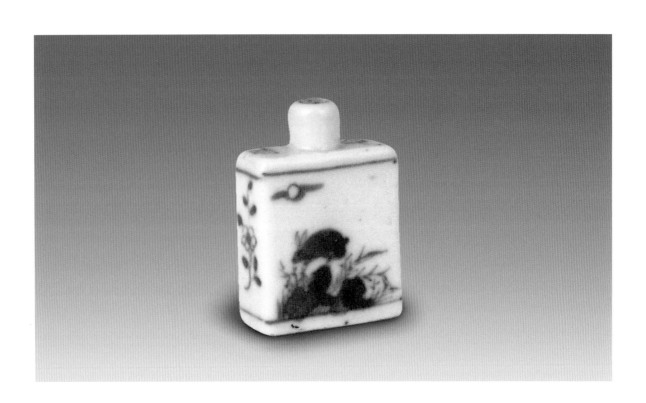

生肖药瓶（卯兔）

清

瓷质

口径 1.4 厘米，宽 4.1 厘米，通高 5.9 厘米，厚 1.9 厘米

Medicine Bottle with Chinese Zodiac Design (Mao Tu)

Qing Dynasty

Porcelain

Mouth Diameter 1.4 cm/ Width 4.1 cm/ Height 5.9 cm/ Thickness 1.9 cm

方瓶形青花瓷瓶，直口，平底，浅圈足。该套药瓶瓶肩分别书有"子鼠""丑牛"等标记，该藏为"卯兔瓶"，工艺精良，美观大方。盛药器具。保存基本完好。1957 年入藏。

中华医学会 / 上海中医药大学医史博物馆藏

This cuboid bottle, beautiful and elegant, belongs to blue-and-white porcelain with delicate workmanship. It has a straight mouth, a flat bottom, and a shallow ring foot. On the shoulder of this set of bottle is inscribed the name of the lunar year such as "Zi Shu" (Rat, the first of the twelve zodiac signs), "Chou Niu" (Ox, the second of the twelve zodiac signs) and so on. This is a "Mao Tu" (Rabbit, the fourth of the twelve zodiac signs) bottle and was used as a medicine container. It is kept basically intact and was collected in 1957.

Preserved in Chinese Medical Association/ Museum of Chinese Medicine, Shanghai University of Traditional Chinese Medicine

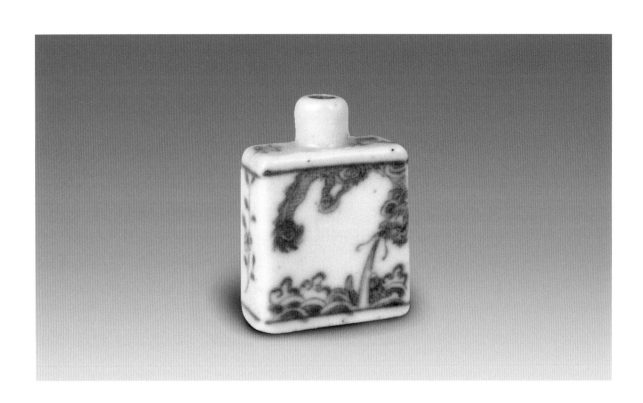

生肖药瓶（辰龙）

清

瓷质

口径 1.4 厘米，宽 4.1 厘米，通高 5.9 厘米，厚 1.9 厘米

Medicine Bottle with Chinese Zodiac Design (Chen Long)

Qing Dynasty

Porcelain

Mouth Diameter 1.4 cm/ Width 4.1 cm/ Height 5.9 cm/ Thickness 1.9 cm

方瓶形青花瓷瓶，直口，平底，浅圈足。该套药瓶瓶肩分别书有"子鼠""丑牛"等标记，该藏为"辰龙瓶"，工艺精良，美观大方。盛药器具。保存基本完好。1957年入藏。

中华医学会/上海中医药大学医史博物馆藏

This cuboid bottle, beautiful and elegant, belongs to blue-and-white porcelain with delicate workmanship. It has a straight mouth, a flat bottom, and a shallow ring foot. On the shoulder of this set of bottle is inscribed the name of the lunar year such as "Zi Shu" (Rat, the first of the twelve zodiac signs), "Chou Niu" (Ox, the second of the twelve zodiac signs) and so on. This is a "Chen Long" (Dragon, the fifth of the twelve zodiac signs) bottle and was used as a medicine container. It is kept basically intact and was collected in 1957.

Preserved in Chinese Medical Association/ Museum of Chinese Medicine, Shanghai University of Traditional Chinese Medicine

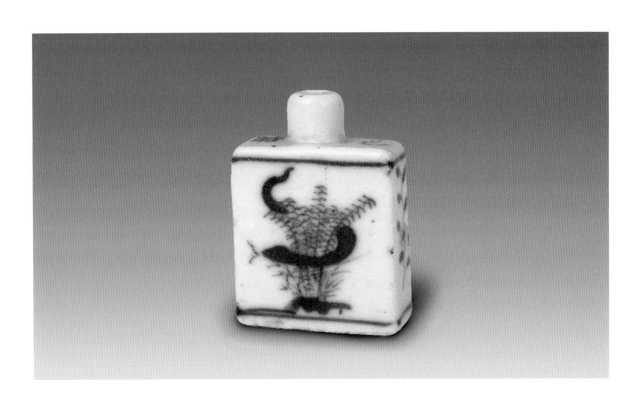

生肖药瓶（巳蛇）

清

瓷质

口径 1.4 厘米，宽 4.1 厘米，通高 5.9 厘米，厚 1.9 厘米

Medicine Bottle with Chinese Zodiac Design (Si She)

Qing Dynasty

Porcelain

Mouth Diameter 1.4 cm/ Width 4.1 cm/ Height 5.9 cm/ Thickness 1.9 cm

方瓶形青花瓷瓶，直口，平底，浅圈足。该套药瓶瓶肩分别书有"子鼠""丑牛"等标记，该藏为"巳蛇瓶"，工艺精良，美观大方。盛药器具。保存基本完好。1957 年入藏。

中华医学会 / 上海中医药大学医史博物馆藏

This cuboid bottle, beautiful and elegant, belongs to blue-and-white porcelain with delicate workmanship. It has a straight mouth, a flat bottom, and a shallow ring foot. On the shoulder of this set of bottle is inscribed the name of the lunar year such as "Zi Shu" (Rat, the first of the twelve zodiac signs), "Chou Niu" (Ox, the second of the twelve zodiac signs) and so on. This is a "Si She" (Snake, the sixth of the twelve zodiac signs) bottle and was used as a medicine container. It is kept basically intact and was collected in 1957.

Preserved in Chinese Medical Association/ Museum of Chinese Medicine, Shanghai University of Traditional Chinese Medicine

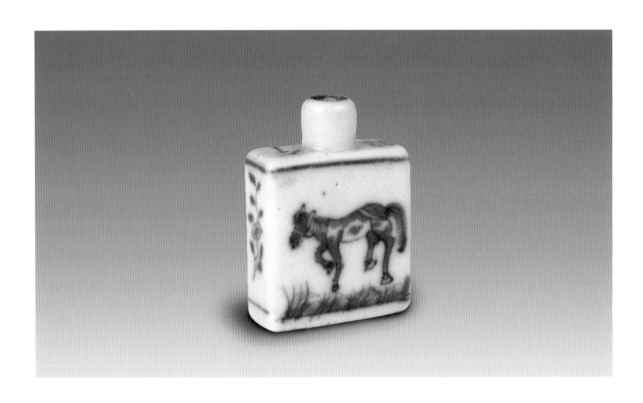

生肖药瓶（午马）

清

瓷质

口径 1.4 厘米，宽 4.1 厘米，通高 5.9 厘米，厚 1.9 厘米

Medicine Bottle with Chinese Zodiac Design (Wu Ma)

Qing Dynasty

Porcelain

Mouth Diameter 1.4 cm/ Width 4.1 cm/ Height 5.9 cm/ Thickness 1.9 cm

方瓶形青花瓷瓶，直口，平底，浅圈足。该套药瓶瓶肩分别书有"子鼠""丑牛"等标记，该藏为"午马瓶"，工艺精良，美观大方。盛药器具。保存基本完好。1957 年入藏。

中华医学会／上海中医药大学医史博物馆藏

This cuboid bottle, beautiful and elegant, belongs to blue-and-white porcelain with delicate workmanship. It has a straight mouth, a flat bottom, and a shallow ring foot. On the shoulder of this set of bottle is inscribed the name of the lunar year such as "Zi Shu" (Rat, the first of the twelve zodiac signs), "Chou Niu" (Ox, the second of the twelve zodiac signs) and so on. This is a "Wu Ma" (Horse, the seventh of the twelve zodiac signs) bottle and was used as a medicine container. It is kept basically intact and was collected in 1957.

Preserved in Chinese Medical Association/ Museum of Chinese Medicine, Shanghai University of Traditional Chinese Medicine

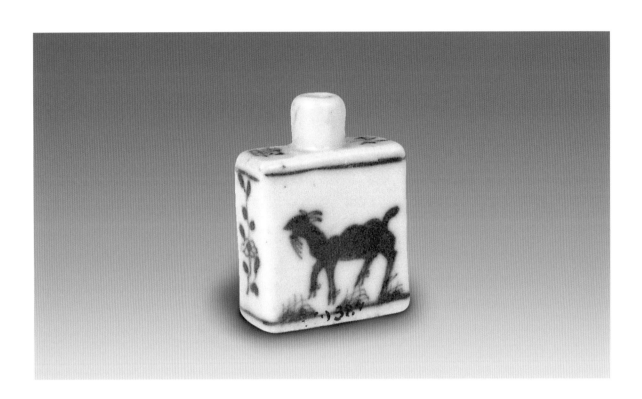

生肖药瓶（未羊）

清

瓷质

口径 1.4 厘米，宽 4.1 厘米，通高 5.9 厘米，厚 1.9 厘米

Medicine Bottle with Chinese Zodiac Design (Wei Yang)

Qing Dynasty

Porcelain

Mouth Diameter 1.4 cm/ Width 4.1 cm/ Height 5.9 cm/ Thickness 1.9 cm

方瓶形青花瓷瓶，直口，平底，浅圈足。该
套药瓶瓶肩分别书有"子鼠""丑牛"等标
记，该藏为"未羊瓶"，工艺精良，美观大方。
盛药器具。保存基本完好。1957 年入藏。

中华医学会 / 上海中医药大学医史博物馆藏

This cuboid bottle, beautiful and elegant, belongs to blue-and-white porcelain with delicate workmanship. It has a straight mouth, a flat bottom, and a shallow ring foot. On the shoulder of this set of bottle is inscribed the name of the lunar year such as "Zi Shu" (Rat, the first of the twelve zodiac signs), "Chou Niu" (Ox, the second of the twelve zodiac signs) and so on. This is a "Wei Yang" (Sheep, the eighth of the twelve zodiac signs) bottle and was used as a medicine container. It is kept basically intact and was collected in 1957.

Preserved in Chinese Medical Association/ Museum of Chinese Medicine, Shanghai University of Traditional Chinese Medicine

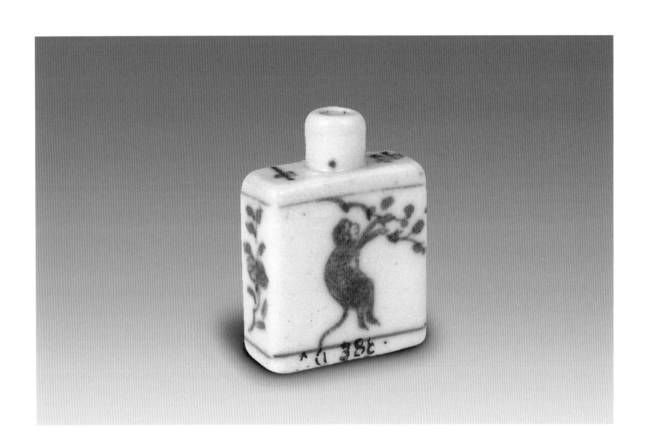

生肖药瓶（申猴）

清

瓷质

口径 1.4 厘米，宽 4.1 厘米，通高 5.9 厘米，厚 1.9 厘米

Medicine Bottle with Chinese Zodiac Design (Shen Hou)

Qing Dynasty

Porcelain

Mouth Diameter 1.4 cm/ Width 4.1 cm/ Height 5.9 cm/ Thickness 1.9 cm

方瓶形青花瓷瓶，直口，平底，浅圈足。该套药瓶瓶肩分别书有"子鼠""丑牛"等标记，该藏为"申猴瓶"，工艺精良，美观大方。盛药器具。保存基本完好。1957 年入藏。

中华医学会 / 上海中医药大学医史博物馆藏

This cuboid bottle, beautiful and elegant, belongs to blue-and-white porcelain with delicate workmanship. It has a straight mouth, a flat bottom, and a shallow ring foot. On the shoulder of this set of bottle is inscribed the name of the lunar year such as "Zi Shu" (Rat, the first of the twelve zodiac signs), "Chou Niu" (Ox, the second of the twelve zodiac signs) and so on. This is a "Shen Hou" (Monkey, the ninth of the twelve zodiac signs) bottle and was used as a medicine container. It is kept basically intact and was collected in 1957.

Preserved in Chinese Medical Association/ Museum of Chinese Medicine, Shanghai University of Traditional Chinese Medicine

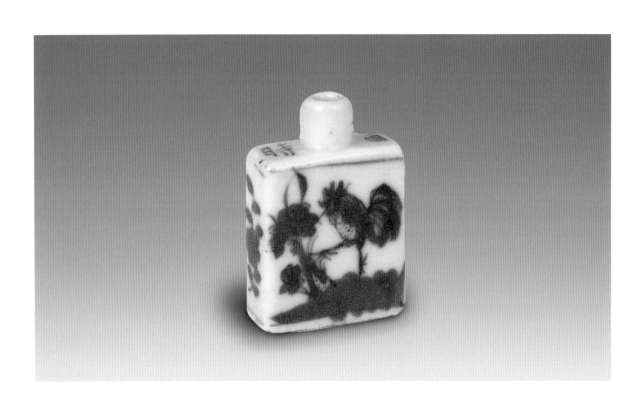

生肖药瓶（酉鸡）

清

瓷质

口径 1.4 厘米，宽 4.1 厘米，通高 5.9 厘米，厚 1.9 厘米

Medicine Bottle with Chinese Zodiac Design (You Ji)

Qing Dynasty

Porcelain

Mouth Diameter 1.4 cm/ Width 4.1 cm/ Height 5.9 cm/ Thickness 1.9 cm

方瓶形青花瓷瓶，直口，平底，浅圈足。该套药瓶瓶肩分别书有"子鼠""丑牛"等标记，该藏为"酉鸡瓶"，工艺精良，美观大方。盛药器具。保存基本完好。1957 年入藏。

中华医学会 / 上海中医药大学医史博物馆藏

This cuboid bottle, beautiful and elegant, belongs to blue-and-white porcelain with delicate workmanship. It has a straight mouth, a flat bottom, and a shallow ring foot. On the shoulder of this set of bottle is inscribed the name of the lunar year such as "Zi Shu" (Rat, the first of the twelve zodiac signs), "Chou Niu" (Ox, the second of the twelve zodiac signs) and so on. This is a "You Ji" (Chicken, the tenth of the twelve zodiac signs) bottle and was used as a medicine container. It is kept basically intact and was collected in 1957.

Preserved in Chinese Medical Association/ Museum of Chinese Medicine, Shanghai University of Traditional Chinese Medicine

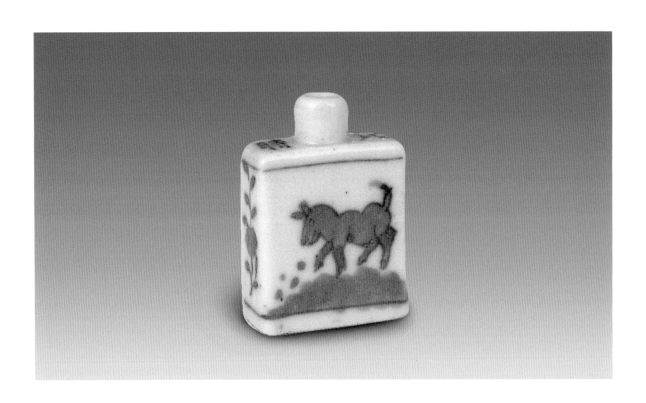

生肖药瓶（戌狗）

清

瓷质

口径 1.4 厘米，宽 4.1 厘米，通高 5.9 厘米，厚 1.9 厘米

Medicine Bottle with Chinese Zodiac Design (Xu Gou)

Qing Dynasty

Porcelain

Mouth Diameter 1.4 cm/ Width 4.1 cm/ Height 5.9 cm/ Thickness 1.9 cm

方瓶形青花瓷瓶，直口，平底，浅圈足。该套药瓶瓶肩分别书有"子鼠""丑牛"等标记，该藏为"戌狗瓶"，工艺精良，美观大方。盛药器具。保存基本完好。1957年入藏。

中华医学会 / 上海中医药大学医史博物馆藏

This cuboid bottle, beautiful and elegant, belongs to blue-and-white porcelain with delicate workmanship. It has a straight mouth, a flat bottom, and a shallow ring foot. On the shoulder of this set of bottle is inscribed the name of the lunar year such as "Zi Shu" (Rat, the first of the twelve zodiac signs), "Chou Niu" (Ox, the second of the twelve zodiac signs) and so on. This is a "Xu Gou" (Dog, the eleventh of the twelve zodiac signs) bottle and was used as a medicine container. It is kept basically intact and was collected in 1957.

Preserved in Chinese Medical Association/ Museum of Chinese Medicine, Shanghai University of Traditional Chinese Medicine

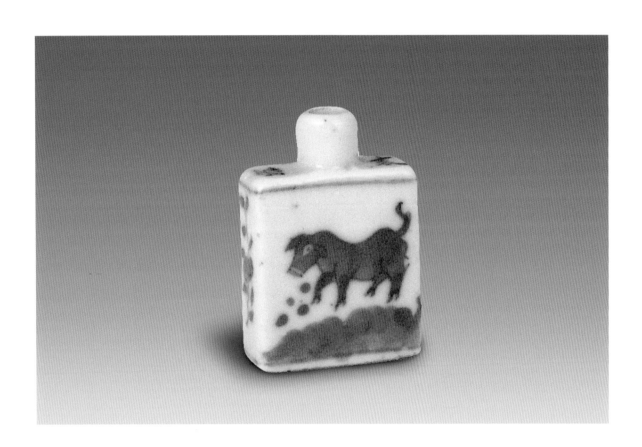

生肖药瓶（亥猪）

清

瓷质

口径 1.4 厘米，宽 4.1 厘米，通高 5.9 厘米，厚 1.9 厘米

Medicine Bottle with Chinese Zodiac Design (Hai Zhu)

Qing Dynasty

Porcelain

Mouth Diameter 1.4 cm/ Width 4.1 cm/ Height 5.9 cm/ Thickness 1.9 cm

方瓶形青花瓷瓶，直口，平底，浅圈足。该套药瓶瓶肩分别书有"子鼠" "丑牛"等标记，该藏为"亥猪瓶"，工艺精良，美观大方。盛药器具。保存基本完好。1957年入藏。

中华医学会 / 上海中医药大学医史博物馆藏

This cuboid bottle, beautiful and elegant, belongs to blue-and-white porcelain with delicate workmanship. It has a straight mouth, a flat bottom, and a shallow ring foot. On the shoulder of this set of bottle is inscribed the name of the lunar year such as "Zi Shu" (Rat, the first of the twelve zodiac signs), "Chou Niu" (Ox, the second of the twelve zodiac signs) and so on. This is a "Hai Zhu" (Pig, the twelfth of the twelve zodiac signs) bottle and was used as a medicine container. It is kept basically intact and was collected in 1957.

Preserved in Chinese Medical Association/ Museum of Chinese Medicine, Shanghai University of Traditional Chinese Medicine

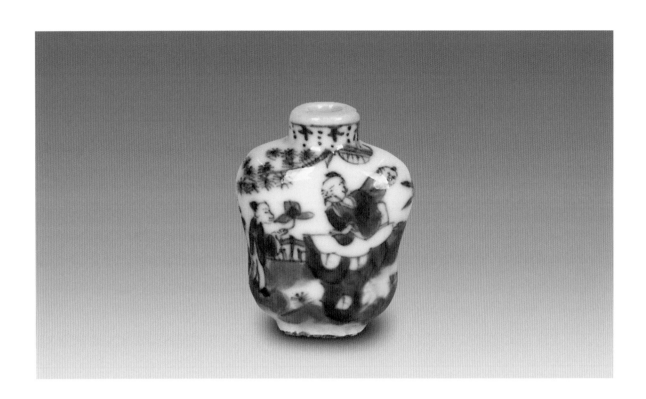

瓷药瓶

清

瓷质

口外径 1.7 厘米，口内径 0.7 厘米，宽 4.2 厘米，高 5.4 厘米，厚 2.2 厘米

Porcelain Medicine Bottle

Qing Dynasty

Porcelain

Mouth Outer Diameter 1.7 cm/ Mouth Inner Diameter 0.7 cm/ Width 4.2 cm/ Height 5.4 cm/ Thickness 2.2 cm

扁瓶状，平底，圈足，瓶身绘青花人物故事
图案，无款识，工艺较好。盛药器具。保存
基本完好。1955 年入藏。

中华医学会 / 上海中医药大学医史博物馆藏

This oblate bottle is decorated with blue-and-white
human figure and scene designs. It has a flat bottom
and a ring foot with no inscription. It was made
with good workmanship and was used as a medicine
container. It is kept basically intact and was collected
in 1955.

Preserved in Chinese Medical Association/ Museum
of Chinese Medicine, Shanghai University of
Traditional Chinese Medicine

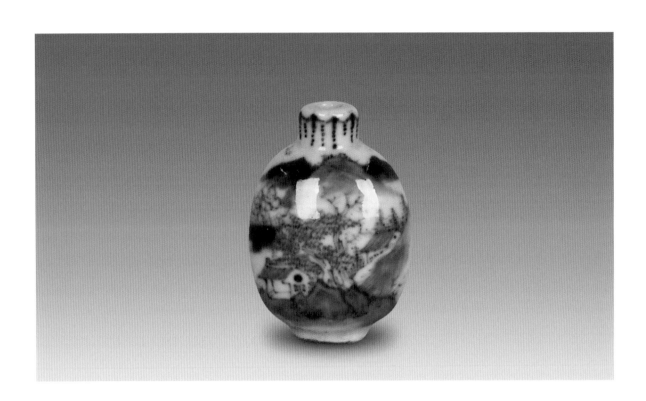

瓷药瓶

清

瓷质

口外径 1.45 厘米，口内径 0.6 厘米，宽 4 厘米，高 5.6 厘米，厚 2.88 厘米

Porcelain Medicine Bottle

Qing Dynasty

Porcelain

Mouth Outer Diameter 1.45 cm/ Mouth Inner Diameter 0.6 cm/ Width 4 cm/ Height 5.6 cm/ Thickness 2.88 cm

扁瓶状，平底，圈足，瓶身绘青花乡间风景图，无款识，工艺较好。盛药器具。保存基本完好。1955 年入藏。

中华医学会 / 上海中医药大学医史博物馆藏

This oblate bottle is decorated with blue-and-white rural landscape designs. It has a flat bottom and a ring foot with no inscription. It was made with good workmanship and was used to contain medicines. It is kept basically intact and was collected in 1955.

Preserved in Chinese Medical Association/ Museum of Chinese Medicine, Shanghai University of Traditional Chinese Medicine

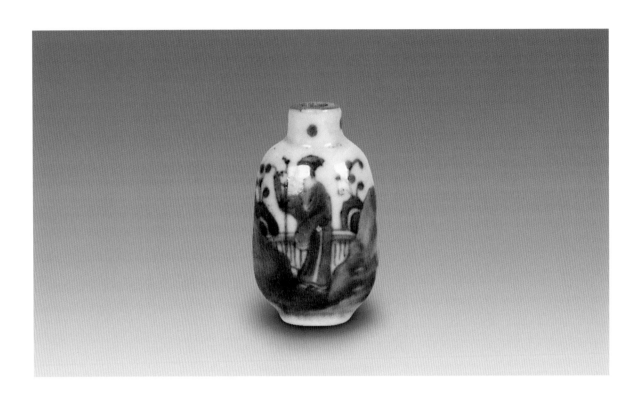

瓷药瓶

清

瓷质

口外径 1.5 厘米，口内径 0.7 厘米，宽 3.45 厘米，高 5.75 厘米，厚 2.5 厘米

Porcelain Medicine Bottle

Qing Dynasty

Porcelain

Mouth Outer Diameter 1.5 cm/ Mouth Inner Diameter 0.7 cm/ Width 3.45 cm/ Height 5.75 cm/ Thickness 2.5 cm

扁瓶状，平底，圈足，瓶身绘青花人物故事
图案，无款识，工艺较好。盛药器具。保存
基本完好。1955 年入藏。

中华医学会 / 上海中医药大学医史博物馆藏

This oblate bottle is decorated with blue-and-white
human figure and scene designs. It has a flat bottom
and a ring foot with no inscription. It was made
with good workmanship and was used as a medicine
container. It is kept basically intact and was collected
in 1955.

Preserved in Chinese Medical Association/ Museum
of Chinese Medicine, Shanghai University of
Traditional Chinese Medicine

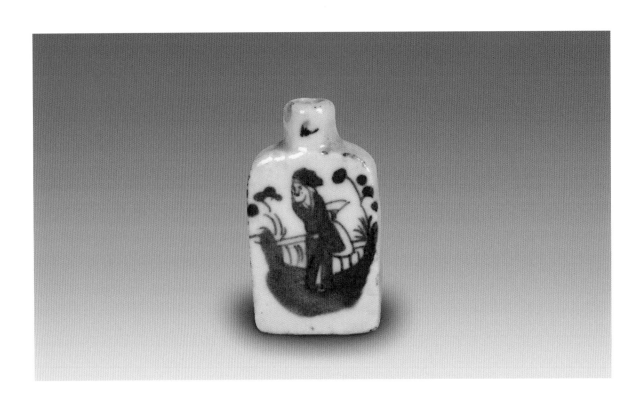

瓷药瓶

清

瓷质

口外径 1.4 厘米，口内径 0.7 厘米，宽 3.4 厘米，高 6.1 厘米，厚 1.6 厘米

Porcelain Medicine Bottle

Qing dynasty

Porcelain

Mouth Outer Diameter 1.4 cm/ Mouth Inner Diameter 0.7 cm/ Width 3.4 cm/ Height 6.1 cm/ Thickness 1.6 cm

方瓶状，青花釉，瓶身一面有人物故事图案，底部无款识，工艺一般。盛药器具。保存基本完好。1955 年入藏。

中华医学会 / 上海中医药大学医史博物馆藏

This cuboid bottle, coated with blue-and-white glaze, was used for storing medicine. One side of its body is decorated with human figure and scene designs. There is no inscription on its bottom. It was made with average workmanship and remains intact. It was collected in 1955.

Preserved in Chinese Medical Association/ Museum of Chinese Medicine, Shanghai University of Traditional Chinese Medicine

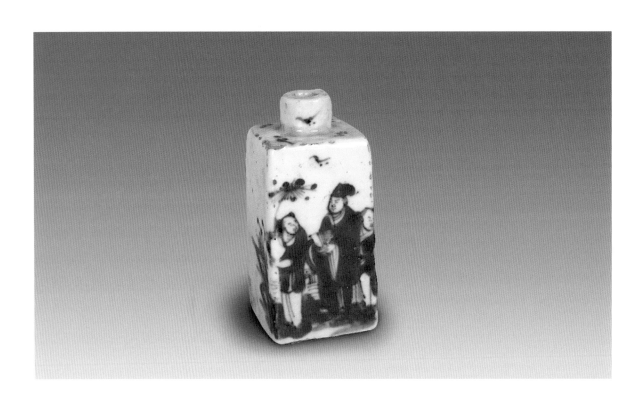

青花药瓶

清

瓷质

口外径 2 厘米，口内径 0.85 厘米，宽 4.4 厘米，高 8.9 厘米

Blue-and-white Medicine Bottle

Qing Dynasty

Porcelain

Mouth Outer Diameter 2 cm/ Mouth Inner Diameter 0.85 cm/ Width 4.4 cm/ Height 8.9 cm

方瓶形，青花釉，瓶身绘人物故事图案，底
部无款识，工艺一般。盛药器具。表面有残。
1955 年入藏。

中华医学会 / 上海中医药大学医史博物馆藏

This cuboid bottle is coated with a blue-and-white
glaze and is embellished with figure and scene
designs. There is no inscription on its bottom. It was
made with average workmanship and was used for
storing medicine. Damaged speckles can be seen on
the surface. It was collected in 1955.

Preserved in Chinese Medical Association/ Museum
of Chinese Medicine, Shanghai University of
Traditional Chinese Medicine

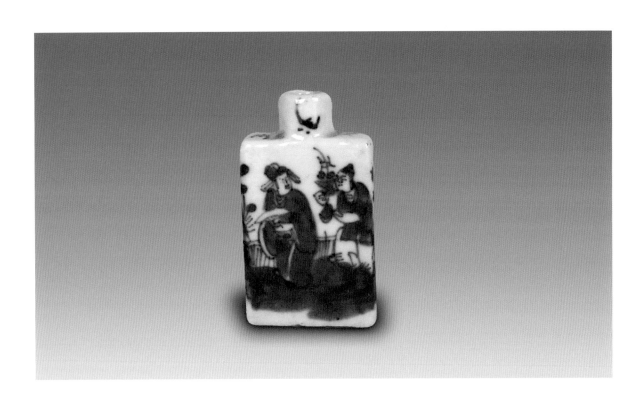

青花药瓶

清

瓷质

口外径 1.65 厘米，口内径 0.85 厘米，宽 4.1 厘米，高 6.9 厘米，厚 1.75 厘米

Blue-and-white Medicine Bottle

Qing Dynasty

Porcelain

Mouth Outer Diameter 1.65 cm/ Mouth Inner Diameter 0.85 cm/ Width 4.1 cm/ Height 6.9 cm/ Thickness 1.75 cm

方瓶形，青花釉，瓶身一面有人物故事图案，
底部无款识，工艺一般。盛药器具。保存基
本完好。1955 年入藏。

中华医学会 / 上海中医药大学医史博物馆藏

This cuboid bottle, coated with blue-and-white glaze,
was used for storing medicine. One side of its body
is decorated with human figure and scene designs.
There is no inscription on its bottom. It was made
with average workmanship and remains intact. It was
collected in 1955.

Preserved in Chinese Medical Association/ Museum
of Chinese Medicine, Shanghai University of
Traditional Chinese Medicine

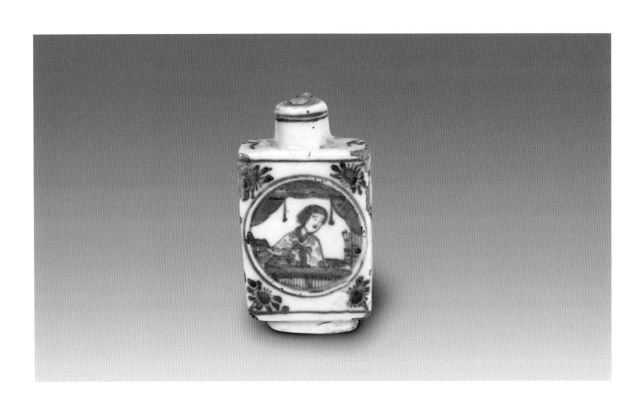

青花药瓶

清

瓷质

口外径 1.6 厘米，口内径 0.7 厘米，宽 3.9 厘米，高 6.7 厘米，厚 1.6 厘米

Blue-and-white Medicine Bottle

Qing Dynasty

Porcelain

Mouth Outer Diameter 1.6 cm/ Mouth Inner Diameter 0.7 cm/ Width 3.9 cm/ Height 6.7 cm/ Thickness 1.6 cm

方瓶形，青花釉，瓶身正、反两面有人物故事图案，底部有"乾隆年制"款识，工艺粗糙。盛药器具。表面残损。1955 年入藏。

中华医学会 / 上海中医药大学医史博物馆藏

This cuboid bottle, coated with blue-and-white glaze, was used for storing medicine. On both sides of its body are painted human figure and scene designs. On its bottom are seen inscriptions of "Qian Long Nian Zhi" (Made during the Reign of Qianlong). It was made with rough workmanship. Damaged specks can be seen on the surface. It was collected in 1955.

Preserved in Chinese Medical Association/ Museum of Chinese Medicine, Shanghai University of Traditional Chinese Medicine

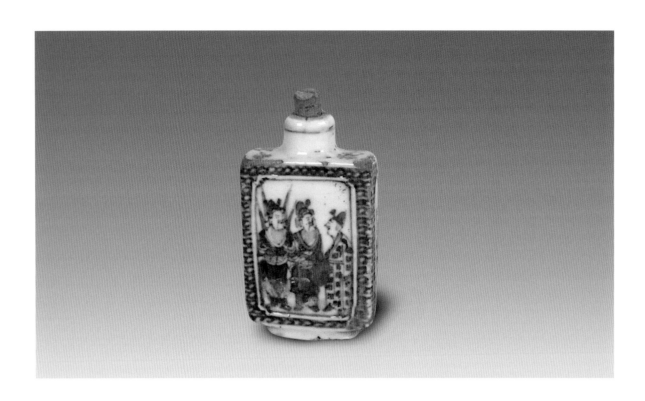

青花药瓶

清

瓷质

□外径 1.5 厘米，□内径 0.6 厘米，宽 3.8 厘米，高 6.65 厘米，厚 1.85 厘米

Blue-and-white Medicine Bottle

Qing Dynasty

Porcelain

Mouth Outer Diameter 1.5 cm/ Mouth Inner Diameter 0.6 cm/ Width 3.8 cm/ Height 6.65 cm/ Thickness 1.85 cm

方瓶形，青花釉，瓶身正、反两面有三才、三杰图案，两侧面分别有"元人笔法汉三杰""三才子岁在梅月林"字样，底部有"乾隆年制"款识，工艺粗糙。盛药器具。表面残损。1955 年入藏。

中华医学会 / 上海中医药大学医史博物馆藏

This cuboid bottle, coated with blue-and-white glaze, was used for storing medicine. The front and back sides of its body are decorated with patterns of Sancai (three talents) and Sanjie (three outstanding figures), and on its left and right sides is respectively painted one line of inscriptions. On its bottom can be seen inscriptions of "Qian Long Nian Zhi" (Made during the Reign of Qianlong). It was made with rough workmanship. Its surface is damaged and it was collected in 1955.

Preserved in Chinese Medical Association/ Museum of Chinese Medicine, Shanghai University of Traditional Chinese Medicine

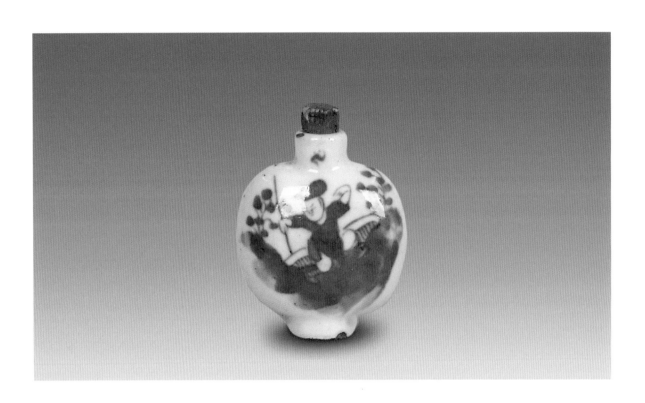

瓷药瓶

清

瓷质

口外径 1.6 厘米，口内径 1 厘米， 宽 5.15 厘米，高 5.85 厘米，厚 2.4 厘米

Porcelain Medicine Bottle

Qing Dynasty

Porcelain

Mouth Outer Diameter 1.6 cm/ Mouth Inner Diameter 1 cm/ Width 5.15 cm/ Height 5.85 cm/ Thickness 2.4 cm

扁瓶状，瓶身绘青花人物故事图案，平底，

圈足，无款识，工艺一般。盛药器具。保存

基本完好。1955 年入藏。

中华医学会 / 上海中医药大学医史博物馆藏

This oblate bottle with blue-and-white human figure
and scene designs was used for storing medicine. It
has a flat bottom and a ring foot without inscription.
It was made with average workmanship and remains
intact. It was collected in 1955.

Preserved in Chinese Medical Association/ Museum
of Chinese Medicine, Shanghai University of
Traditional Chinese Medicine

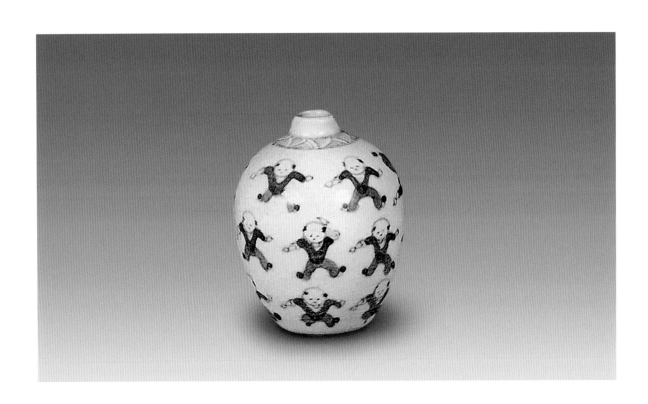

青花百子小药瓶

清

底径 5 厘米，高 6 厘米

直口，溜肩，鼓腹，平底，圈足，上有青花幼子
图案，形态各异。

上海中医药博物馆藏

Small Blue-and-white Medicine Bottle with a Hundred Children Design

Qing Dynasty

Bottom Diameter 5 cm/ Height 6 cm

The medicine bottle has a straight mouth, a sloping shoulder, a drum-like belly, a flat bottom, and a ring foot. It is decorated with blue-and-white designs of children in different shapes.

Preserved in Shanghai Museum of Traditional Chinese Medicine

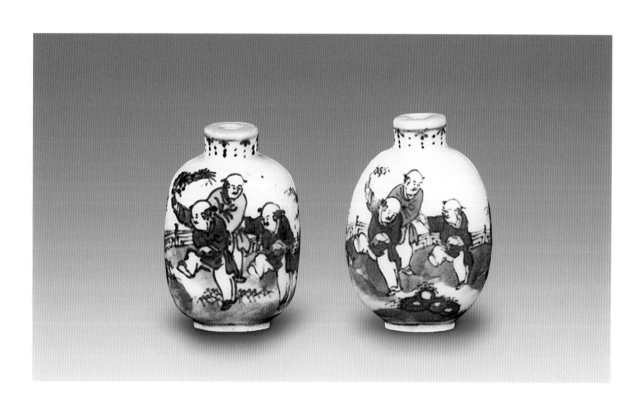

青花婴戏图药瓶

清

瓷质

底径 3 厘米，高 7 厘米

直口，平沿，溜肩，平底，圈足，表面以青花绘
婴戏图案，活泼可爱。盛药器具。

上海中医药博物馆藏

Blue-and-white Medicine Bottle with Design of Children at Play

Qing Dynasty

Porcelain

Bottom Diameter 3 cm/ Height 7 cm

This bottle has a straight mouth, a flat mouth rim, a
sloping shoulder, a flat bottom, and a ring foot.On this
medicine bottle are painted designs of lovely children at
play. It was used for storing medicine.

Preserved in Shanghai Museum of Traditional Chinese
Medicine

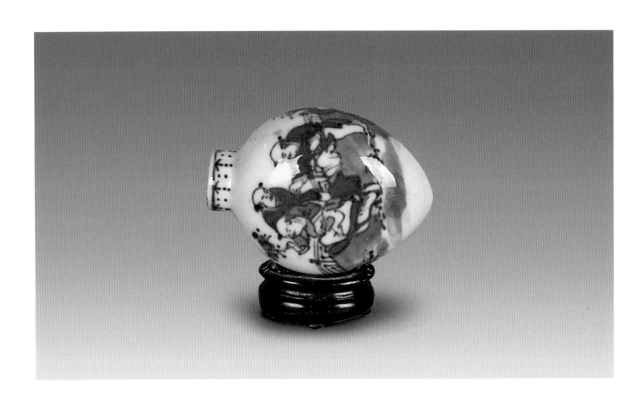

青花药瓶

清

瓷质

口外径 1.63 厘米，口内径 0.5 厘米，宽 4.5 厘米，高 6.4 厘米，厚 2.9 厘米

Blue-and-white Medicine Bottle

Qing Dynasty

Porcelain

Mouth Outer Diameter 1.63 cm/ Mouth Inner Diameter 0.5 cm/ Width 4.5 cm/ Height 6.4 cm/ Thickness 2.9 cm

扁瓶形，直口，尖底，涂釉均匀，表面光亮，瓶身绘童子郊外嬉戏图，工艺较好。盛药器具。保存基本完好。1955 年入藏。

中华医学会 / 上海中医药大学医史博物馆藏

This is an oblate medicine bottle with a straight mouth and a pointed bottom. It is glazed evenly and sheds bright lustre. On its surface are painted designs of children playing in the suburbs. It was made with good workmanship and remains intact. It was collected in 1955.

Preserved in Chinese Medical Association/ Museum of Chinese Medicine, Shanghai University of Traditional Chinese Medicine

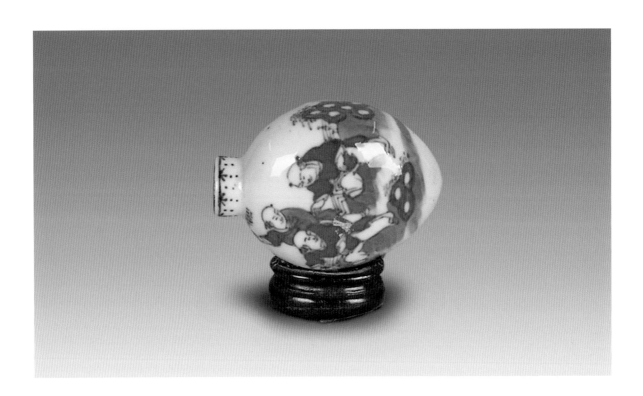

青花药瓶

清

瓷质

口外径 1.65 厘米，口内径 0.75 厘米，宽 4.6 厘米，高 6.4 厘米，厚 2.85 厘米

Blue-and-white Medicine Bottle

Qing Dynasty

Porcelain

Mouth Outer Diameter 1.65 cm/ Mouth Inner Diameter 0.75 cm/ Width 4.6 cm/ Height 6.4 cm/ Thickness 2.85 cm

扁瓶形，直口，尖底，涂釉均匀，表面光亮，瓶身绘童子郊外嬉戏图，工艺较好。盛药器具。保存基本完好。1955 年入藏。

中华医学会 / 上海中医药大学医史博物馆藏

This is an oblate medicine bottle with a straight mouth and a pointed bottom. It is glazed evenly and sheds bright lustre. On its surface are painted designs of children playing in the suburbs. It was made with good workmanship and remains intact. It was collected in 1955.

Preserved in Chinese Medical Association/ Museum of Chinese Medicine, Shanghai University of Traditional Chinese Medicine

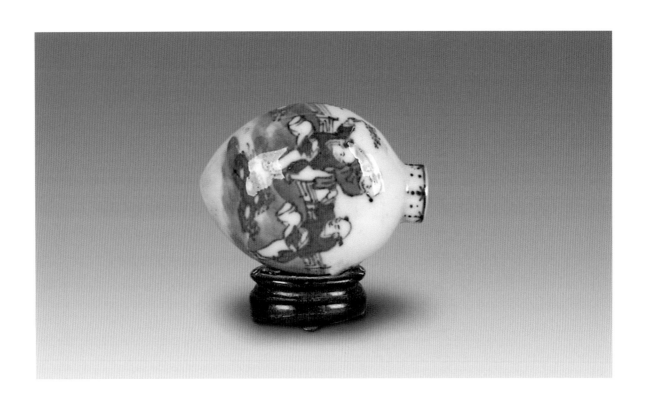

青花药瓶

清

瓷质

□外径 1.65 厘米，□内径 0.5 厘米，宽 4.55 厘米，高 6.35 厘米，厚 2.8 厘米

Blue-and-white Medicine Bottle

Qing Dynasty

Porcelain

Mouth Outer Diameter 1.65 cm/ Mouth Inner Diameter 0.5 cm/ Width 4.55 mm/ Height 6.35 cm/ Thickness 2.8 cm

扁瓶形，直口，尖底，涂釉均匀，表面光亮，瓶身绘童子郊外嬉戏图，工艺较好。盛药器具。保存基本完好。1955 年入藏。

中华医学会 / 上海中医药大学医史博物馆藏

This is an oblate medicine bottle with a straight mouth and a pointed bottom. It is glazed evenly and sheds bright lustre. On its surface are painted designs of children playing in the suburbs. It was made with good workmanship and remains intact. It was collected in 1955.

Preserved in Chinese Medical Association/ Museum of Chinese Medicine, Shanghai University of Traditional Chinese Medicine

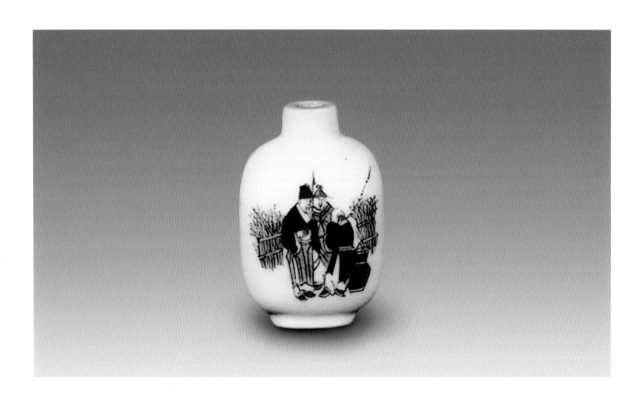

青花人物小药瓶

清

瓷质

底径 3 厘米，高 7 厘米

直口，平沿，溜肩，平底，圈足，瓶身绘青花人
物图，三人似交谈状。

上海中医药博物馆藏

Small Blue-and-white Medicine Bottle with Figure Design

Qing Dynasty

Porcelain

Bottom Diameter 3 cm/ Height 7 cm

This bottle has a straight mouth, a flat mouth rim, a sloping shoulder, a flat bottom, and a ring foot. On its body is the blue-and-white pattern of three figures, who look like talking with each other.

Preserved in Shanghai Museum of Traditional Chinese Medicine

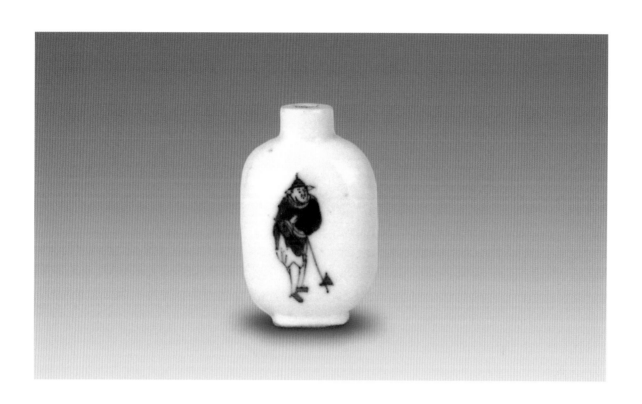

药瓶

Medicine Bottle

清

瓷质

口径 1.6 厘米，宽 4.1 厘米，通高 6 厘米，厚 2.6 厘米

扁瓶状，瓶身饰青花人物故事图，直口，平底，圈足，小巧玲珑，造型美观。盛药器具。保存基本完好。1954 年入藏。

中华医学会 / 上海中医药大学医史博物馆藏

Qing Dynasty

Porcelain

Mouth Diameter 1.6 cm/ Width 4.1 cm/ Height 6 cm/ Thickness 2.6 cm

It is an oblate medicine bottle with human figure and scene designs. It is shaped exquisitely and beautifully with a straight mouth, a flat bottom and a ring foot. It is kept intact and was collected in 1954.

Preserved in Chinese Medical Association/ Museum of Chinese Medicine, Shanghai University of Traditional Chinese Medicine

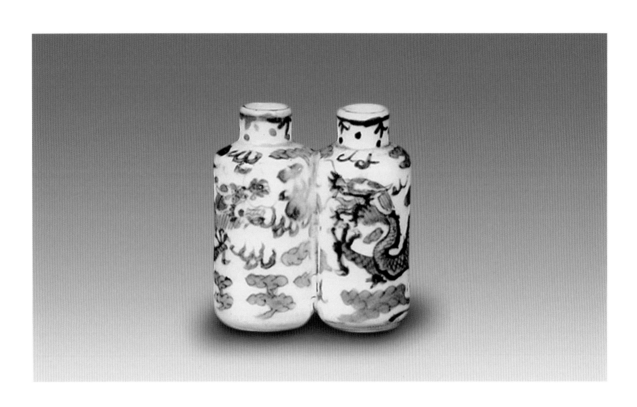

青花双龙戏珠双连药瓶

清

瓷质

底径 4 厘米，高 7 厘米

两瓶相连接，上为双龙戏珠图案。

上海中医药博物馆藏

Double Blue-and-white Medicine Bottles with Design of Two Dragons Playing with a Ball

Qing Dynasty

Porcelain

Bottom Diameter 4 cm/ Height 7 cm

The two bottles are connected together and decorated with designs of two dragons playing with a ball.

Preserved in Shanghai Museum of Traditional Chinese Medicine

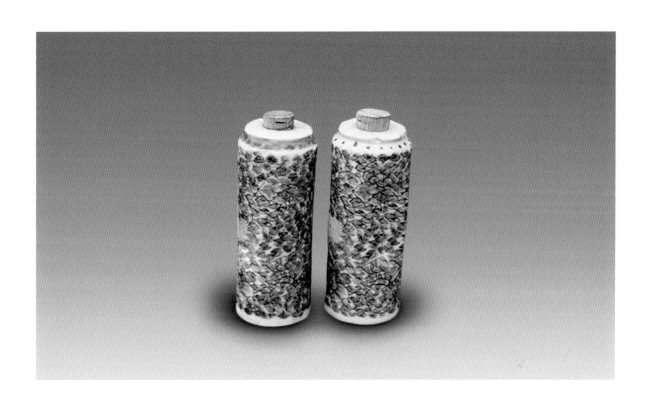

青花圆形药瓶

清

瓷质

左：口外径 1.15 厘米，底径 3.21 厘米，通高
7.17 厘米，重 45 克

右：口外径 1.25 厘米，底径 3.18 厘米，通高
7.22 厘米，重 55 克

两件。圆柱形，平口，平底，青花。装药用。

广东中医药博物馆藏

Round Blue-and-white Porcelain Medicine Bottles

Qing Dynasty

Porcelain

Left: Mouth Outer Diameter 1.15 cm/ Bottom Diameter
3.21 cm/ Height 7.17 cm/ Weight 45 g

Right: Mouth Outer Diameter 1.25cm/ Bottom Diameter
3.18 cm/ Height 7.22 cm/ Weight 55 g

The two bottles, used as medicine containers, are
cylindrical in shape with flat mouths and flat bottoms.
They are decorated with blue-and-white designs.

Preserved in Guangdong Chinese Medicine Museum

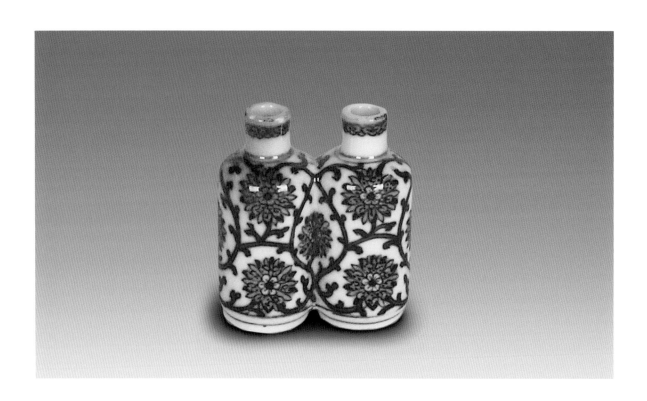

联体瓷药瓶

清

瓷质

圆瓶形，通身绘菊花缠枝纹，为双瓶联体，底部书"雅致"二字，无盖，制作工艺较好。盛药器具。保存基本完好。1958 年入藏。

中华医学会／上海中医药大学医史博物馆藏

Conjoined Porcelain Medicine Bottles

Qing Dynasty

Porcelain

This vessel is conjoined twin bottles with no lid, each of which is round and decorated with designs of interlocking branches of chrysanthemum. On its bottom are written two Chinese characters"Ya Zhi" (elegant). It was used for storing medicine and is kept intact. It was collected in 1958.

Preserved in Chinese Medical Association/ Museum of Chinese Medicine, Shanghai University of Traditional Chinese Medicine

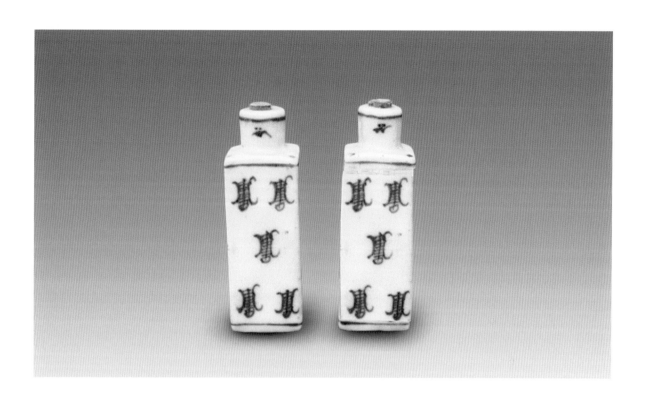

青花"寿"字方形药瓶

清

瓷质

口外径 1.55 厘米，通高 7.3 厘米，瓶身长 2.34 厘米，瓶身宽 2.35 厘米，瓶身高 5.9 厘米，两瓶共重 72 克

两件。方形，平口，细直颈，平底，上绘"寿"字。用于装药。

广东中医药博物馆藏

Cubic Blue-and-white Medicine Bottles with Chinese Character "Shou"

Qing Dynasty

Porcelain

Mouth Outer Diameter 1.55 cm/ Height 7.3 cm/ Body Length 2.34 cm/ Body Width 2.35 cm/ Body Height 5.9 cm/ Weight (the two bottles) 72 g

The two cubic medicine bottle have flat mouths, narrow and straight necks, and flat bottoms, decorated with Chinese characters "Shou"(longevity). It was used for storing medicine.

Preserved in Guangdong Chinese Medicine Museum

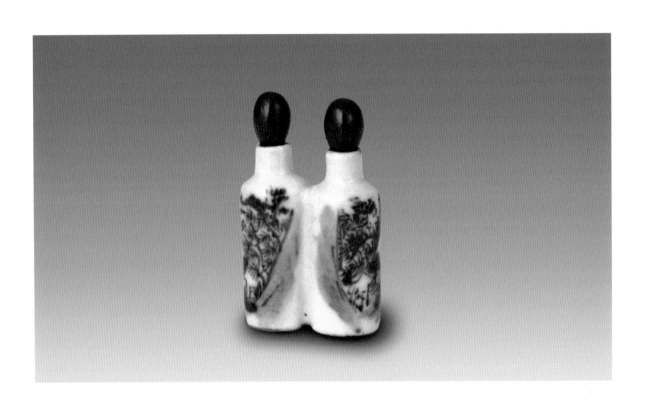

双连药瓶

清

瓷质

口径 1.1 厘米，宽 4.4 厘米，高 5.3 厘米，厚 2.2 厘米

Two Conjoined Medicine Bottles

Qing Dynasty

Porcelain

Mouth Diameter 1.1 cm/ Width 4.4 cm/ Height 5.3 cm/ Thickness 2.2 cm

圆瓶连体，表面绘青花松石图，直口，平底，双连，配木塞，小巧玲珑，工艺较好。盛药器具。保存基本完好。1955 年入藏。

中华医学会 / 上海中医药大学医史博物馆藏

This is a round conjoined double bottles with blue-and-white designs of pine and stone. They have straight mouths, flat bottoms and wooden plugs. It is shaped exquisitely with good workmanship and was used for storing medicine. It is kept basically intact and was collected in 1955.

Preserved in Chinese Medical Association/ Museum of Chinese Medicine, Shanghai University of Traditional Chinese Medicine

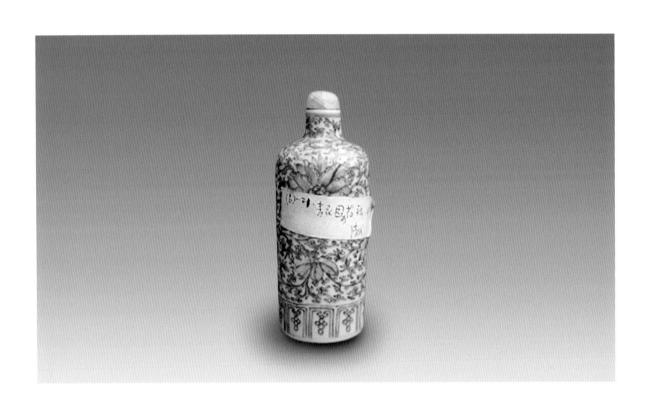

青花圆形药用瓶

清

瓷质

口外径 2 厘米，底径 5.27 厘米，通高 13.64 厘米，瓶深 11.5 厘米，重 165 克

Round Blue-and-white Medicine Bottle

Qing Dynasty

Porcelain

Mouth Outer Diameter 2 cm/ Bottom Diameter 5.27 cm/ Height 13.64 cm/ Depth 11.5 cm/ Weight 165 g

一式四件。圆柱形，直口，平沿，溜肩，直
腹，平底，圈足，颈、腹部饰缠枝芍药花纹。
用于盛药。

广东中医药博物馆藏

This set of porcelain ware comprises four bottles
of the same style. Each has a straight mouth, a flat
mouth rim, a sloping shoulder, a straight cylindrical
belly, a flat bottom, and a ring foot. Patterns of
interlocking peonies are painted on its body and
neck. They were used as medicine container.

Preserved in Guangdong Chinese Medicine Museum

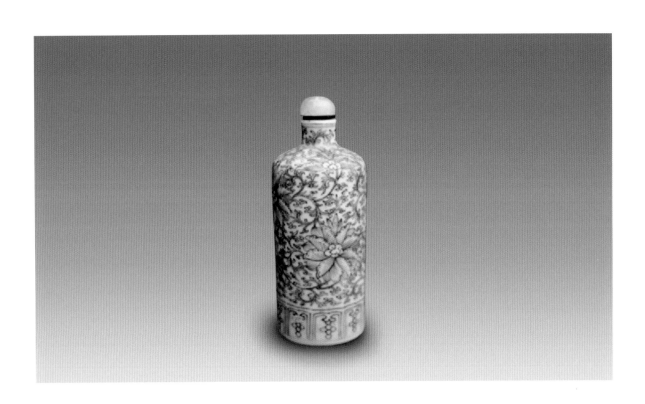

青花圆形药用瓶

清

瓷质

口外径 2 厘米，底径 5.4 厘米，通高 13.6 厘米，

瓶深 11.4 厘米，重 180 克

一式四件。用于盛药。

广东中医药博物馆藏

Round Blue-and-white Medicine Bottle

Qing Dynasty

Porcelain

Mouth Outer Diameter 2.0 cm/ Bottom Diameter 5.4 cm/ Height 13.6 cm/ Depth 11.4 cm/ Weight 180 g

This set of porcelain ware comprises four bottles of the same style. It was used as a medicine container.

Preserved in Guangdong Chinese Medicine Museum

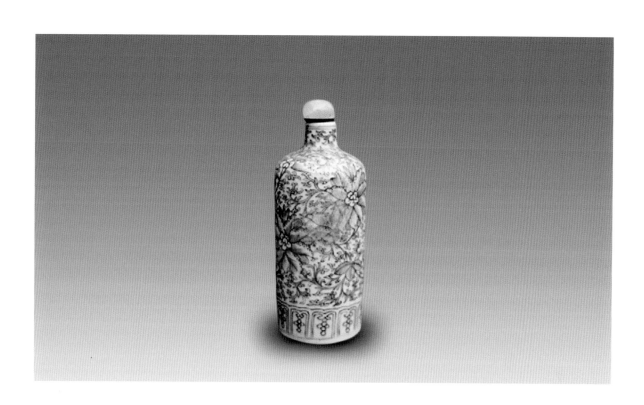

青花圆形药用瓶

清

瓷质

口外径 1.92 厘米，底径 5.42 厘米，通高 13.77 厘米，瓶深 11.6 厘米，重 180 克

一式四件。用于盛药。

广东中医药博物馆藏

Round Blue-and-white Medicine Bottle

Qing Dynasty

Porcelain

Mouth Outer Diameter 1.92 cm/ Bottom Diameter 5.42 cm/ Height 13.77 cm/ Depth 11.6 cm/ Weight 180 g

This set of porcelain ware comprises four bottles of the same style. It was used as a medicine container.

Preserved in Guangdong Chinese Medicine Museum

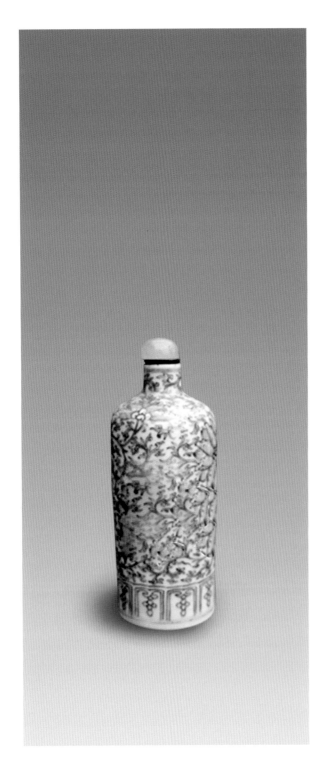

青花圆形药用瓶

清

瓷质

口外径 1.94 厘米，底径 5.23 厘米，通高 13.55 厘米，瓶深 11.5 厘米，重 195 克

一式四件。用于盛药。

广东中医药博物馆藏

Round Blue-and-white Medicine Bottle

Qing Dynasty

Porcelain

Mouth Outer Diameter 1.94 cm/ Bottom Diameter 5.23 cm/ Height 13.55 cm/ Depth 11.5 cm/ Weight 195 g

This set of porcelain ware comprises four bottles of the same style. It was used as a medicine container.

Preserved in Guangdong Chinese Medicine Museum

瓷药瓶

清

瓷质

腹径 3.6 厘米，通高 8.2 厘米

圆瓶形，青花瓷，瓶身饰人物故事图案，瓶底无
款识。盛药器具。保存基本完好，口沿有残。
1955 年入藏。

中华医学会 / 上海中医药大学医史博物馆藏

Porcelain Medicine Bottle

Qing Dynasty

Porcelain

Belly Diameter 3.6 cm/ Height 8.2 cm

This round blue-and-white medicine bottle, used to
contain medicine, is decorated with motifs of human
figures and landscape with no inscription on the bottom.
Except the damaged mouth rim, it is basically kept intact.
It was collected in 1955.

Preserved in Chinese Medical Association/ Museum of
Chinese Medicine, Shanghai University of Traditional
Chinese Medicine

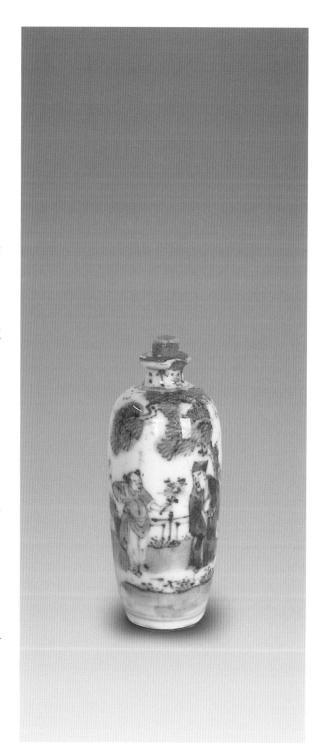

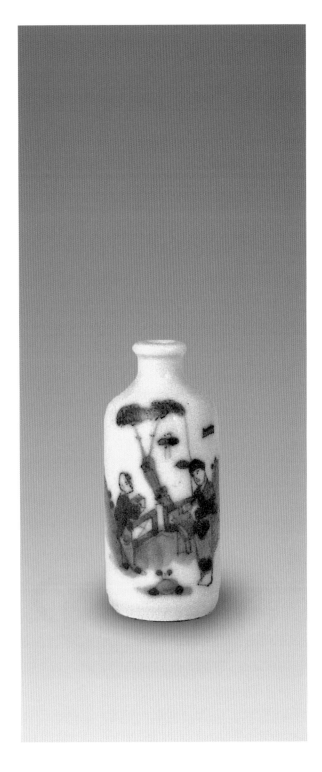

药瓶

清

瓷质

口径 1.5 厘米，腹径 3.1 厘米，通高 7 厘米

圆瓶形，表面饰青花人物故事图，直口，翻沿，平底，小巧玲珑，工艺精良。盛药器具。保存基本完好。1954 年入藏。

中华医学会 / 上海中医药大学医史博物馆藏

Medicine Bottle

Qing Dynasty

Porcelain

Mouth Diameter 1.5 cm/ Belly Diameter 3.1 cm/ Height 7 cm

The round medicine bottle, with blue-and-white motifs of human figures and landscape, has a straight mouth with scrolled rim and a flat bottom. The exquisite bottle with delicate craftsmanship was used for storing medicine. It is basically well-preserved and was collected in 1954.

Preserved in Chinese Medical Association/ Museum of Chinese Medicine, Shanghai University of Traditional Chinese Medicine

瓷药瓶

清

瓷质

腹径 2.7 厘米，通高 7.3 厘米

圆瓶形青花瓷，瓶身有朱绘双龙云海图案，金属盖连带一象牙药勺。香具。保存基本完好。1955 年入藏。

中华医学会 / 上海中医药大学医史博物馆藏

Porcelain Medicine Bottle

Qing Dynasty

Porcelain

Belly Diameter 2.7 cm/ Height 7.3 cm

This round blue-and-white porcelain bottle has a metal lid and an ivory medicine spoon. Its belly is decorated with patterns of twin dragons and clouds. It is an incense container, which is still in good condition. It was collected in 1955.

Preserved in Chinese Medical Association/ Museum of Chinese Medicine, Shanghai University of Traditional Chinese Medicine

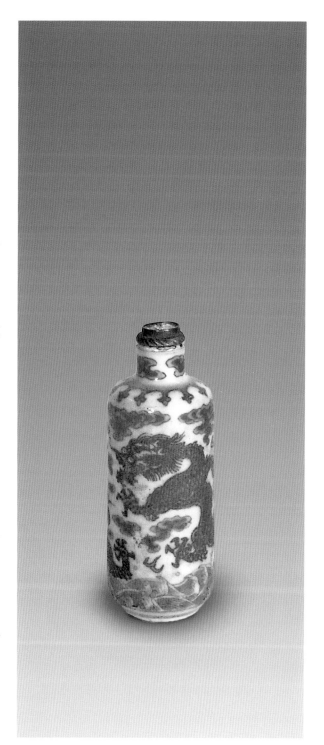

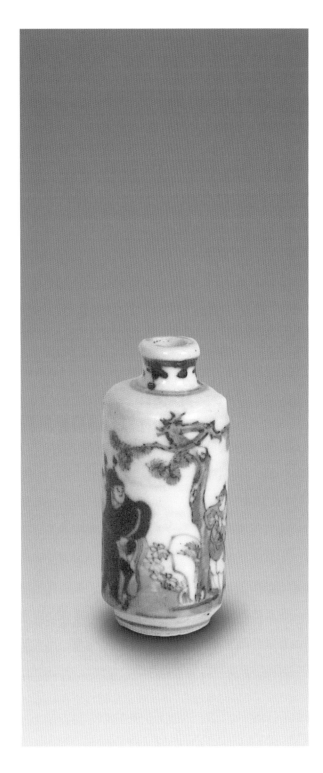

瓷药瓶

清

瓷质

腹径 3.3 厘米，通高 7.2 厘米

圆瓶形青花瓷，瓶身绘有人物故事图案，瓶底有"雍正年制"款识。盛药器具。保存基本完好。1955 年入藏。

中华医学会 / 上海中医药大学医史博物馆藏

Porcelain Medicine Bottle

Qing Dynasty

Porcelain

Belly Diameter 3.3 cm/ Height 7.2 cm

This round blue-and-white bottle was used for storing medicine. The basically well-preserved bottle has motifs of human figure and landscape on the body, and on its bottom is found the inscription of "Yong Zheng Nian Zhi" (Made during the Reign of Yongzheng). It was collected in 1955.

Preserved in Chinese Medical Association/ Museum of Chinese Medicine, Shanghai University of Traditional Chinese Medicine

瓷药瓶

清

瓷质

腹径 3.1 厘米，通高 8.15 厘米

圆瓶形青花瓷，瓶身绘有动物图案，瓶底有"雍正年制"款识。盛药器具。保存基本完好。1955 年入藏。

中华医学会 / 上海中医药大学医史博物馆藏

Porcelain Medicine Bottle

Qing Dynasty

Porcelain

Belly Diameter 3.1 cm/ Height 8.15 cm

This round blue-and-white bottle was used for storing medicine. The basically well-preserved bottle has animal motifs on the body, and on its bottom is found the inscription of "Yong Zheng Nian Zhi" (Made during the Reign of Yongzheng). It was collected in 1955.

Preserved in Chinese Medical Association/ Museum of Chinese Medicine, Shanghai University of Traditional Chinese Medicine

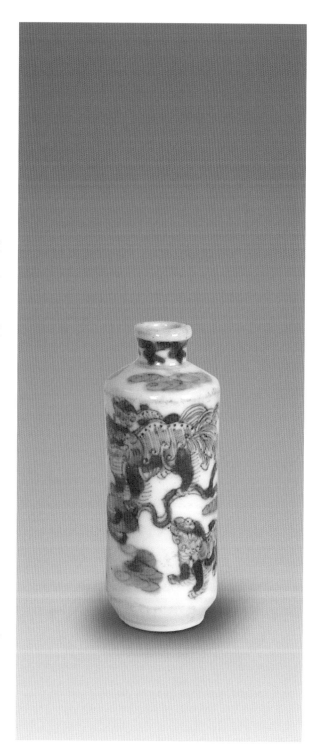

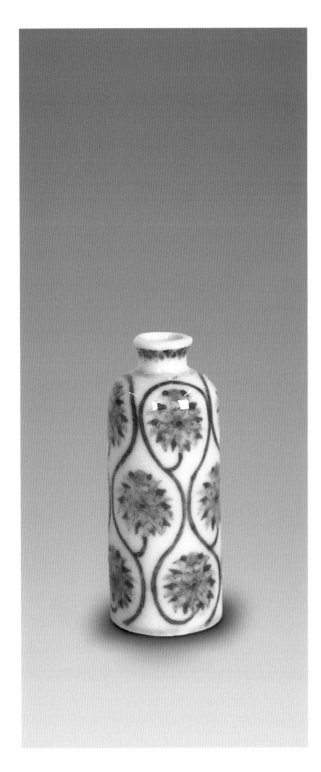

瓷药瓶

清

瓷质

腹径 2.7 厘米，通高 6.7 厘米

圆瓶形青花瓷，瓷胎细腻，烧制上乘，瓶身绘有菊花缠枝图案，瓶底有"大清乾隆年制"款识。盛药器具。保存基本完好。1955 年入藏。

中华医学会 / 上海中医药大学医史博物馆藏

Porcelain Medicine Bottle

Qing Dynasty

Porcelain

Belly Diameter 2.7 cm/ Height 6.7 cm

The bottle is a round blue-and-white medicine container. Its body is fine and smooth, and was fired with superior technique. It is decorated with interlocking chrysanthemum designs, and on the bottom is found the inscription of "Da Qing Qian Long Nian Zhi" (Made during the Reign of Qianlong in the Qing Dynasty). It is basically kept intact and was collected in 1955.

Preserved in Chinese Medical Association/ Museum of Chinese Medicine, Shanghai University of Traditional Chinese Medicine

瓷药瓶

清

瓷质

口外径 2 厘米，口内径 1.1 厘米，直径 4.7 厘米，

通高 10.2 厘米

圆瓶形，施乳白釉，为小开片青花瓷药瓶，瓶身

绘有菊花缠枝图案，瓶底无款识，制作工艺一般。

盛药器具。保存基本完好。1958 年入藏。

中华医学会 / 上海中医药大学医史博物馆藏

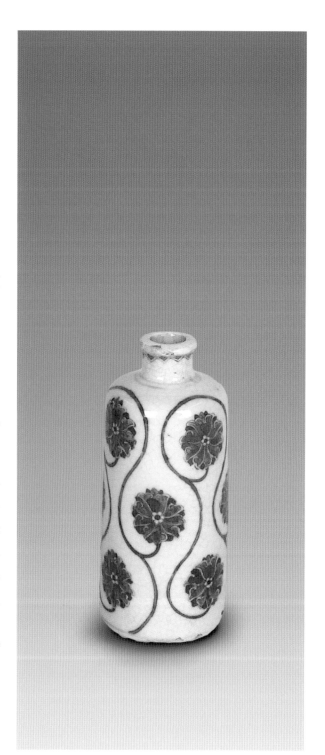

Porcelain Medicine Bottle

Qing Dynasty

Porcelain

Mouth Outer Diameter 2 cm/ Mouth Inner Diameter 1.1 cm/

Diameter 4.7 cm/ Height 10.2 cm

This round blue-and-white bottle, used to contain
medicine, is coated with milk-white glaze, with small
crackles. The body is decorated with interlocking
chrysanthemum designs and there is no inscription
on the bottom. This medicine container is of average
workmanship and is basically kept intact. It was collected
in 1958.

Preserved in Chinese Medical Association/ Museum of
Chinese Medicine, Shanghai University of Traditional
Chinese Medicine

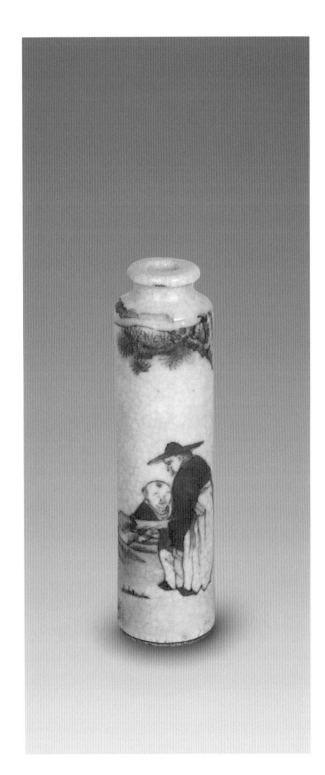

瓷药瓶

清

瓷质

腹径 2.2 厘米，通高 8.3 厘米

圆瓶形，为青花小开片药瓶，瓶身绘有老叟给童子上课的青花图案，瓶底无款识，绘制精细，制作工艺较好。盛药器具。保存基本完好，瓶肩有残。

中华医学会／上海中医药大学医史博物馆藏

Porcelain Medicine Bottle

Qing Dynasty

Porcelain

Belly Diameter 2.2 cm/ Height 8.3 cm

This round blue-and-white medicine bottle with small crackles has a motif of an old man teaching a child painted delicately on its body, and there is no inscription on the bottom. The bottle, used to contain medicine, is of exquisite workmanship. It is basically preserved well, with the shoulder slightly damaged.

Preserved in Chinese Medical Association/ Museum of Chinese Medicine, Shanghai University of Traditional Chinese Medicine

青花药瓶

清

瓷质

口外径 1.35 厘米，口内径 0.85 厘米，腹径 2.6 厘米，高 7.6 厘米

圆瓶形，表面绘青花人物泛舟风景画，平底，圈足，无款识，工艺精良。盛药器具。保存基本完好。1955 年入藏。

中华医学会 / 上海中医药大学医史博物馆藏

Blue-and-white Medicine Bottle

Qing Dynasty

Porcelain

Mouth Outer Diameter 1.35 cm/ Mouth Inner Diameter 0.85 cm/ Belly Diameter 2.6 cm/ Height 7.6 cm

The round bottle has a flat bottom and a ring foot, on which is found no inscription. With exquisite workmanship, its body is decorated with blue-and-white scenic motifs of a figure rowing a boat. It was used for storing medicine and is basically kept intact. It was collected in 1955.

Preserved in Chinese Medical Association/ Museum of Chinese Medicine, Shanghai University of Traditional Chinese Medicine

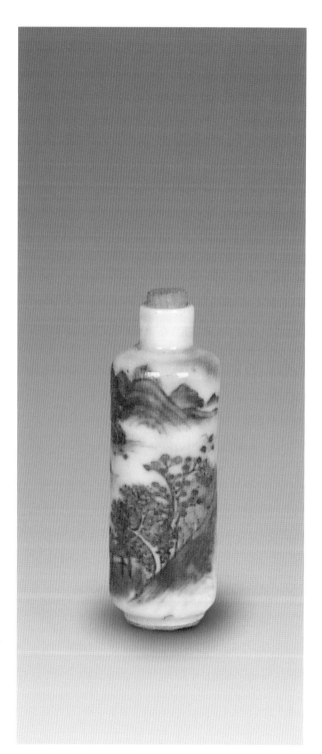

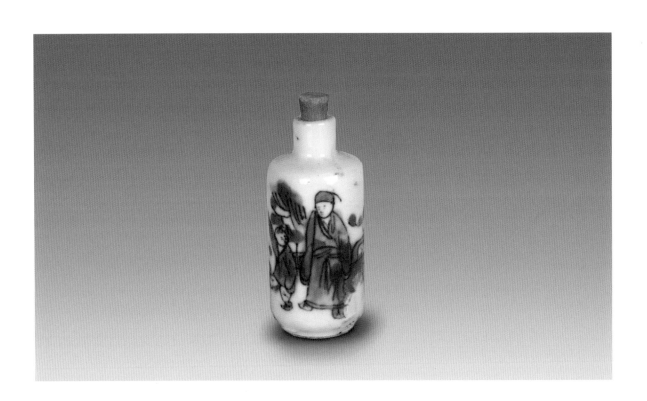

瓷药瓶

清

瓷质

口外径 1.2 厘米，口内径 0.7 厘米，腹径 2.75 厘米，高 6.15 厘米

Porcelain Medicine Bottle

Qing Dynasty

Porcelain

Mouth Outer Diameter 1.2 cm/ Mouth Inner Diameter 0.7 cm/ Belly Diameter 2.75 cm/ Height 6.15 cm

圆瓶形，表面绘青花父子采芝图，平底，圈足，无款识，工艺精良。盛药器具。保存基本完好。1955 年入藏。

中华医学会 / 上海中医药大学医史博物馆藏

This round bottle, with exquisite workmanship, has a flat bottom and a ring foot, on which is found no inscription. On its body is painted a blue-and-white motif of a father and his son picking ganoderma lucidum. It remains basically intact. It was used for storing medicine and was collected in 1955.

Preserved in Chinese Medical Association/ Museum of Chinese Medicine, Shanghai University of Traditional Chinese Medicine

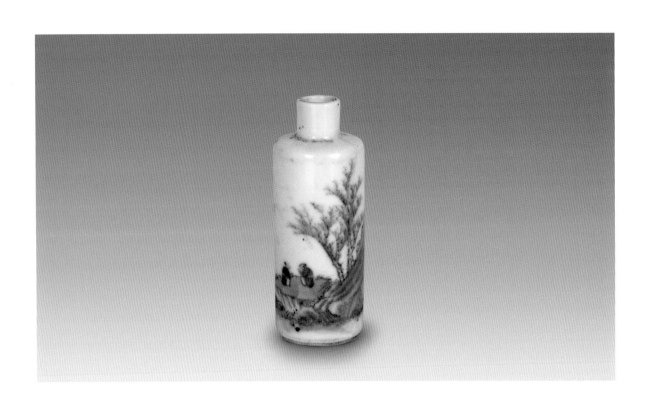

瓷药瓶

清

瓷质

口外径 1.35 厘米，口内径 0.9 厘米，腹径 2.8 厘米，高 7.5 厘米

Porcelain Medicine Bottle

Qing Dynasty

Porcelain

Mouth Outer Diameter 1.35 cm/ Mouth Inner Diameter 0.9 cm/ Belly Diameter 2.8 cm/ Height 7.5 cm

圆瓶形，表面绘青花人物故事图案，平底，圈足，无款识，工艺精良。盛药器具。保存基本完好。1955 年入藏。

中华医学会 / 上海中医药大学医史博物馆藏

This round bottle, used to contain medicine, has a flat bottom and a ring foot, on which is found no inscription. On its body are painted blue-and-white motifs of human figure and landscape, with fine workmanship. It is basically kept intact and was collected in 1955.

Preserved in Chinese Medical Association/ Museum of Chinese Medicine, Shanghai University of Traditional Chinese Medicine

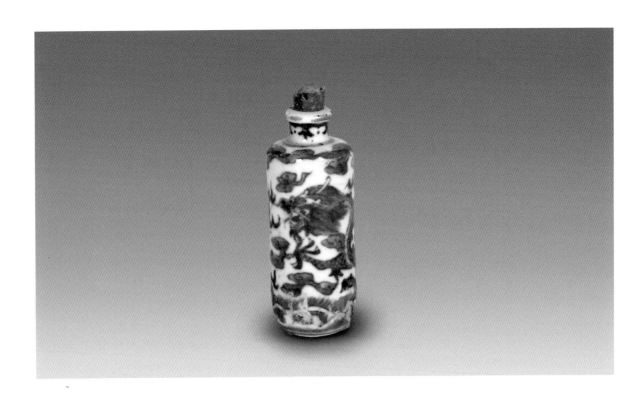

青花药瓶

清

瓷质

口外径 1.65 厘米，口内径 0.95 厘米，腹径 3 厘米，高 7.6 厘米

Blue-and-white Medicine Bottle

Qing Dynasty

Porcelain

Mouth Outer Diameter 1.65 cm/ Mouth Inner Diameter 0.95 cm/ Belly Diameter 3 cm/ Height 7.6 cm

圆瓶形，表面绘青花双龙云海图案，平底，
圈足，无款识，工艺较好。盛药器具。保存
基本完好，釉有脱落。1955 年入藏。

中华医学会／上海中医药大学医史博物馆藏

The round bottle, used to contain medicine, has a
flat bottom and a ring foot, on which is found no
inscription. On the body of the bottle are painted
blue-and-white motifs of double dragons among
clouds. The basically well-preserved bottle is of good
workmanship with some of its glaze peeled off. It
was collected in 1955.

Preserved in Chinese Medical Association/ Museum
of Chinese Medicine, Shanghai University of
Traditional Chinese Medicine

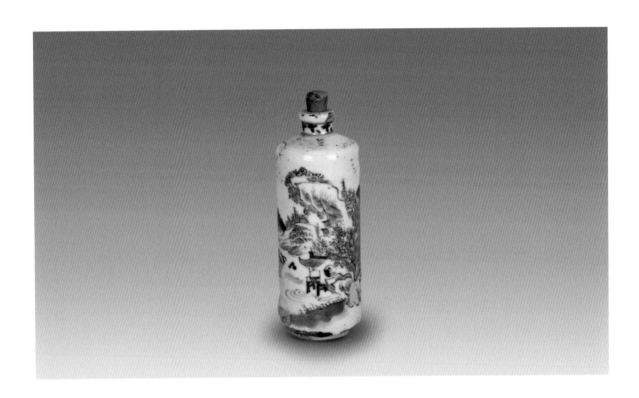

青花药瓶

清

瓷质

口外径 1.5 厘米，口内径 0.65 厘米，腹径 3.4 厘米，高 8.9 厘米

Blue-and-white Medicine Bottle

Qing Dynasty

Porcelain

Mouth Outer Diameter 1.5 cm/ Mouth Inner Diameter 0.65 cm/ Belly Diameter 3.4 cm/ Height 8.9 cm

圆瓶形，平底，圈足，表面绘青花人物垂钓

山水风景画，有"乾隆年制"款识，工艺精良。

盛药器具。口沿有残，釉有脱落。1955年入藏。

中华医学会 / 上海中医药大学医史博物馆藏

This round bottle, used to contain medicine, has a flat bottom and a ring foot with an inscription of "Qian Long Nian Zhi" (Made during the Reign of Qianlong). Its body, with exquisite workmanship, is decorated with blue-and-white scenic motifs of landscapes and a fishing figure. The mouth rim is damaged and some of its glaze is peeled off. It was collected in 1955.

Preserved in Chinese Medical Association/ Museum of Chinese Medicine, Shanghai University of Traditional Chinese Medicine

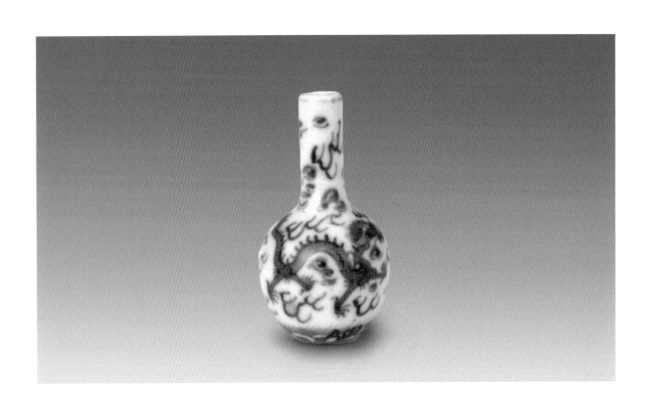

药瓶

清

瓷质

口径 1.3 厘米，腹径 3.9 厘米，通高 6.9 厘米

Medicine Bottle

Qing Dynasty

Porcelain

Mouth Diameter 1.3 cm/ Belly Diameter 3.9 cm/ Height 6.9 cm

圆瓶形，表面绘青花云龙纹，直口，长颈，
平底，圈足，底有"乾隆年制"款识，小巧
玲珑，工艺精良。盛药器具。保存基本完好。
1954年入藏。

中华医学会/上海中医药大学医史博物馆藏

This round bottle, used to contain medicine, has
a straight mouth, a long neck, a flat bottom, and a
ring foot. The bottom is inscribed with "Qian Long
Nian Zhi" (Made during the Reign of Qianlong). It
is decorated with blue-and-white designs of a dragon
among clouds. The bottle is small and exquisite with
fine workmanship. The well-preserved bottle was
collected in 1954.

Preserved in Chinese Medical Association/ Museum of
Chinese Medicine, Shanghai University of Traditional
Chinese Medicine

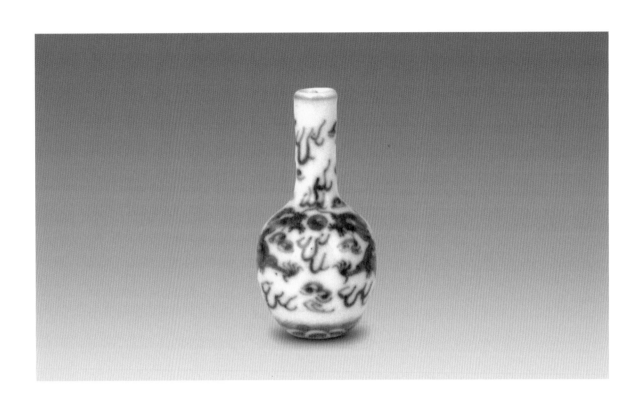

药瓶

清

瓷质

口径 1.4 厘米，腹径 3.8 厘米，通高 7.2 厘米

Medicine Bottle

Qing Dynasty

Porcelain

Mouth Diameter 1.4 cm/ Belly Diameter 3.8 cm/ Height 7.2 cm

圆瓶形，直口，长颈，平底，圈足，表面绘青花云龙纹，底有"乾隆年制"款识，小巧玲珑，工艺精良。盛药器具。保存基本完好。1954 年入藏。

中华医学会 / 上海中医药大学医史博物馆藏

This round medicine bottle, used to contain medicine, has a straight mouth, a long neck, a flat bottom, and a ring foot, and an inscription on the bottom that reads, "Qian Long Nian Zhi" (Made during the Reign of Qianlong). It is decorated with blue-and-white designs of a dragon among clouds. The bottle is small and exquisite with fine workmanship. The well-preserved bottle was collected in 1954.

Preserved in Chinese Medical Association/ Museum of Chinese Medicine, Shanghai University of Traditional Chinese Medicine

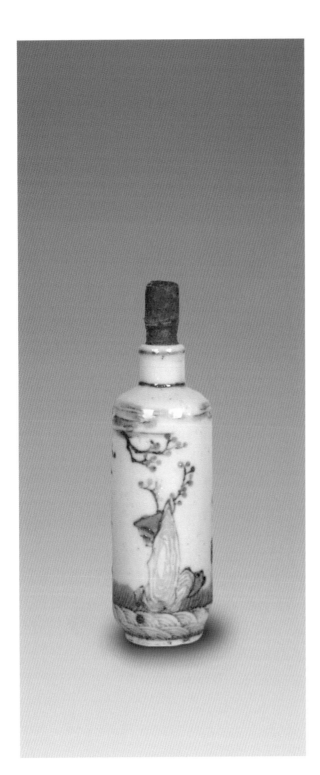

瓷药瓶

清

瓷质

口外径 1.5 厘米，口内径 0.9 厘米，腹径 3.2 厘米，通高 8.95 厘米

圆瓶形，表面粗糙，瓶身绘有青花朱绘梅石图案，有纸卷盖，瓶底无款识，制作工艺一般。盛药器具。保存基本完好。1958 年入藏。

中华医学会 / 上海中医药大学医史博物馆藏

Porcelain Medicine Bottle

Qing Dynasty

Porcelain

Mouth Outer Diameter 1.5 cm/ Mouth Inner Diameter 0.9 cm/ Belly Diameter 3.2 cm/ Height 8.95 cm

This round bottle with average workmanship has a rough surface. Its body is decorated with a blue-and-white motifs of plum branches and stones. It has a lid made by rolled paper, and a bottom without inscription. The basically well-preserved bottle was used for storing medicine. It was collected in 1958.

Preserved in Chinese Medical Association/ Museum of Chinese Medicine, Shanghai University of Traditional Chinese Medicine

瓷药瓶

清

瓷质

宽 2.2 厘米，通高 6.1 厘米，厚 2 厘米

方形，瓷瓶表面有残疵坑点，瓶身绘有童子戏草青花图案，配有木塞为盖，瓶底无款识，制作工艺一般。盛药器具。保存基本完好，瓶肩有残。

中华医学会 / 上海中医药大学医史博物馆藏

Porcelain Medicine Bottle

Qing Dynasty

Porcelain

Width 2.2 cm/ Height 6.1 cm/ Thickness 2 cm

This cubic bottle, with average workmanship, has a wood lid and a bottom without inscription. There are pit defects on the surface. On the body of the bottle are painted blue-and-white motifs of a boy playing with grass. It is basically well-preserved, except the damaged shoulder. It was used for storing medicine.

Preserved in Chinese Medical Association/ Museum of Chinese Medicine, Shanghai University of Traditional Chinese Medicine

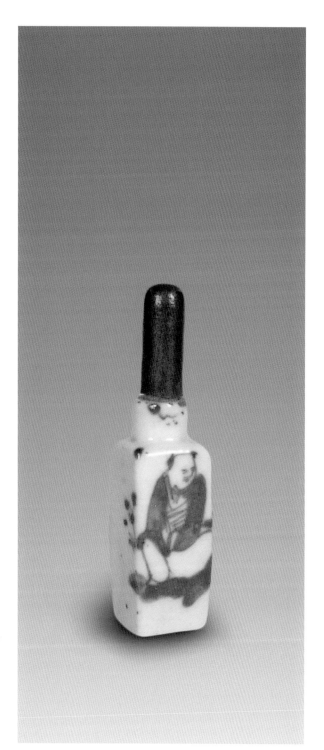

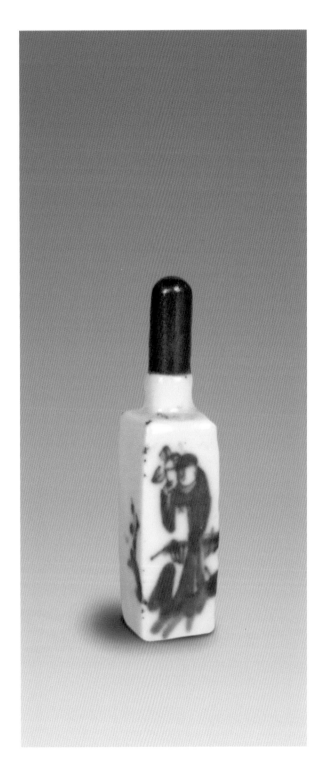

瓷药瓶

清

瓷质

口外径 1.3 厘米，宽 2.1 厘米，通高 6.5 厘米

方形，瓷瓶表面有残疵坑点，瓶身绘有人物采芝青花图案，配有木塞为盖，瓶底无款识，制作工艺一般。盛药器具。保存基本完好。1958 年入藏。

中华医学会 / 上海中医药大学医史博物馆藏

Porcelain Medicine Bottle

Qing Dynasty

Porcelain

Mouth Outer Diameter 1.3 cm/ Width 2.1 cm/ Height 6.5 cm

This cubic bottle, made with average workmanship, has pit defects on its surface. On its body is painted a blue-and-white motif of a figure picking ganoderma lucidum. It has a wood lid and a bottom without inscription. It was used for storing medicine and is basically well preserved. It was collected in 1958.

Preserved in Chinese Medical Association/ Museum of Chinese Medicine, Shanghai University of Traditional Chinese Medicine

瓷药瓶

清

瓷质

口外径 1 厘米，宽 2.1 厘米，通高 6.25 厘米

方形，瓷瓶表面有残疵坑点，瓶身绘有童子青花

图案，配有木塞为盖，瓶底无款识，制作工艺一

般。盛药器具。保存基本完好。1958 年入藏。

中华医学会 / 上海中医药大学医史博物馆藏

Porcelain Medicine Bottle

Qing Dynasty

Porcelain

Mouth Outer Diameter 1cm/ Width 2.1 cm/ Height 6.25 cm

This cubic bottle, made with average workmanship, has

pit defects on its surface and no inscription on its bottom.

On its body is painted a blue-and-white kid motif. The

bottle, with a wooden lid, was used for storing medicine.

It is basically well preserved and was collected in 1958.

Preserved in Chinese Medical Association/ Museum of

Chinese Medicine, Shanghai University of Traditional

Chinese Medicine

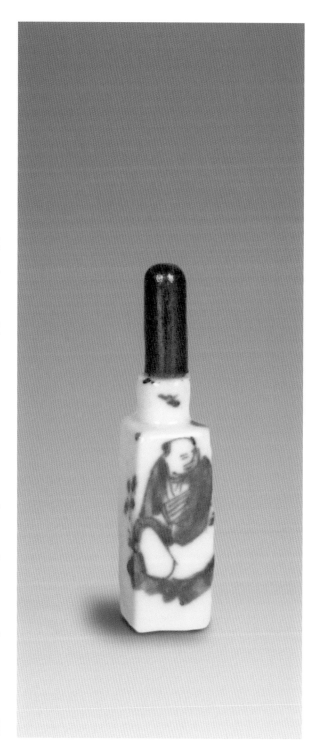

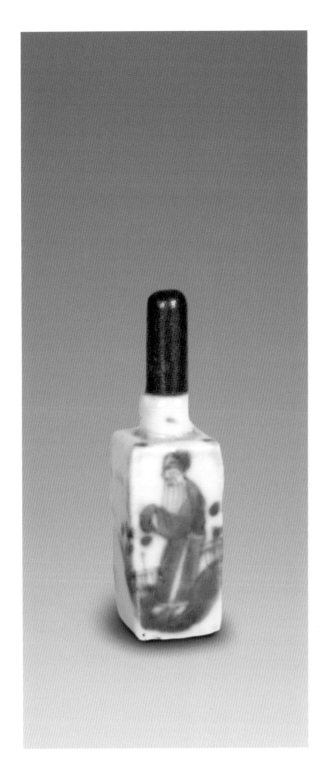

瓷药瓶

清

瓷质

口外径 1.4 厘米，宽 2.5 厘米，通高 6.2 厘米

方形，瓷瓶表面有残疵坑点，瓶身绘有长须老翁青花图案，配有木塞为盖，瓶底无款识，制作工艺一般。盛药器具。保存基本完好。1958 年入藏。

中华医学会 / 上海中医药大学医史博物馆藏

Porcelain Medicine Bottle

Qing Dynasty

Porcelain

Mouth Outer Diameter 1.4 cm/ Width 2.5 cm/ Height 6.2 cm

This cubic bottle, made with average workmanship, has pit defects on its surface and no inscription on its bottom. On its body is painted a blue-and-white motif of a long-bearded old man. The bottle, with a wooden lid, was used for storing medicine. It is basically well preserved and was collected in 1958.

Preserved in Chinese Medical Association/ Museum of Chinese Medicine, Shanghai University of Traditional Chinese Medicine

瓷药瓶

清

瓷质

口外径 1.4 厘米，宽 2.3 厘米，通高 5.75 厘米
方形，瓷瓶表面有残疵坑点，瓶身有青花图案，
配有木塞为盖，瓶底无款识，制作工艺一般。盛
药器具。保存基本完好。1958 年入藏。

中华医学会 / 上海中医药大学医史博物馆藏

Porcelain Medicine Bottle

Qing Dynasty

Porcelain

Mouth Outer Diameter 1.4 cm/ Width 2.3 mm/ Height 5.75 cm

This cubic bottle, made with average workmanship, has
pit defects on its surface and no inscription on its bottom.
On its body are painted blue-and-white motifs. The bottle,
with a wooden lid, was used for storing medicine. It is
basically well preserved and was collected in 1958.

Preserved in Chinese Medical Association/ Museum of
Chinese Medicine, Shanghai University of Traditional
Chinese Medicine

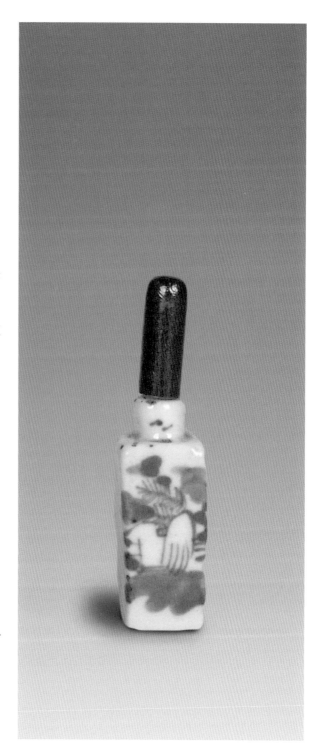

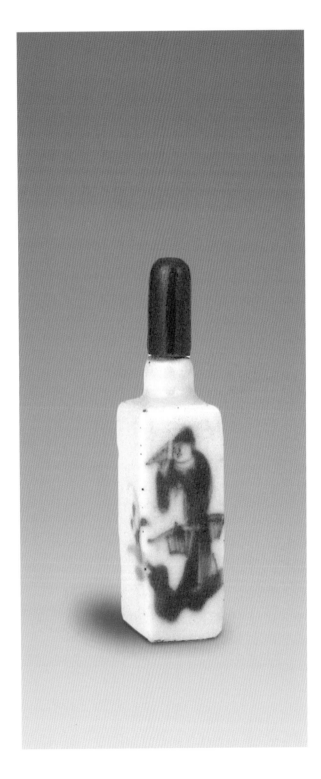

瓷药瓶

清

瓷质

口径 1.3 厘米，宽 2.2 厘米，高 6.5 厘米

方形，表面绘有青花人物故事图，直口，翻沿，平底，小巧玲珑，工艺精良。盛药器具。保存基本完好。1958 年入藏。

中华医学会 / 上海中医药大学医史博物馆藏

Porcelain Medicine Bottle

Qing Dynasty

Porcelain

Mouth Diameter 1.3 cm/ Width 2.2 cm/ Height 6.5 cm

The cubic bottle has a straight mouth with an everted rim and a flat bottom. On its body are painted motifs of a human figure and landscape. The bottle is small and exquisite with delicate workmanship. It was basically well preserved and was collected in 1958.

Preserved in Chinese Medical Association/ Museum of Chinese Medicine, Shanghai University of Traditional Chinese Medicine

青花百寿药瓶

清

瓷质

通高 16.5 厘米

敞口，长颈，溜肩，直腹。上有不同写法的"寿"字。有盖，盖上亦书"寿"字。

广东中医药博物馆藏

Blue-and-white Medicine Bottle with a Hundred "Shou" (Longevity)

Qing Dynasty

Porcelain

Height 16.5 cm

This bottle has a flared mouth, a lid, a long neck, a sloping shoulder, a straight belly. The Chinese character "Shou" (longevity) is written in different calligraphic styles all over the bottle body, and a "Shou" is on its lid.

Preserved in Guangdong Chinese Medicine Museum

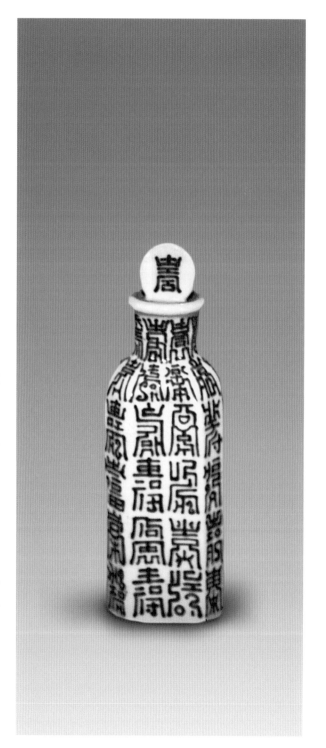

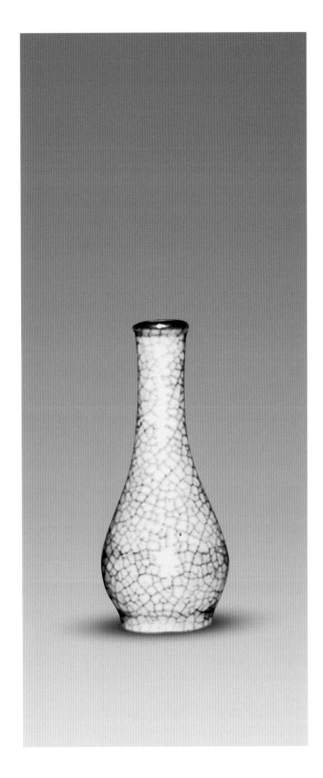

冰碴纹小药瓶

清

瓷质

口径 2.2 厘米，底径 3 厘米，通高 10 厘米，重 50 克

小喇叭口，长颈，垂腹，圈足，表面饰浅灰色冰碴纹。贮药器具。完整无损。

陕西医史博物馆藏

Small Medicine Bottle with Ice Crackles

Qing Dynasty

Porcelain

Mouth Diameter 2.2 cm/ Bottom Diameter 3 cm/ Height 10 cm/ Weight 50 g

The bottle with light grey ice crackles has a flared mouth, a long neck, a droop belly, and a ring foot. It was used for storing medicine and is kept intact.

Preserved in Shaanxi Museum of Medical History

青花药瓶

清

瓷质

口径 8 厘米，底径 8.5 厘米，通高 23 厘米，重 800 克

盘口，颈部有双耳，腹稍直，圈足，表面绘蝴蝶采蜜图。贮药器具。一耳有残。陕西省汉中市公兴大药店征集。

陕西医史博物馆藏

Blue-and-white Medicine Bottle

Qing Dynasty

Porcelain

Mouth Diameter 8 cm/ Bottom Diameter 8.5 cm/ Height 23 cm/ Weight 800 g

This bottle, used to contain medicine, has a dish-shaped mouth, two ears on the shoulder with one damaged, a slightly straight belly, and a ring foot. The bottle is decorated with a motif of butterflies collecting honey. It was collected from the Gongxing Pharmacy, Hanzhong City, Shaanxi Province.

Preserved in Shaanxi Museum of Medical History

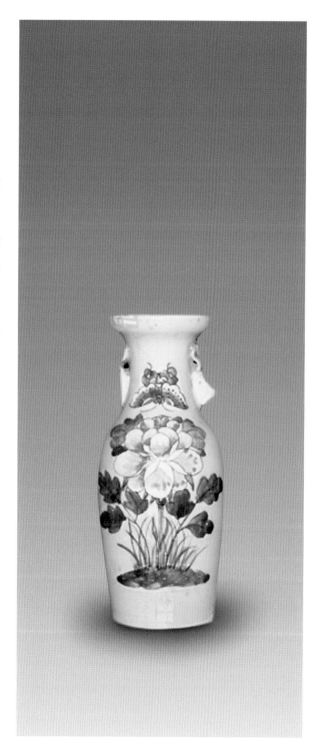

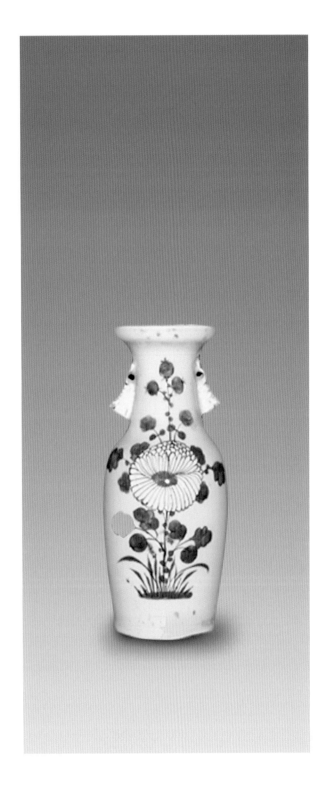

青花药瓶

清

瓷质

口径 8 厘米，底径 8.5 厘米，通高 23 厘米，重 800 克

盘口，颈部有双耳，腹稍直，圈足，表面绘菊花图。贮药器具。完整无损。陕西省汉中市公兴大药店征集。

陕西医史博物馆藏

Blue-and-white Medicine Bottle

Qing Dynasty

Porcelain

Mouth Diameter 8 cm/ Bottom Diameter 8.5 cm/ Height 23 cm/ Weight 800 g

The bottle, used to contain medicine, has a dish-shaped mouth, two ears on the shoulder, a slightly straight belly, and a ring foot. It is decorated with chrysanthemum design. It is kept intact and was collected from Gongxing Pharmacy, Hanzhong City, Shaanxi Province.

Preserved in Shaanxi Museum of Medical History

双耳瓷药瓶

清

瓷质

口径 1.6 厘米，底径 2.6 厘米，高 6.5 厘米，重 50 克

影青，平口，扁腹，平底，颈肩处有双耳，腹部雕有花卉图案。贮药器具。完整无损。2001 年 9 月入藏，陕西省西安市古玩市场征集。

陕西医史博物馆藏

Porcelain Medicine Bottle with Two Ears

Qing Dynasty

Porcelain

Mouth Diameter 1.6 cm/ Bottom Diameter 2.6 cm/ Height 6.5 cm/ Weight 50 g

The misty-blue bottle, used to contain medicine, has a flat mouth, an oblate belly, a flat bottom, and two ears on the neck. On the belly are carved floral designs. It is kept intact and was collected from the Antique Market in Xi'an, Shaanxi Province, in September 2001.

Preserved in Shaanxi Museum of Medical History

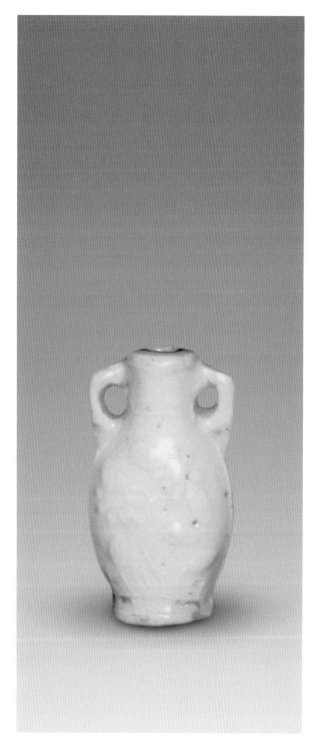

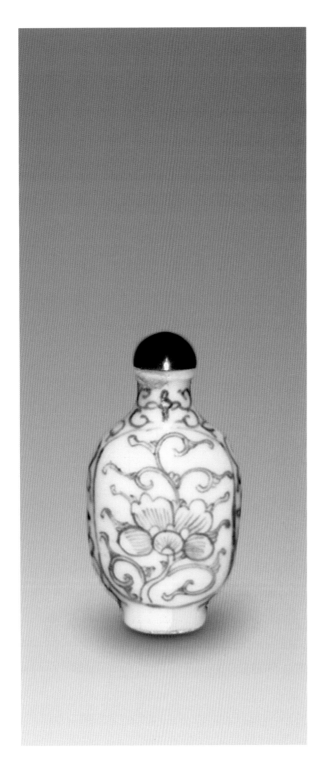

瓷药瓶

清

瓷质

口径 1.5 厘米，底径 2.5 厘米 ×1.9 厘米，带盖
高 8.1 厘米，高 7.1 厘米，重 39 克

平口，扁腹，圈足，通体为缠枝花卉纹，带一红
色小盖。贮药器具。完整无损。2001 年 9 月入藏，
陕西省西安市古玩市场征集。

陕西医史博物馆藏

Porcelain Medicine Bottle

Qing Dynasty

Porcelain

Mouth Diameter 1.5 cm/ Bottom Diameter 2.5 cm×1.9 cm/
Height (with a lid) 8.1 cm/ Height 7.1 cm/ Weight 39 g

This bottle, used to contain medicine, has a flat mouth, an
oblate belly, a ring foot, and a small red lid. The whole
body is decorated with interlocking floral designs. It is
kept intact and was collected from the Antique Market in
Xi'an, Shaanxi Province, in September 2001.

Preserved in Shaanxi Museum of Medical History

瓷药瓶

清

瓷质

口径 3.5 厘米，底径 3.8 厘米，通高 10 厘米，
重 100 克

喇叭口，长颈，扁腹，圈足。贮药器具。完整无损。

陕西医史博物馆藏

Porcelain Medicine Bottle

Qing Dynasty

Porcelain

Mouth Diameter 3.5 cm/ Bottom Diameter 3.8 cm/
Height 10 cm/ Weight 100 g

The bottle, used to contain medicine, has a flared mouth,
a long neck, an oblate belly, and a ring foot. It remains
intact.

Preserved in Shaanxi Museum of Medical History

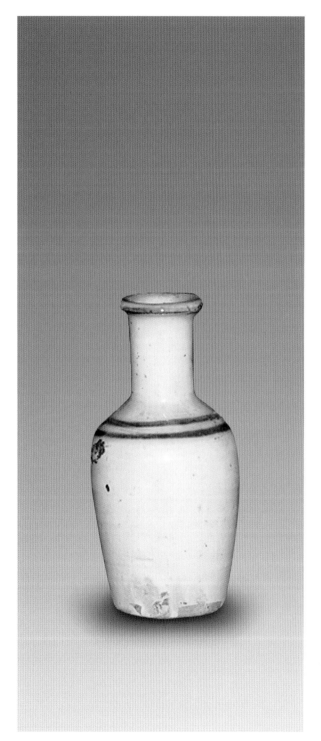

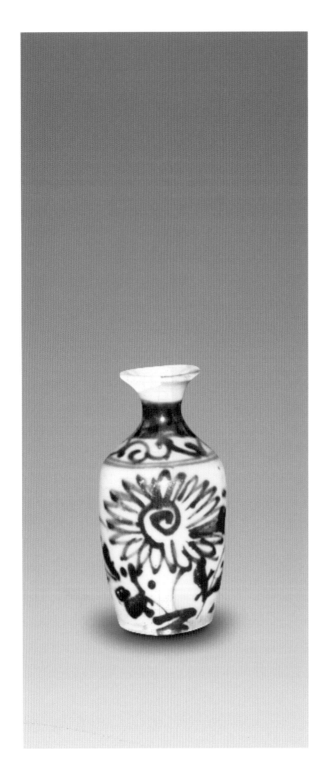

瓷药瓶

清

瓷质

口径 3.5 厘米，底径 4 厘米，通高 10 厘米，重 100 克

喇叭口，折肩，直腹，圈足，表面绘菊花图。贮药器具。口沿有修补。

陕西医史博物馆藏

Porcelain Medicine Bottle

Qing Dynasty

Porcelain

Mouth Diameter 3.5 cm/ Bottom Diameter 4 cm/ Height 10 cm/ Weight 100 g

This bottle has a flared mouth, an angular shoulder, a straight belly, and a ring foot. It is decorated with chrysanthemum designs. It was used to contain medicine. Its mouth rim has been restored.

Preserved in Shaanxi Museum of Medical History

瓷药瓶

清

瓷质

口径 5 厘米，底径 5.4 厘米，通高 17 厘米，重 600 克

喇叭口，圆腹，圈足，表面饰双 "喜" 缠枝图，标签名为 "神效疟疾丸"。医药器具。口沿有修补。

陕西医史博物馆藏

Porcelain Medicine Bottle

Qing Dynasty

Porcelain

Mouth Diameter 5 cm/ Bottom Diameter 5.4 cm/ Height 17 cm/ Weight 600 g

This medicine bottle has a flared mouth, a rounded belly, and a ring foot. The bottle is covered with designs of interlocking branches together with two Chinese characters "Xi" (happiness). To the bottle is attached a label of the name of the medicine "Shen Xiao Nüe Ji Wan". Its mouth rim has been restored.

Preserved in Shaanxi Museum of Medical History

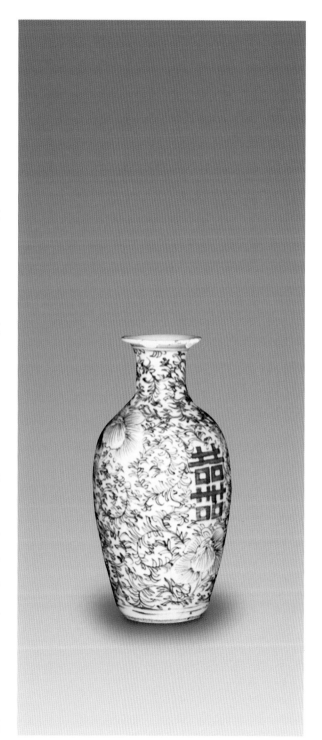

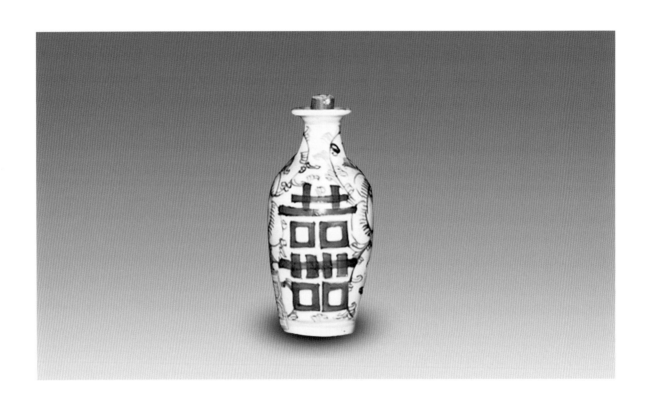

瓷药瓶

清

瓷质

口径 3 厘米，底径 3.8 厘米，通高 11.5 厘米，
重 150 克

喇叭口，圆肩，斜腹，圈足，表面饰缠枝双"喜"
图。贮药器具。完整无损。

陕西医史博物馆藏

Porcelain Medicine Bottle

Qing Dynasty

Porcelain

Mouth Diameter 3 cm/ Bottom Diameter 3.8 cm/ Height
11.5 cm/ Weight 150 g

This bottle has a flared mouth, a rounded shoulder, an
oblique belly, and a ring foot. It is decorated with designs
of interlocking branches together with two Chinese
characters "Xi" (happiness). It is kept intact and was
used for storing medicine.

Preserved in Shaanxi Museum of Medical History

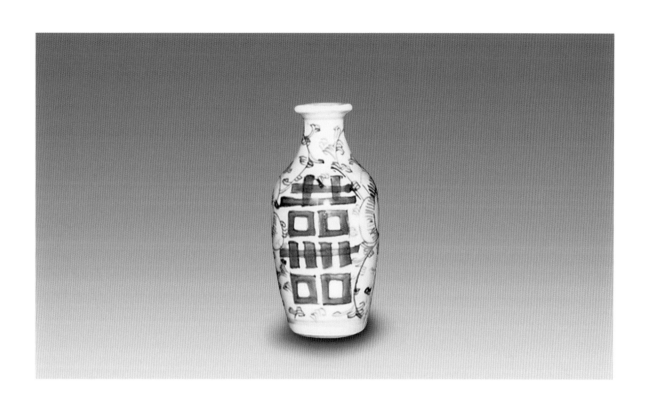

瓷药瓶

清

瓷质

口径 3 厘米，底径 3.8 厘米，通高 11.5 厘米，
重 150 克

喇叭口，斜腹，圈足，表面饰双"喜"缠枝图。
贮药器物。完整无损。

陕西医史博物馆藏

Porcelain Medicine Bottle

Qing Dynasty

Porcelain

Mouth Diameter 3 cm/ Bottom Diameter 3.8 cm/ Height
11.5 cm/ Weight 150 g

This bottle has a flared mouth, an oblique belly, and a ring
foot. It is decorated with designs of interlocking branches
together with two Chinese characters "Xi" (happiness). It
is kept intact and was used for storing medicine.

Preserved in Shaanxi Museum of Medical History

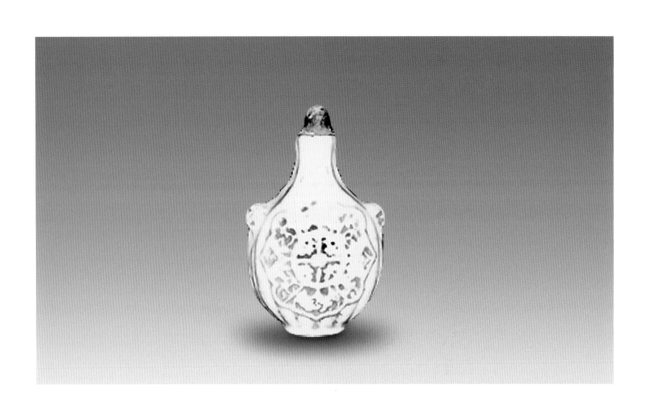

小瓷药瓶

清

瓷质

口径 1 厘米，底径 1.7 厘米，通高 5.5 厘米，重 50 克

直口，双耳，扁腹，圈足，白瓷，腹部雕刻瓜棱纹，上有"寿"字。贮药器具。完整无损。

陕西医史博物馆藏

Small Porcelain Medicine Bottle

Qing Dynasty

Porcelain

Mouth Diameter 1 cm/ Bottom Diameter 1.7 cm/ Height 5.5 cm/ Weight 50 g

This bottle has a straight mouth, two ears, an oblate belly, and a ring foot. It is coated with white glaze. On its belly are carved melon-ribbed patterns as well as a Chinese character "Shou" (longevity). It is kept intact and was used for storing medicine.

Preserved in Shaanxi Museum of Medical History

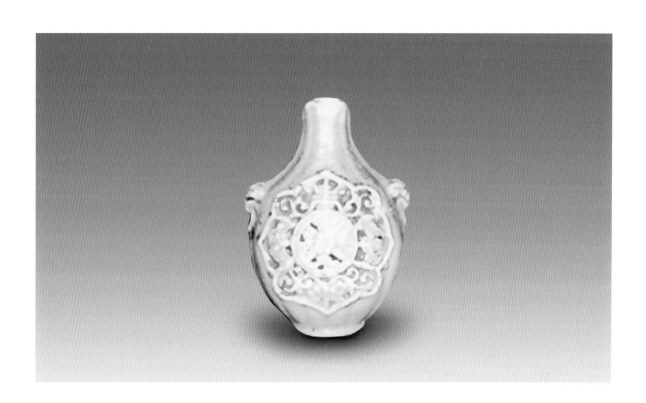

小瓷药瓶

清

瓷质

口径 1 厘米，底径 1.7 厘米，通高 5.5 厘米，重 50 克

直口，双耳，扁腹，圈足，施绿釉，腹部雕刻瓜棱纹，上有"寿"字。贮药器具。口沿小残。

陕西医史博物馆藏

Small Porcelain Medicine Bottle

Qing Dynasty

Porcelain

Mouth Diameter 1 cm/ Bottom Diameter 1.7 cm/ Height 5.5 cm/ Weight 50 g

This bottle has a straight mouth, two ears, an oblate belly, and a ring foot. It is glazed green with melon ribbed patterns. A Chinese character "Shou" (longevity) can be seen on it. It was used for storing medicine. Its mouth rim is slightly damaged.

Preserved in Shaanxi Museum of Medical History

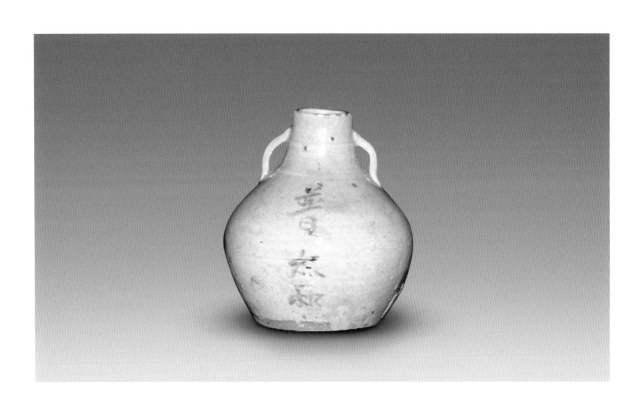

双耳瓷瓶

清

瓷质

口径 2.7 厘米，底径 5.4 厘米，通高 9 厘米，重 200 克

直口，双贯耳，鼓腹，圈足，粗瓷，腹有"普太和"字。贮药器具。完整无损。陕西省汉中市公兴大药店征集。

陕西医史博物馆藏

Porcelain Bottle with Two Ears

Qing Dynasty

Porcelain

Mouth Diameter 2.7 cm/ Bottom Diameter 5.4 cm/ Height 9 cm/ Weight 200 g

This coarse porcelain bottle, used to contain medicine, has a straight mouth, two tube-shaped ears, a drum-like belly, and a ring foot. On its gritty belly can be seen the name of the pharmacy "Pu Tai He". It is kept intact. It was collected from Gongxing Pharmacy, Hanzhong City, Shaanxi Province.

Preserved in Shaanxi Museum of Medical History

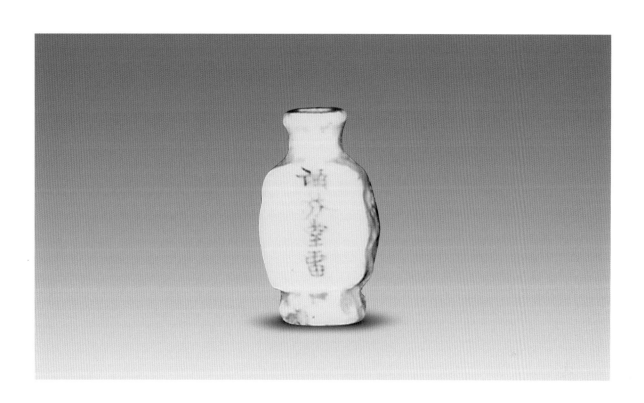

小瓷药瓶

清

瓷质

口径 1.5 厘米，底径 2 厘米，通高 5 厘米，重 50 克

小喇叭口，扁腹，腹稍折，平底，腹有 "诵芬堂雷" 字样。贮药器具。完整无损。江苏省苏州市雷允上中药店专用贮药瓶。

陕西医史博物馆藏

Small Porcelain Medicine Bottle

Qing Dynasty

Porcelain

Mouth Diameter 1.5 cm/ Bottom Diameter 2 cm/ Height 5 cm/ Weight 50 g

This bottle has a small flared mouth, an oblate belly, and a flat bottom. On its belly are written the name of the pharmacy "Song Fen Tang Lei" (Song Fen Tang indicates the name of a drugstore and Lei is the surname of the storekeeper). It is kept intact. It was a medicine container used at Leiyunshang Chinese Medicinal Herbs Store in Suzhou, Jiangsu Province.

Preserved in Shaanxi Museum of Medical History

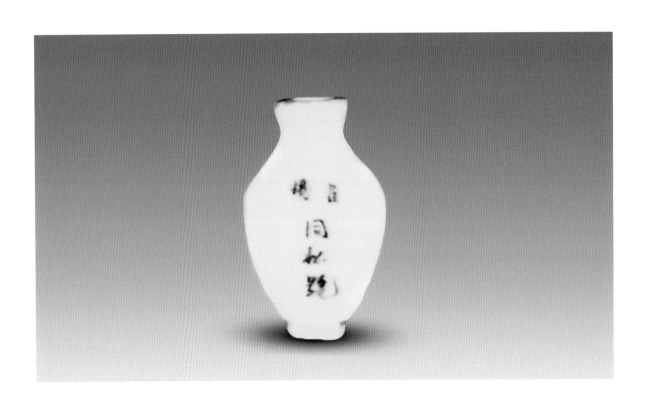

小瓷药瓶

清

瓷质

口径 1.5 厘米，底径 1.2 厘米，通高 5 厘米，重 50 克

Small Porcelain Medicine Bottle

Qing Dynasty

Porcelain

Mouth Diameter 1.5 cm/ Bottom Diameter 1.2 cm/ Height 5 cm/ Weight 50 g

小喇叭口，斜扁腹，圈足，上有"扬淮同松号"字样。贮药器具。完整无损。江苏省苏州市雷允上中药店专用贮药瓶。

陕西医史博物馆藏

This bottle has a small flared mouth, an oblate and oblique belly, and a ring foot. On its belly are written the name of the pharmacy "Yang Huai Tong Song Hao". It is kept intact. It was a medicine container used at Leiyunshang Chinese Medicinal Herbs Store in Suzhou, Jiangsu Province.

Preserved in Shaanxi Museum of Medical History

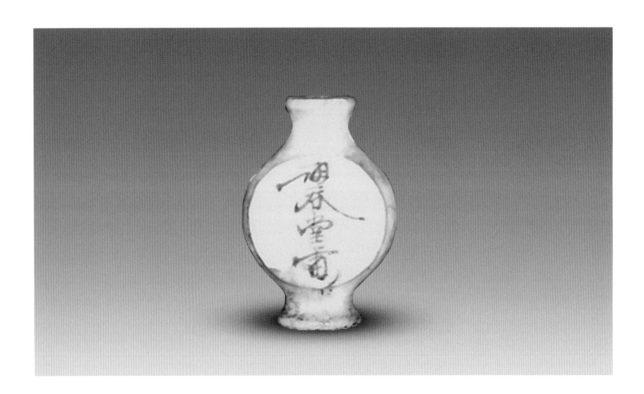

小瓷药瓶

清

瓷质

口径 2 厘米，底径 2.5 厘米，通高 6.5 厘米，重 50 克

Small Porcelain Medicine Bottle

Qing Dynasty

Porcelain

Mouth Diameter 2 cm/ Bottom Diameter 2.5 cm/ Height 6.5 cm/ Weight 50 g

小喇叭口，扁圆腹，平底，腹有"诵芬堂雷"
字样。贮药器具。完整无损。江苏省苏州市
雷允上中药店专用贮药瓶。

陕西医史博物馆藏

This bottle has a small flared mouth, an oblate belly, and a flat bottom. On its belly are written four Chinese characters "Song Fen Tang Lei" (Song Fen Tang indicates the name of a drugstore and Lei is the surname of the storekeeper). It is kept intact. And it was a medicine container used at Leiyunshang Chinese Medicinal Herbs Store in Suzhou, Jiangsu Province.

Preserved in Shaanxi Museum of Medical History

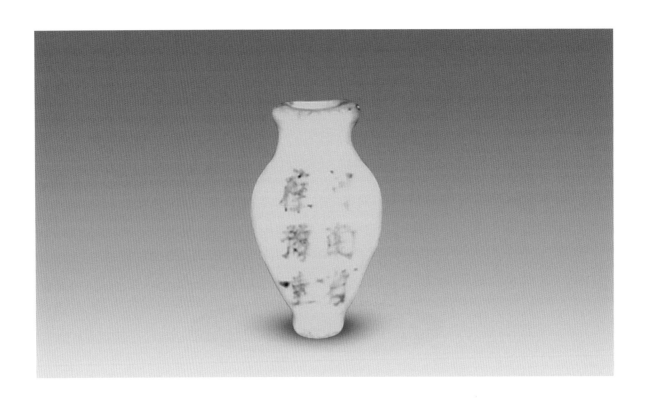

小药瓶

清

瓷质

口径 1.5 厘米，底径 0.9 厘米，高 4 厘米，重 12 克

Small Medicine Bottle

Qing Dynasty

Porcelain

Mouth Diameter 1.5 cm/ Bottom Diameter 0.9 cm/ Height 4 cm/ Weight 12 g

平口沿,扁腹,平底,腹部有"河南省葆豫堂",另一面为"痧气丹"字样。贮药器具。完整无损。2001年9月入藏，陕西省西安市古玩市场征集。

陕西医史博物馆藏

This bottle, used to contain medicine, has a flat mouth rim, an oblate belly, and a flat bottom. On one side of its belly is written the name of the pharmacy "He Nan Sheng Bao Yu Tang" with the name of the medicine "Sha Qi Dan" on the other side. It is kept intact and was collected from the Antique Market in Xi'an, Shaanxi Province, in September 2001.

Preserved in Shaanxi Museum of Medical History

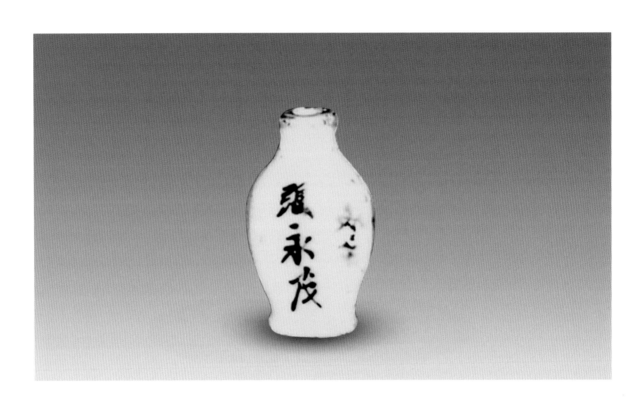

小瓷药瓶

清

瓷质

口径 1 厘米，底径 1.5 厘米，高 3.8 厘米，重 12 克

Small Porcelain Medicine Bottle

Qing Dynasty

Porcelain

Mouth Diameter 1 cm/ Bottom Diameter 1.5 cm/ Height 3.8 cm/ Weight 12 g

平口沿，扁圆腹，浅圈足，腹部两面有"张永茂"字样。贮药器具。保存完整。2001年9月入藏，陕西省西安市古玩市场征集。

陕西医史博物馆藏

This bottle, used to contain medicine, has a flat mouth rim, an oblate belly, and a shallow ring foot. On the two sides of its belly is written the name of the pharmacy "Zhang Yong Mao". It is kept intact and was collected from the Antique Market in Xi'an, Shaanxi Province, in September 2001.

Preserved in Shaanxi Museum of Medical History

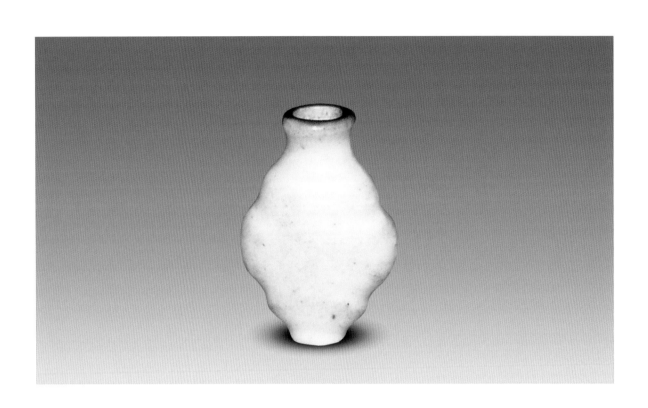

瓷药瓶

清

瓷质

口径 1.4 厘米，底径 1 厘米，高 4.5 厘米，重 16 克

平口沿，扁腹，平底，青瓷，素面。贮药器具。保存完整。2001 年 9 月入藏，陕西省西安市古玩市场征集。

陕西医史博物馆藏

Porcelain Medicine Bottle

Qing Dynasty

Porcelain

Mouth Diameter 1.4 cm/ Bottom Diameter 1 cm/ Height 4.5 cm/ Weight 16 g

This bottle, with a flat mouth rim, an oblate belly and a flat bottom, is coated with celadon glaze. It was a plain drug container with no decoration. It is kept intact and was collected from the Antique Market in Xi'an City, Shaanxi Province, in September 2001.

Preserved in Shaanxi Museum of Medical History

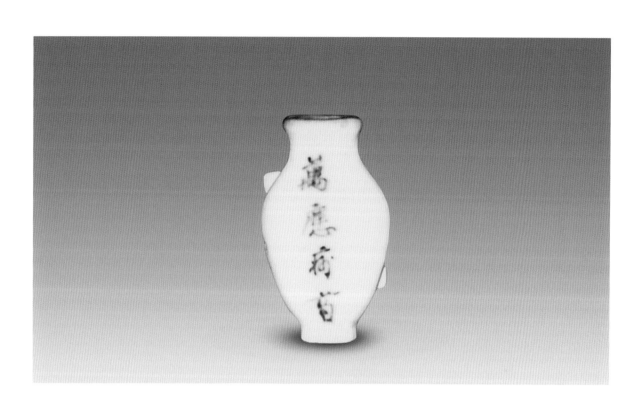

小瓷药瓶

清

瓷质

口径 1.7 厘米，底径 0.8 厘米，通高 5 厘米，重 50 克

小喇叭口，扁腹，圈足，腹上有"景镇种德堂""万应痧药"名。贮药器具。完整无损。

陕西医史博物馆藏

Small Porcelain Medicine Bottle

Qing Dynasty

Porcelain

Mouth Diameter 1.7 cm/ Bottom Diameter 0.8 cm/ Height 5 cm/ Weight 50 g

The bottle, used to contain medicine, has a small flared mouth, an oblate belly, and a ring foot. On one side of its belly is written the name of the pharmacy "Jing Zhen Zhong De Tang" with the name of the medicine "Wan Ying Sha Yao" on the other side. It is kept intact.

Preserved in Shaanxi Museum of Medical History

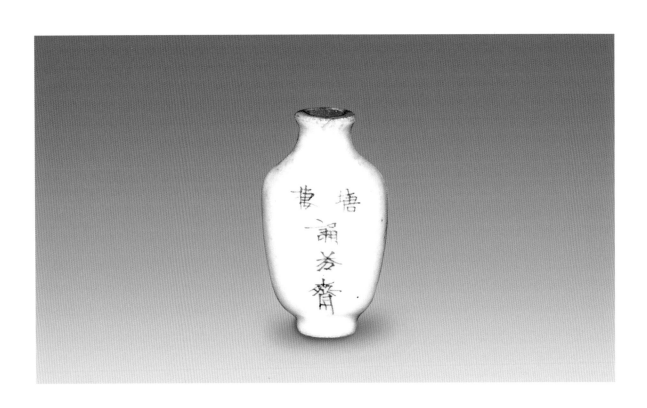

瓷药瓶

清

瓷质

口径1.4厘米,底径1.4厘米×1.2厘米,高5.3厘米,重19克

平口沿，扁腹，圈足，腹一面有"姚制隐壶处卧龙丹"，一面有"塘曹诵芬斋"。贮药器具。口沿略残。2001年9月入藏，陕西省西安市古玩市场征集。

陕西医史博物馆藏

Porcelain Medicine Bottle

Qing Dynasty

Porcelain

Mouth Diameter 1.4 cm/ Bottom Diameter 1.4 cm×1.2 cm/ Height 5.3 cm/ Weight 19 g

This bottle, used to contain medicine, has a flat mouth rim, which is slightly damaged, an oblate belly, and a ring foot. On one side of its belly is written the name of the medicine "Yao Zhi Yin Hu Chu Wo Long Dan" with the name of the pharmacy "Tang Cao Song Fen Zhai" on the other side. It was collected from the Antique Market in Xi'an, Shaanxi Province, in September 2001.

Preserved in Shaanxi Museum of Medical History

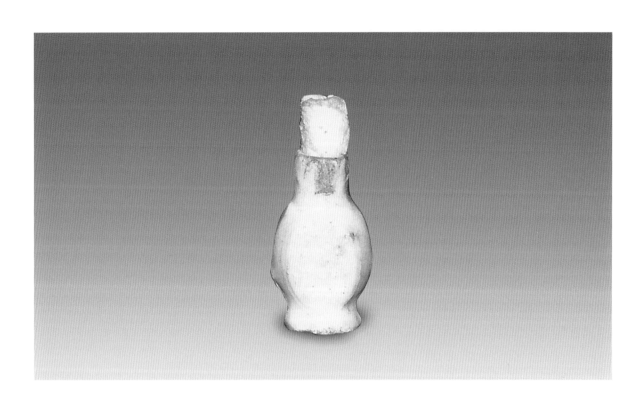

瓷药瓶

清

瓷质

口径 1.1 厘米，底径 1.6 厘米，高 4 厘米，重 15 克

直口，扁腹，平底，青瓷，瓶内有药。贮药器具。口、底略残。2001 年 9 月入藏，陕西省西安市古玩市场征集。

陕西医史博物馆藏

Porcelain Medicine Bottle

Qing Dynasty

Porcelain

Mouth Diameter 1.1 cm/ Bottom Diameter 1.6 cm/ Height 4 cm/ Weight 15 g

This bottle, used to contain medicine, has a straight mouth, an oblate belly, and a flat bottom. It is coated with celadon glaze. There is some medicine in the bottle. The mouth and bottom of the bottle are broken slightly. It was collected from the Antique Market in Xi'an, Shaanxi Province, in September 2001.

Preserved in Shaanxi Museum of Medical History

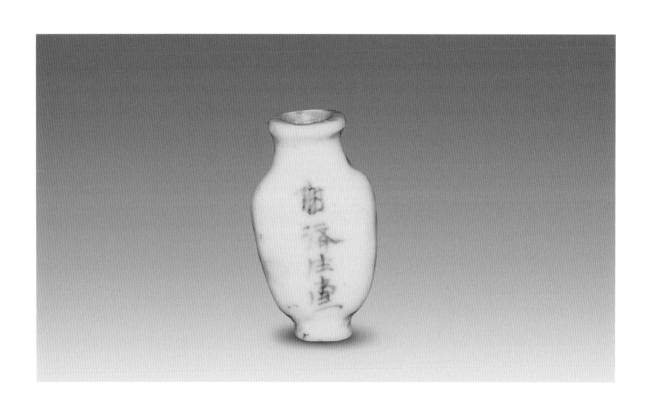

瓷药瓶

清

瓷质

口径 1.4 厘米，底径 1 厘米，高 4.4 厘米，重
10 克

平口沿，扁腹，浅圈足，腹一面有"卧龙丹"，
另一面有"谢济生堂"字样。贮药器具。保存完整。
2001 年 9 月入藏，陕西省西安市古玩市场征集。

陕西医史博物馆藏

Porcelain Medicine Bottle

Qing Dynasty

Porcelain

Mouth Diameter 1.4 cm/ Bottom Diameter 1 cm/ Height
4.4 cm/ Weight 10 g

This bottle, used to contain medicine, has a flat mouth rim,
an oblate belly, and a shallow ring foot. On one side of its
belly is written the name of the medicine "Wo Long Dan"
with the name of the pharmacy "Xie Ji Sheng Tang" on
the other side. It is kept intact and was collected from the
Antique Market in Xi'an, Shaanxi Province, in September
2001.

Preserved in Shaanxi Museum of Medical History

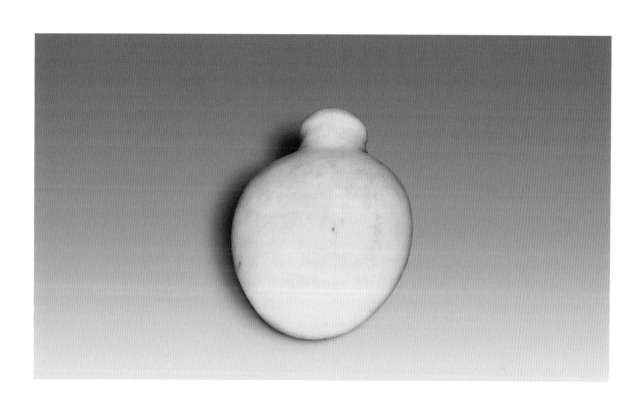

瓷药瓶

清

瓷质

口径 1.2 厘米，高 4.7 厘米，重 16 克

直口，椭圆腹、底，腹中有一黑点，口沿施黄釉。

贮药器具。保存完整。2001 年 9 月入藏，陕西
省西安市古玩市场征集。

陕西医史博物馆藏

Porcelain Medicine Bottle

Qing Dynasty

Porcelain

Mouth Diameter 1.2 cm/ Height 4.7 cm/ Weight 16 g

This bottle has a straight mouth, an oval belly and bottom,
a black spot inside of the belly, and a yellow-glazed
mouth rim. This well-preserved medicine container was
collected from the Antique Market in Xi'an, Shaanxi
Province, in September 2001.

Preserved in Shaanxi Museum of Medical History

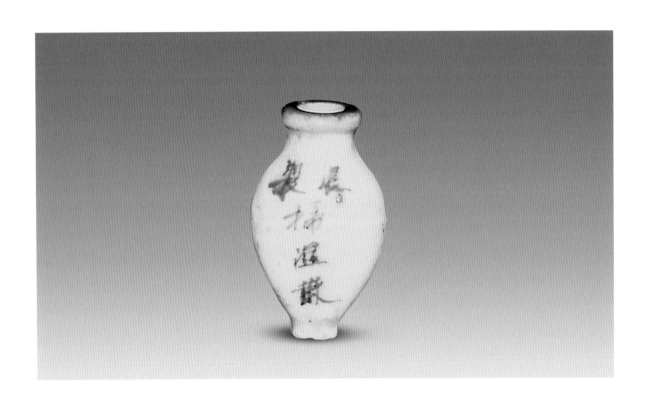

小瓷药瓶

清

瓷质

口径 1.6 厘米，底径 1 厘米，高 5.4 厘米，重 23 克

Small Porcelain Medicine Bottle

Qing Dynasty

Porcelain

Mouth Diameter 1.6 cm/ Bottom Diameter 1 cm/ Height 5.4 cm/ Weight 23 g

平口沿，口沿施黄釉，束颈，溜肩，扁腹，
小平底，腹部一面有"苏城吴署前"，另一
面为"张制扫湿散"字样。药具。2001 年 9 月
入藏，陕西省西安市古玩市场征集。

陕西医史博物馆藏

This bottle has a yellow glazed flat mouth rim,
a contracted neck, a sloping shoulder, an oblate
belly，and a flat bottom. Its belly is inscribed with
the address of the pharmacy in Chinese characters
"Su Cheng Wu Shu Qian" on one side and the name
of the drug "Zhang Zhi Sao Shi San" on the other
side. This medicine container was collected from
the Antique Market in Xi'an, Shaanxi Province, in
September 2001.

Preserved in Shaanxi Museum of Medical History

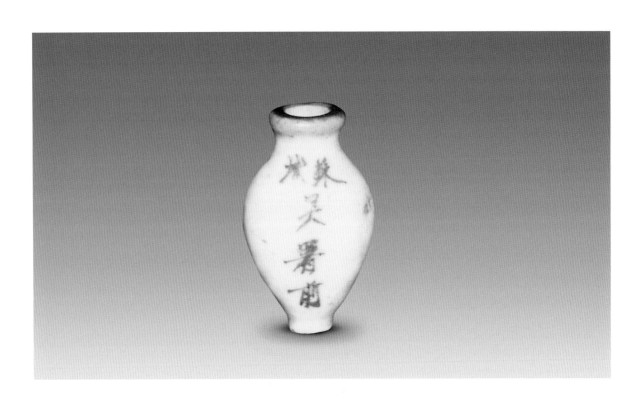

小瓷药瓶

清

瓷质

口径 1.7 厘米，底径 1 厘米，高 5.3 厘米，重 23 克

Small Porcelain Medicine Bottle

Qing Dynasty

Porcelain

Mouth Diameter 1.7 cm/ Bottom Diameter 1 cm/ Height 5.3 cm/ Weight 23 g

平口沿，口沿施黄釉，短颈，扁腹，小平底，腹部一面有"苏城吴署前"，另一面为"张制扫湿散"。贮药器具。完整无损。2002 年入藏，陕西省咸阳市征集。

陕西医史博物馆藏

This bottle has a yellow glazed flat mouth rim, a short neck, an oblate belly, and a small flat bottom. Its belly is inscribed with the address of the pharmacy in Chinese characters "Su Cheng Wu Shu Qian" on one side and the name of the drug "Zhang Zhi Sao Shi San" on the other side. This well-preserved medicine container was collected from Xianyang City, Shaanxi Province, in 2002.

Preserved in Shaanxi Museum of Medical History

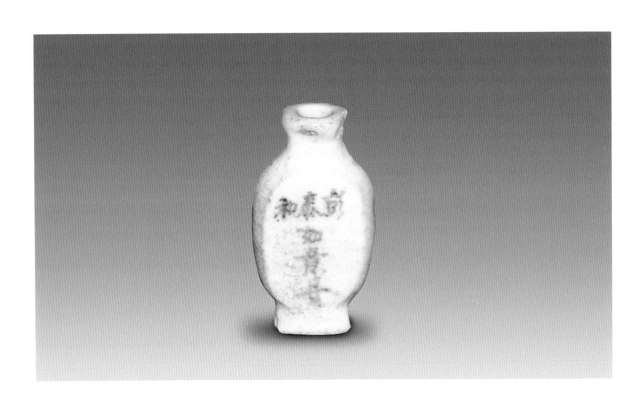

小瓷药瓶

清

瓷质

口径 1.8 厘米，底径 1.8 厘米 ×1.4 厘米，高 5.1 厘米，重 19 克

Small Porcelain Medicine Bottle

Qing Dynasty

Porcelain

Mouth Diameter 1.8 cm/ Bottom Diameter 1.8 cm × 1.4 cm/ Height 5.1 cm/ Weight 19g

平口沿，短颈，扁腹，浅圈足，腹部有"彭
泰和如意丹"字样。药具。口沿残。2001 年
9 月入藏，陕西省西安市古玩市场征集。

陕西医史博物馆藏

The bottle has a flat mouth rim, a short neck, an
oblate belly, and a shallow ring foot. Its belly
is inscribed with the name of the drug and the
pharmacy in Chinese characters "Peng Tai He Ru Yi
Dan". This medical utensil is slightly damaged on the
mouth rim. It was collected from the Antique Market
in Xi'an, Shaanxi Province, in September 2001.

Preserved in Shaanxi Museum of Medical History

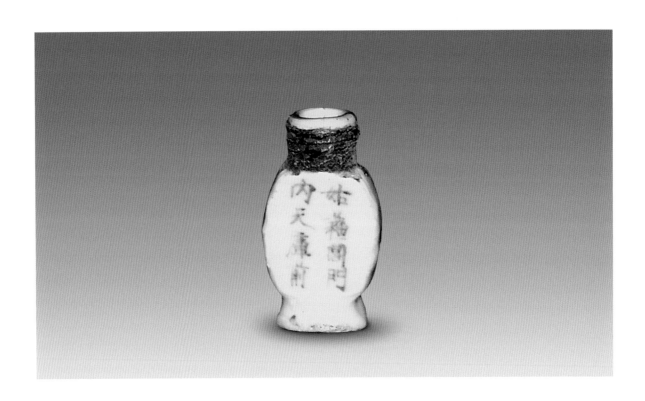

小瓷药瓶

清

瓷质

口径 1.7 厘米，底径 2.4 厘米 ×2 厘米，高 5.5 厘米，重 32 克

Small Porcelain Medicine Bottle

Qing Dynasty

Porcelain

Mouth Diameter 1.7 cm/ Bottom Diameter 2.4 cm ×2 cm/ Height 5.5 cm/ Weight 32 g

直口，扁腹，平底，腹部一面有"诵芬堂雷"，另一面为"姑苏阊门内天库前"字样。贮药器具。口沿有残。2001 年 9 月入藏，陕西省西安市古玩市场征集。

陕西医史博物馆藏

The bottle has a straight mouth, an oblate belly, and a flat bottom. Its belly is inscribed with the name of the pharmacy in Chinese characters "Song Fen Tang Lei" on one side and the address of the pharmacy "Gu Su Lü Men Nei Tian Ku Qian" on the other side. This medical utensil is slightly damaged on the mouth rim. It was collected from the Antique Market in Xi'an, Shaanxi Province, in September 2001.

Preserved in Shaanxi Museum of Medical History

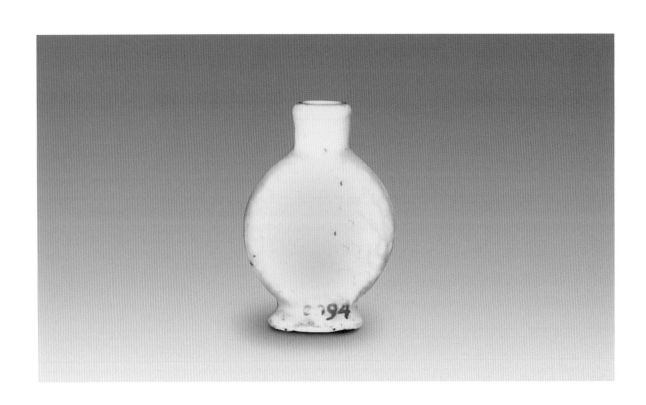

小瓷药瓶

清

瓷质

口径 1.5 厘米，底径 2.6 厘米，通高 6 厘米，重 50 克

直口，扁腹，平底，腹上有菊花图，豆绿瓷。贮药器具。完整无损。

陕西医史博物馆藏

Small Porcelain Medicine Bottle

Qing Dynasty

Porcelain

Mouth Diameter 1.5 cm/ Bottom Diameter 2.6 cm/ Height 6 cm/ Weight 50 g

This pea green glazed bottle has a straight mouth, an oblate belly, and a flat bottom. On its belly is painted a chrysanthemum design. This medicine container remains intact.

Preserved in Shaanxi Museum of Medical History

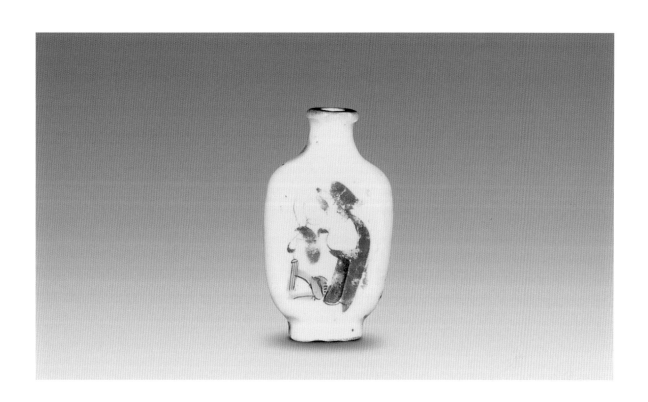

小瓷药瓶

清

瓷质

口径 1.7 厘米，底径 2.3 厘米，通高 7 厘米，重 50 克

直口，扁腹，圈足，腹上有彩色人物图。贮药器具。完整无损。

陕西医史博物馆藏

Small Porcelain Medicine Bottle

Qing Dynasty

Porcelain

Mouth Diameter 1.7 cm/ Bottom Diameter 2.3 cm/ Height 7 cm/ Weight 50 g

This bottle has a straight mouth, an oblate belly, and a ring foot. On its belly is painted coloured figures. This medicine container remains intact.

Preserved in Shaanxi Museum of Medical History

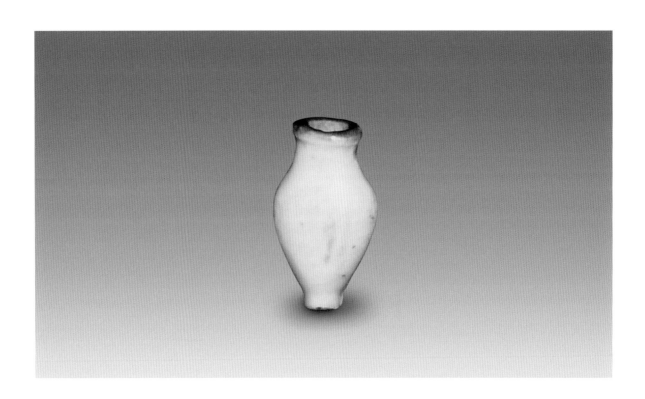

小白药瓶

清

瓷质

口径 1.7 厘米，底径 0.8 厘米，高 3.5 厘米，重 9 克

Small White Medicine Bottle

Qing Dynasty

Porcelain

Mouth Diameter 1.7 cm/ Bottom Diameter 0.8 cm/ Height 3.5 cm/ Weight 9 g

平口沿，束颈，扁腹，浅圈足，青白瓷，素
面。医药器具。完整无损。2001 年 9 月入藏，
陕西省西安市古玩市场征集。

陕西医史博物馆藏

This porcelain bottle has a flat mouth rim, a contacted
neck, an oblate belly, and a shallow ring foot, with no
decoration. This well-preserved medicine container
was collected from the Antique Market in Xi'an,
Shaanxi Province, in September 2001.

Preserved in Shaanxi Museum of Medical History

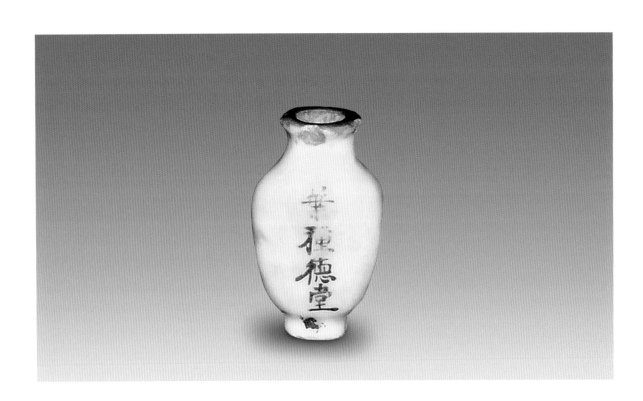

小白瓷药瓶

清

瓷质

口径 1.4 厘米，底径 1 厘米，高 4.4 厘米，重 17 克

Small White Porcelain Medicine Bottle

Qing Dynasty

Porcelain

Mouth Diameter 1.4 cm/ Bottom Diameter 1 cm/ Height 4.4 cm/ Weight 17 g

平口沿，口沿施黄釉，扁腹，浅圈足，腹一
面有"杭城"，另一面为"叶种德堂"字样。
贮药器具。口沿略残。2001 年 9 月入藏，陕
西省西安市古玩市场征集。

陕西医史博物馆藏

This bottle has a yellow-glazed flat mouth rim, an
oblate belly, and a shallow ring foot. Its belly is
inscribed with "Hang Cheng" (Hangzhou City) on
one side and the name of the pharmacy "Ye Zhong
De Tang" on the other side. This medicine container,
with the mouth rim slightly damaged, was collected
from the Antique Market in Xi'an, Shaanxi Province,
in September 2001.

Preserved in Shaanxi Museum of Medical History

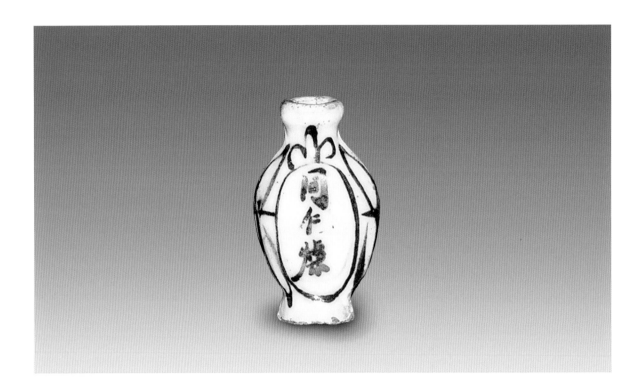

小瓷药瓶

清

瓷质

口径 1.3 厘米，底径 1.7 厘米 ×1.2 厘米，高 5.1 厘米，重 19 克

Small Porcelain Medicine Bottle

Qing Dynasty

Porcelain

Mouth Diameter 1.3 cm/ Bottom Diameter 1.7 cm×1.2 cm/ Height 5.1 cm/ Weight 19 g

平口沿，束颈，扁腹，圈足，腹部有"痧气丹"，
另一面有"同仁□"字样，两侧有蓝色条纹。
贮药器具。保存完整。2001 年 9 月入藏，陕
西省西安市古玩市场征集。

陕西医史博物馆藏

This bottle has a flat mouth rim, a contracted neck,
an oblate belly, and a ring foot. Its belly is inscribed
with the name of the drug "Sha Qi Dan" on one side
and the name of the pharmacy "Tong Ren □ " on the
other side. The two sides of the body arc decorated
with blue stripe patterns. This well-preserved medicine
container was collected from the Antique Market in
Xi'an, Shaanxi Province, in September 2001.

Preserved in Shaanxi Museum of Medical History

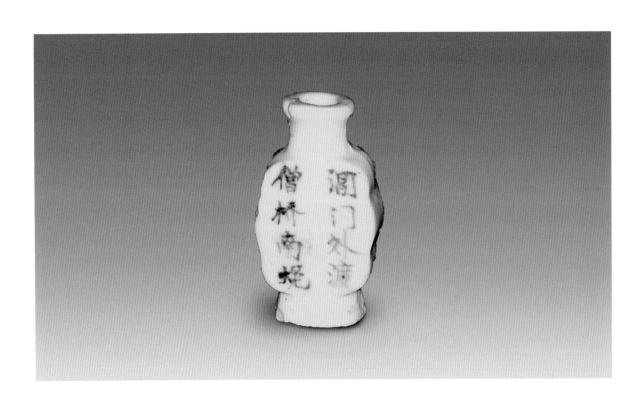

小瓷药瓶

清

瓷质

口径 1.5 厘米，底径 1.9 厘米 ×1.7 厘米，高 5 厘米，重 25 克

Small Porcelain Medicine Bottle

Qing Dynasty

Porcelain

Mouth Diameter 1.5 cm/ Bottom Diameter 1.9 cm × 1.7 cm/ Height 5 cm/ Weight 25 g

平口沿，束颈，扁方形腹，平底，腹部有"阊门外渡，僧桥南堍（堍，释为桥的南头）"及"姑苏沐泰堂"字样。贮药器具。保存完整。2001 年 9 月入藏，陕西省西安市古玩市场征集。

陕西医史博物馆藏

The bottle has a flat mouth rim, a contracted neck, an oblate and square belly, and a flat bottom. On one side of its belly is inscribed the address of the pharmacy in Chinese characters "Lü Men Wai Du, Seng Qiao Nan Tu", while the name of the pharmacy "Gu Su Mu Tai Tang" on the other side. This well-preserved medical utensil was collected from the Antique Market in Xi'an, Shaanxi Province, in September 2001.

Preserved in Shaanxi Museum of Medical History

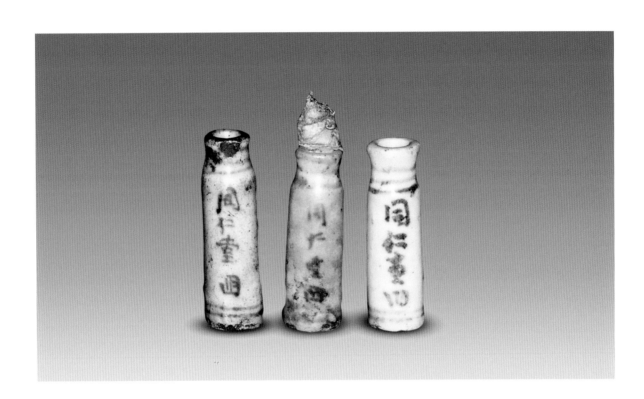

瓷药瓶

清

瓷质

口径 1.4 厘米，底径 1.5 厘米，高 5.1 厘米，重 14 克

Porcelain Medicine Bottles

Qing Dynasty

Porcelain

Mouth Diameter 1.4 cm/ Bottom Diameter 1.5 cm/ Height 5.1 cm/ Weight 14 g

圆柱状，平口沿，直腹，平底，腹部有"同
仁堂四，平安散四"字样，颈部、底部有两
道弦纹。贮药器具。保存完整。2001 年 9 月
入藏，陕西省西安市八仙庵市场征集。

陕西医史博物馆藏

The bottle has a flat mouth rim, a straight belly, a flat
bottom, and a cylindrical body. Its belly is inscribed
with the name of the pharmacy "Tong Ren Tang Si",
and the name of the drug "Ping An San Si". Its neck
and bottom are decorated with two string patterns.
This well-preserved medical utensil was collected
from the Baxian'an Market in Xi'an, Shaanxi
Province, in September 2001.

Preserved in Shaanxi Museum of Medical History

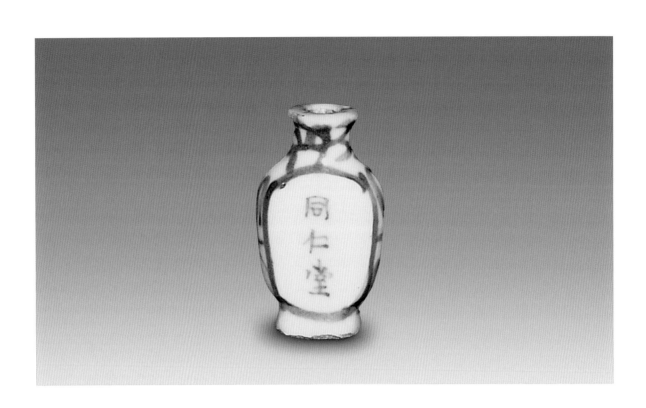

同仁堂药瓶

清

瓷质

口径1.4厘米,底径1.8厘米×1.5厘米,高4.9厘米,
重18克

平口沿,扁腹,浅圈足,腹部有"同仁堂"字样,
颈和两侧有条纹。贮药器具。保存完整。2001年
9月入藏,陕西省西安市八仙庵市场征集。

陕西医史博物馆藏

Medicine Bottle with Inscription of "Tong Ren Tang"

Qing Dynasty

Porcelain

Mouth Diameter 1.4 cm/ Bottom Diameter 1.8 cm×1.5 cm/
Height 4.9 cm/ Weight 18g

The bottle has a flat mouth rim, an oblate belly, and a
shallow ring foot. Its belly is inscribed with the name of
the pharmacy "Tong Ren Tang". Its neck and sides of
the body are decorated with stripe patterns. This well-
preserved medical utensil was collected from Baxian'an
Market in Xi'an, Shaanxi Province, in September 2001.

Preserved in Shaanxi Museum of Medical History

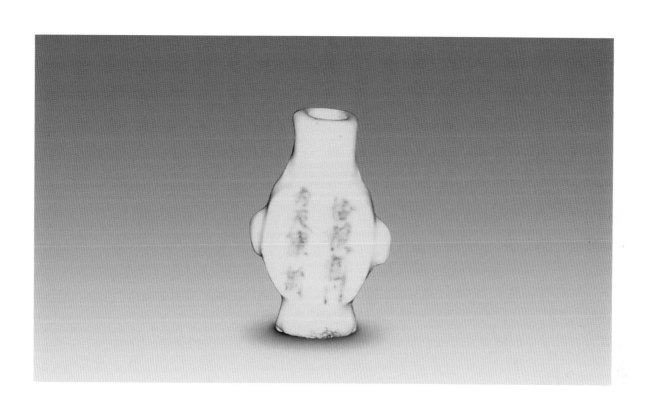

小瓷药瓶

清

瓷质

口径 1 厘米，底径 1.5 厘米，高 4.2 厘米，重 15 克

直口，扁腹，平底，腹两侧有一对称双耳，腹一面有"姑苏阊门内天库前"字样。药具。完整无损。2001 年 9 月入藏，陕西省西安市古玩市场征集。

陕西医史博物馆藏

Small Porcelain Medicine Bottle

Qing Dynasty

Porcelain

Mouth Diameter 1 cm/ Bottom Diameter 1.5 cm/ Height 4.2 cm/ Weight 15 g

The bottle has a straight mouth, an oblate belly, and a flat bottom. To the sides of the body are attached a pair of lugs, while on its belly is inscribed the address of the pharmacy "Gu Su Lü Men Nei Tian Ku Qian". This well-preserved medical utensil was collected from the Antique Market in Xi'an, Shaanxi Province, in September 2001.

Preserved in Shaanxi Museum of Medical History

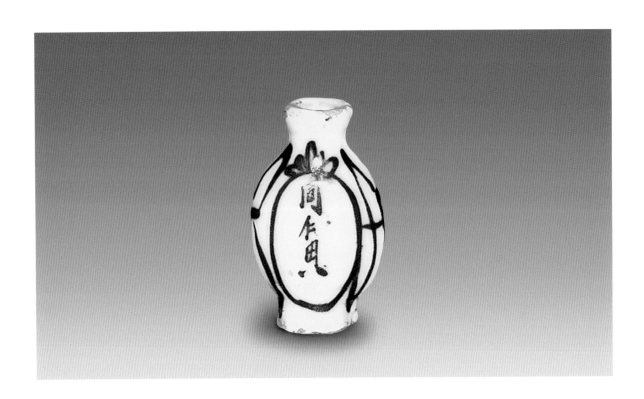

小瓷药瓶

清

瓷质

口径 1.5 厘米，底径 1.9 厘米 ×1.5 厘米，高 5.1 厘米，重 17 克

Small Porcelain Medicine Bottle

Qing Dynasty

Porcelain

Mouth Diameter 1.5 cm/ Bottom Diameter 1.9 cm ×1.5 cm/ Height 5.1 cm/ Weight 17 g

平口沿，束颈，扁腹，圈足，腹一面有"痧气丹"，另一面有"同仁思"字样，两侧为条纹。贮药器具。完整无损。2001年9月入藏，陕西省西安市古玩市场征集。

陕西医史博物馆藏

This bottle has a flat mouth rim, a contracted neck, an oblate belly, and a ring foot. Its belly is inscribed with the name of the drug "Sha Qi Dan" on one side and the name of the pharmacy "Tong Ren Si" on the other side. The two sides of the body are decorated with stripe patterns. This well-preserved medicine container was collected from the Antique Market in Xi'an, Shaanxi Province, in September 2001.

Preserved in Shaanxi Museum of Medical History

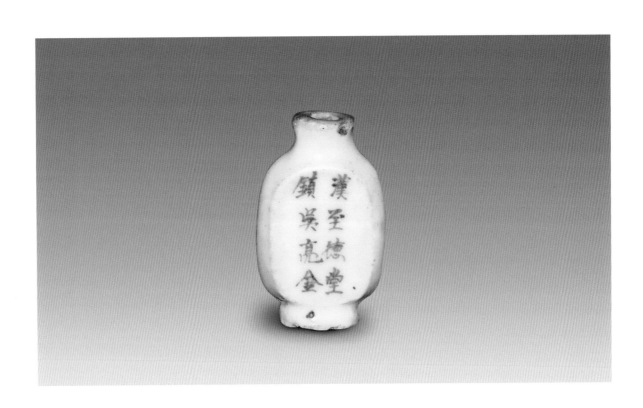

瓷药瓶

清

瓷质

口径 1.5 厘米，底径 2 厘米 ×1.6 厘米，高 5.5 厘米，重 30 克

平口沿，扁腹，平底，腹部有"汉镇至德堂吴亮金"字样。贮药器具。口沿残。陕西省西安市古玩市场征集。

陕西医史博物馆藏

Porcelain Medicine Bottle

Qing Dynasty

Porcelain

Mouth Diameter 1.5 cm/ Bottom Diameter 2 cm×1.6 cm/ Height 5.5 cm/ Weight 30 g

The medicine bottle has a flat mouth rim, an oblate belly, and a flat bottom. The belly is inscribed with the name of the pharmacy together with the doctor's name "Han Zhen Zhi De Tang Wu Liang Jin". With damaged mouth rim, the medical instrument was collected from the Antique Market in Xi'an, Shaanxi Province.

Preserved in Shaanxi Museum of Medical History

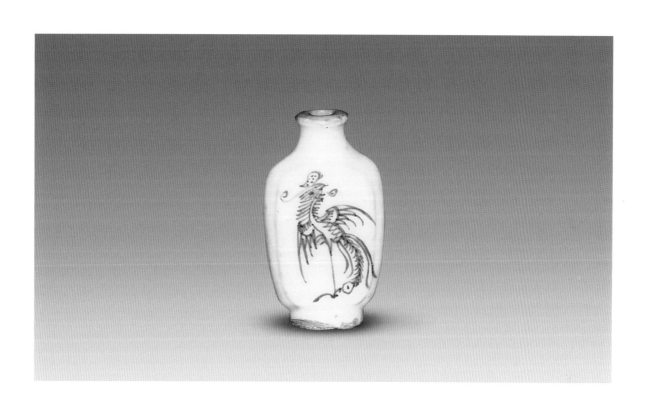

凤鸟瓷药瓶

清

瓷质

口径 1.5 厘米，底径 2.3 厘米 ×1.8 厘米，通高 6.8 厘米，重 42 克

平口沿，短颈，扁腹，腹一面有"朱德生凤记老店"字样。贮药器具。完整无损。2001 年 9 月入藏，陕西省西安市古玩市场征集。

陕西医史博物馆藏

Porcelain Medicine Bottle with Phoenix Design

Qing Dynasty

Porcelain

Mouth Diameter 1.5 cm/ Bottom Diameter 2.3 cm×1.8 cm/ Height 6.8 cm/ Weight 42 g

The bottle has a flat mouth rim, a short neck, and an oblate belly. On one side of the belly is inscribed the name of the pharmacy "Zhu De Sheng Feng Ji Lao Dian". This well-preserved medical utensil was collected from the Antique Market in Xi'an, Shaanxi Province, in September 2001.

Preserved in Shaanxi Museum of Medical History

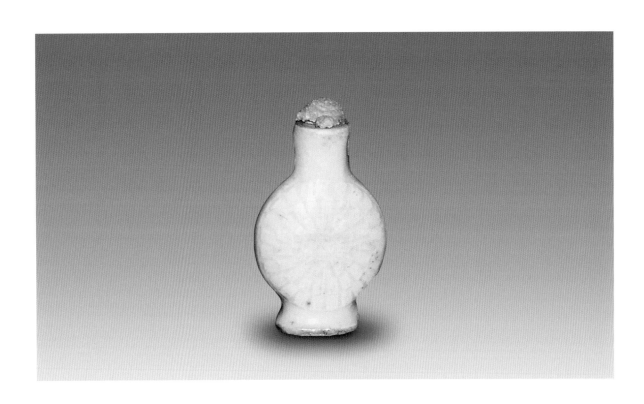

瓷药瓶

清

瓷质

口径 1.5 厘米，底径 1.9 厘米 ×2.5 厘米，高 5.9 厘米，重 34 克

Porcelain Medicine Bottle

Qing Dynasty

Porcelain

Mouth Diameter 1.5 cm/ Bottom Diameter 1.9 cm ×2.5 cm/ Height 5.9 cm/ Weight 34 g

直口，扁腹，平底，青瓷，腹面饰浅浮雕图
案。贮药器具。口沿残。2001 年 9 月入藏，
陕西省西安市古玩市场征集。

陕西医史博物馆藏

This blue-and-white glazed bottle has a straight
mouth, an oblate belly, and a flat bottom. Its belly
is decorated with thin relief patterns. This medicine
container is slightly damaged on the mouth rim. It
was collected from the Antique Market in Xi'an,
Shaanxi Province, in September 2001.

Preserved in Shaanxi Museum of Medical History

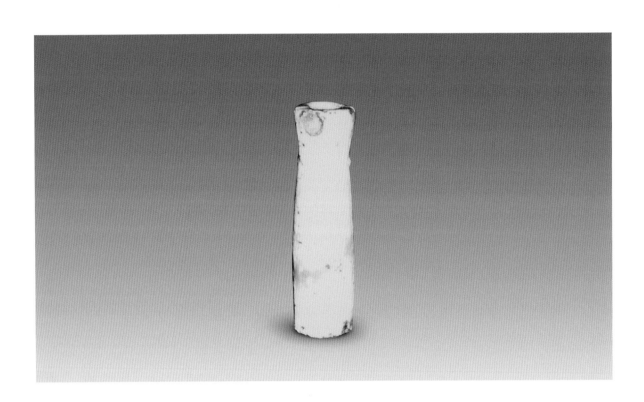

瓷药瓶

清

瓷质

口径 1.2 厘米，底径 1.2 厘米，高 4.9 厘米，重 11 克

Porcelain Medicine Bottle

Qing Dynasty

Porcelain

Mouth Diameter 1.2 cm/ Bottom Diameter 1.2 cm/ Height 4.9 cm/ Weight 11 g

圆柱状，平口沿，直口，直腹，平底，素面
白瓷。贮药器具。口沿略残。2001年9月入藏，
陕西省西安市古玩市场征集。

陕西医史博物馆藏

This white-glazed cylindrical bottle has a flat mouth
rim, a straight mouth, a straight belly, and a flat
bottom, with no decoration. This medicine container
is slightly damaged on the mouth rim. It was collected
from the Antique Market in Xi'an, Shaanxi Province,
in September 2001.

Preserved in Shaanxi Museum of Medical History

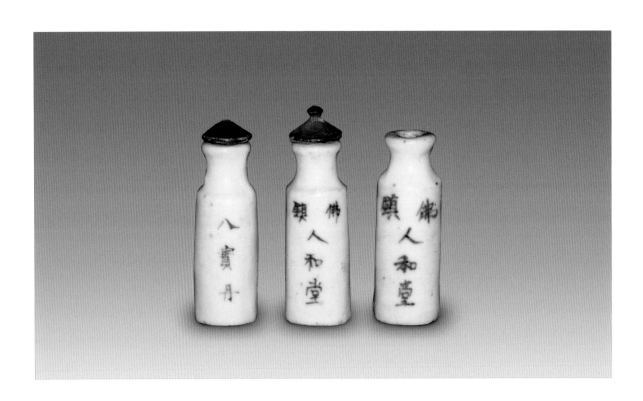

瓷药瓶

清

瓷质

口径 1.6 厘米，底径 2.1 厘米，高 6.3 厘米，重 30 克

Porcelain Medicine Bottles

Qing Dynasty

Porcelain

Mouth Diameter 1.6 cm/ Bottom Diameter 2.1 cm/ Height 6.3 cm/ Weight 30 g

圆柱状，平口沿，束颈，折肩，直腹，平底，
腹上有"佛镇人和堂""八宝丹"字样，并
带一小木盖。贮药器具。保存完整。2001 年
9 月入藏，陕西省西安市古玩市场征集。

陕西医史博物馆藏

These cylindrical medicine bottles have flat mouth
rims with wooden corks, contracted necks, angular
shoulders, straight bellies, and flat bottoms. Their
bellies are inscribed with the name of the pharmacy
"Fo Zhen Ren He Tang""Ba Bao Dan". These well-
preserved medical instruments were collected from
the Antique Market in Xi'an, Shaanxi Province, in
September 2001.

Preserved in Shaanxi Museum of Medical History

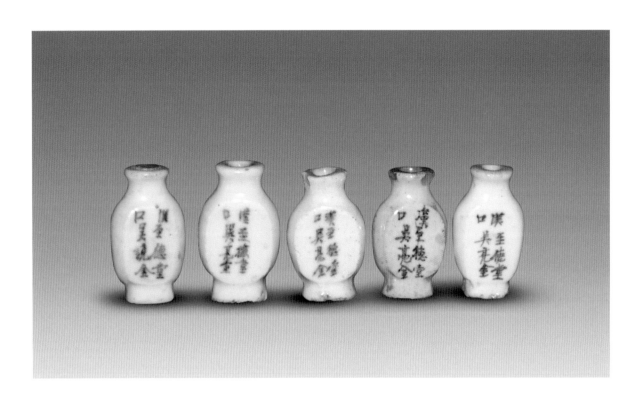

小瓷药瓶

清

瓷质

重 26 克

平口沿，扁腹，圈足，腹一面有"汉口至德堂吴
亮金"字样。贮药器具。苏州文物市场征集。

陕西医史博物馆藏

Small Porcelain Medicine Bottles

Qing Dynasty

Porcelain

Weight 26 g

These medicine bottles have flat mouth rims, ring feet and oblate bellies which are inscribed with the name of the pharmacy together with the name of the doctor "Han Kou Zhi De Tang Wu Liang Jin" on one side. These medical instruments were collected from the Antique Market in Suzhou, Jiangsu Province.

Preserved in Shaanxi Museum of Medical History

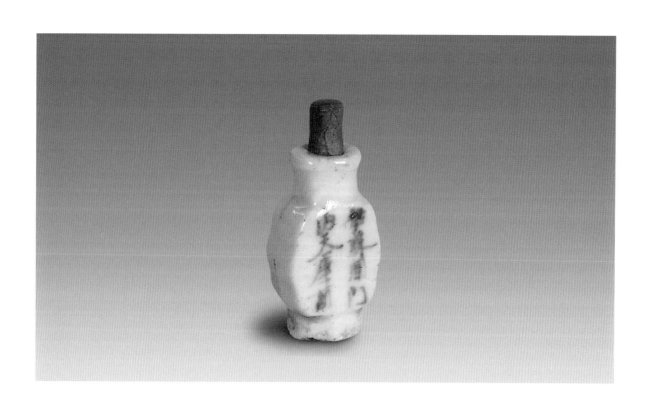

瓷药瓶

清

瓷质

口外径 1.55 厘米，口内径 0.7 厘米，宽 2.35 厘米，

通高 4.05 厘米，厚 1.45 厘米

扁瓶状，通身施乳白釉，瓶身有"姑苏阊门内天库前"蓝色字样，表面较粗糙，底部缺釉。盛药器具。保存基本完好。1955 年入藏。

中华医学会 / 上海中医药大学医史博物馆藏

Porcelain Medicine Bottle

Qing Dynasty

Porcelain

Mouth Outer Diameter 1.55 cm/ Mouth Inner Diameter 0.7 cm/ Width 2.35 cm/ Height 4.05 cm/ Thickness 1.45 cm

The opalescent-glazed bottle has an oblate body with an inscription "Gu Su Lü Men Nei Tian Ku Qian" in blue on the rough surface, and an unglazed bottom. This basically well-preserved medicine container was collected in 1955. Preserved in Chinese Medical Association/ Museum of Chinese Medicine, Shanghai University of Traditional Chinese Medicine

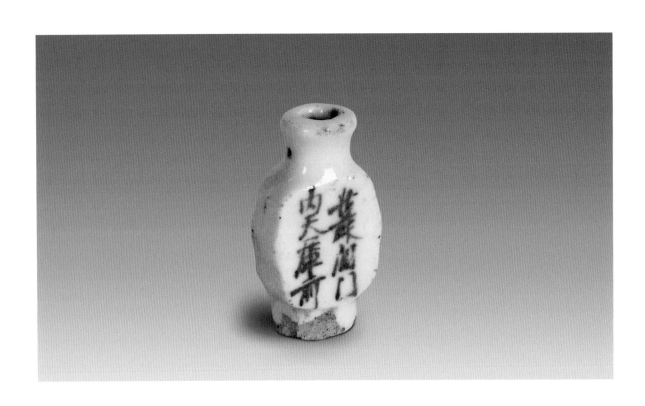

瓷药瓶

清

瓷质

口外径 1.6 厘米，口内径 0.65 厘米，宽 2.65 厘米，通高 4.6 厘米，厚 1.5 厘米

扁瓶状，通身施乳白釉，瓶身有"姑苏阊门内天库前"蓝字色样，瓷瓶表面较粗糙，底部缺釉。盛药器具。保存基本完好。1955 年入藏。

中华医学会 / 上海中医药大学医史博物馆藏

Porcelain Medicine Bottle

Qing Dynasty

Porcelain

Mouth Outer Diameter 1.6 cm/ Mouth Inner Diameter 0.65 cm/ Width 2.65 cm/ Height 4.6 cm/ Thickness 1.5 cm

The opalescent-glazed bottle has an oblate body with an inscription "Gu Su Lü Men Nei Tian Ku Qian" in blue on the rough surface, and an unglazed bottom. This basically well-preserved medicine container was collected in 1955. Preserved in Chinese Medical Association/ Museum of Chinese Medicine, Shanghai University of Traditional Chinese Medicine

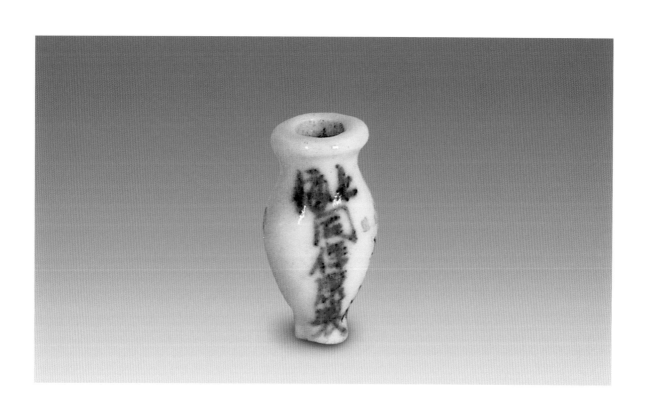

瓷药瓶

清

瓷质

宽 3.85 厘米，通高 3.6 厘米，厚 1.4 厘米

扁瓶状，通身施乳白釉，瓶身有 "上海同保康制"
蓝色字样。盛药器具。保存基本完好。1955 年
入藏。

中华医学会 / 上海中医药大学医史博物馆藏

Porcelain Medicine Bottle

Qing Dynasty

Porcelain

Width 3.85 cm/ Height 3.6 cm/ Thickness 1.4 cm

The opalescent-glazed bottle has an oblate body with
the name of the pharmacy "Shang Hai Tong Bao Kang
Zhi" inscribed in blue on the surface. This basically well-
preserved medicine container was collected in 1955.

Preserved in Chinese Medical Association/ Museum of
Chinese Medicine, Shanghai University of Traditional
Chinese Medicine

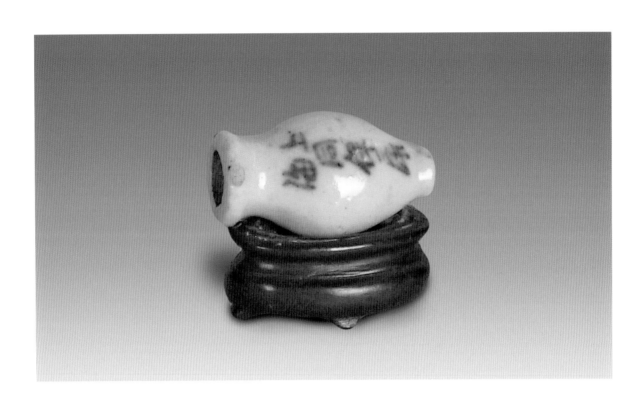

瓷药瓶

清

瓷质

口外径 1.5 厘米，口内径 0.8 厘米，宽 2.05 厘米，

通高 3.55 厘米，厚 1.4 厘米

扁瓶状，上有"上海同保康""卧龙丹"字样。

盛药器具。保存基本完好，上口有残。1955 年

入藏。

中华医学会 / 上海中医药大学医史博物馆藏

Porcelain Medicine Bottle

Qing Dynasty

Porcelain

Mouth Outer Diameter 1.5 cm/ Mouth Inner Diameter 0.8 cm/

Width 2.05 cm/ Height 3.55 cm/ Thickness 1.4 cm

The bottle has an oblate body with the name of the

pharmacy "Shang Hai Tong Bao Kang" and the name

of the drug "Wo Long Dan" inscribed on the surface.

Collected in 1955, this medicine container was almost

well-preserved except a crack on the mouth.

Preserved in Chinese Medical Association/ Museum of

Chinese Medicine, Shanghai University of Traditional

Chinese Medicine

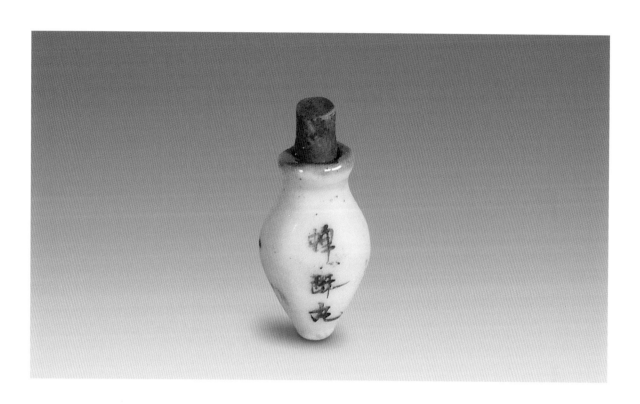

瓷药瓶

清

瓷质

宽 2.3 厘米，通高 4.05 厘米，厚 1.55 厘米

扁瓶状，通身施乳白釉，口沿施棕黄釉，瓶身书
有"上洋王大吉""蝉酥丸"黑色字样，瓶口内
有纸塞。盛药器具。保存基本完好。1955 年入藏。

中华医学会 / 上海中医药大学医史博物馆藏

Porcelain Medicine Bottle

Qing Dynasty

Porcelain

Width 2.3 cm/ Height 4.05 cm/ Thickness 1.55 cm

This oblate bottle has an opalescent-glazed body and a
yellowish brown glazed mouth rim where a paper cork
can be found. On the surface of the body are inscribed the
name of the pharmacy "Shang Yang Wang Da Ji" and the
name of the drug "Chan Su Wan" in ink. This basically well-
preserved medicine container was collected in 1955.

Preserved in Chinese Medical Association/ Museum of
Chinese Medicine, Shanghai University of Traditional
Chinese Medicine

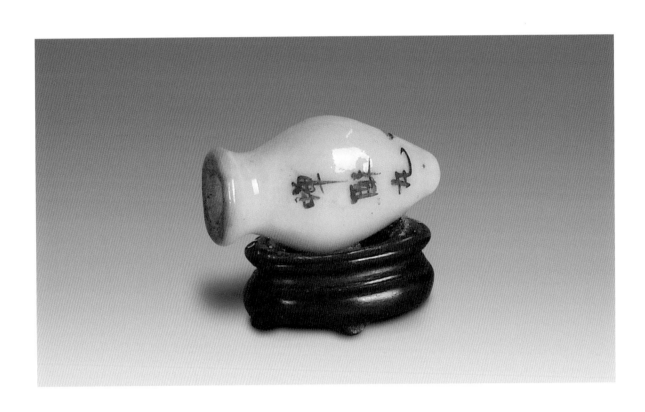

瓷药瓶

清

瓷质

宽 2.3 厘米，通高 4.1 厘米，厚 1.5 厘米

扁瓶状，通身施乳白釉，口沿施棕黄釉，瓶身书有"上洋王大吉""蝉酥丸"黑色字样。盛药器具。保存基本完好。1955 年入藏。

中华医学会 / 上海中医药大学医史博物馆藏

Porcelain Medicine Bottle

Qing Dynasty

Porcelain

Width 2.3 cm/ Height 4.1 cm/ Thickness 1.5 cm

This oblate bottle has an opalescent-glazed body and a yellowish-brown glazed mouth rim. On the surface of the body are inscribed the name of the pharmacy "Shang Yang Wang Da Ji"and the name of the drug "Chan Su Wan" (Chan Su Pills) in ink on the surface. This basically well-preserved medicine container was collected in 1955.

Preserved in Chinese Medical Association/ Museum of Chinese Medicine, Shanghai University of Traditional Chinese Medicine

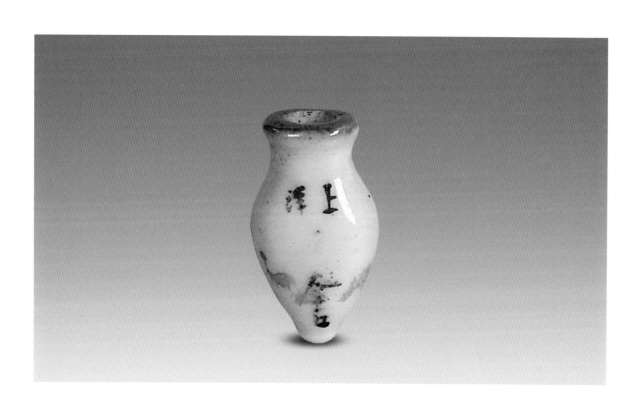

瓷药瓶

清

瓷质

宽 2.3 厘米，通高 4.1 厘米，厚 1.5 厘米

扁瓶状，通身施乳白釉，口沿涂棕黄色釉，瓶身有黑字，个别字模糊。盛药器具。保存基本完好。1955 年入藏。

中华医学会 / 上海中医药大学医史博物馆藏

Porcelain Medicine Bottle

Qing Dynasty

Porcelain

Width 2.3 cm/ Height 4.1 cm/ Thickness 1.5 cm

This oblate bottle has an opalescent-glazed body and a yellowish-brown glazed mouth rim with ink inscriptions, some of which are vague, on the surface. The bottle was used as a medicine container. This basically well-preserved medicine container was collected in 1955.

Preserved in Chinese Medical Association/ Museum of Chinese Medicine, Shanghai University of Traditional Chinese Medicine

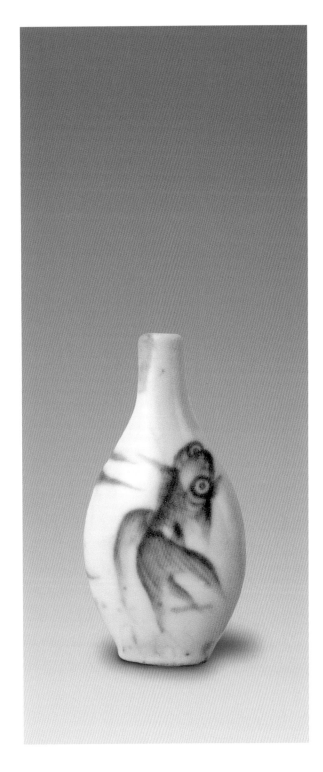

药瓶

清

瓷质

口径 1.1 厘米，宽 4.1 厘米，通高 7.4 厘米，
厚 1.9 厘米

Medicine Bottle

Qing Dynasty

Porcelain

Mouth Diameter 1.1 cm/ Width 4.1 cm/ Height 7.4 cm/

Thickness 1.9 cm

扁瓶状，直口，平底，施白釉，瓶身两面分别彩绘黑、红金鱼，制作精细，造型美观。盛药器具。口有残。1955 年入藏。

中华医学会 / 上海中医药大学医史博物馆藏

This white-glazed bottle has a straight mouth, a flat bottom, and an oblate body. On one side of the body is painted a black golden fish, with a red one on the other. This medicine container is exquisite in workmanship and elegant in design. The bottle was collected in 1955, and its mouth rim is damaged. Preserved in Chinese Medical Association/ Museum of Chinese Medicine, Shanghai University of Traditional Chinese Medicine

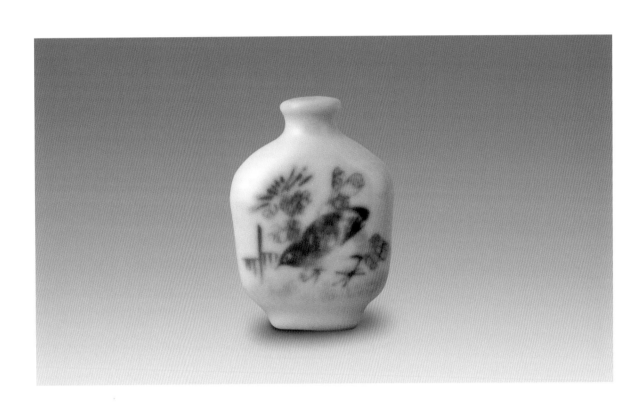

药瓶

清

瓷质

口径 1.5 厘米，宽 3.9 厘米，通高 5.4 厘米，厚 1.9 厘米

Medicine Bottle

Qing Dynasty

Porcelain

Mouth Diameter 1.5 cm/ Width 3.9 cm/ Height 5.4 cm/ Thickness 1.9 cm

扁瓶状，直口，平底，圈足，施白釉，彩绘花鸟人物骑马图案，制作精细，造型美观。盛药器具。保存基本完好。1954 年入藏。

中华医学会 / 上海中医药大学医史博物馆藏

This white-glazed bottle, decorated with designs of plants, birds and people on horseback, has a straight mouth, an oblate body, a flat bottom, and a ring foot. This medicine container is exquisite in workmanship and elegant in design. It was collected in 1954, and it is basically well-preserved.

Preserved in Chinese Medical Association/ Museum of Chinese Medicine, Shanghai University of Traditional Chinese Medicine

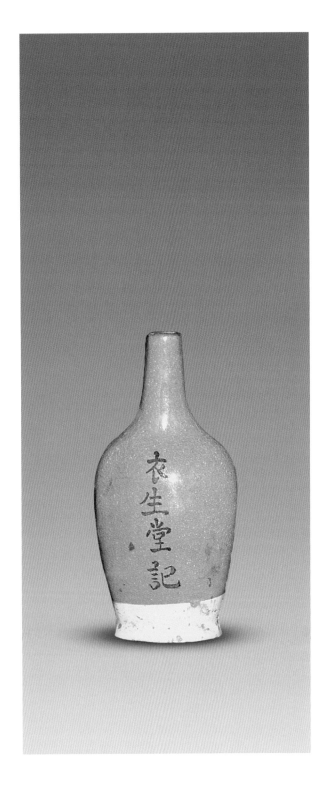

酱釉药瓶

清

瓷质

口径 1.5 厘米，底径 5 厘米，高 13.3 厘米，重 100 克

Brown-glazed Medicine Bottle

Qing Dynasty

Porcelain

Mouth Diameter 1.5 cm/ Bottom Diameter 5 cm/ Height 13.3 cm/ Weight 100 g

直口，扁腹，圈足，酱釉，底部白釉，瓶腹
有"衣生堂记"字样。医药器具。完整无损。
2001 年 9 月入藏，陕西省西安市古玩市场
征集。

陕西医史博物馆藏

This brown-glazed medicine bottle has a straight
mouth, an oblate belly, a ring foot, and a white-
glazed bottom. On the belly is vertically inscribed the
name of the pharmacy "Yi Sheng Tang Ji". This well-
preserved medicine container was collected from
the Antique Market in Xi'an, Shaanxi Province, in
September 2001.

Preserved in Shaanxi Museum of Medical History

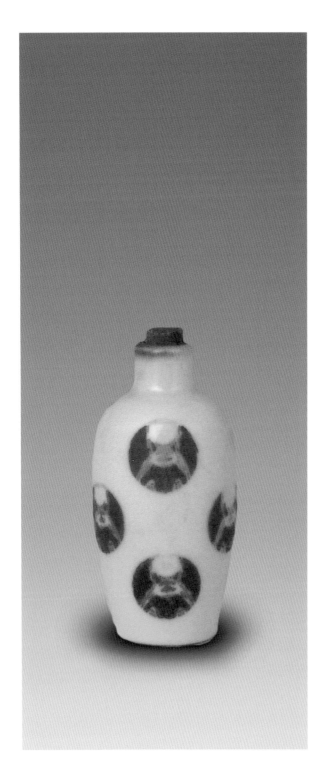

瓷药瓶

清

瓷质

口径 1.4 厘米，腹径 3.3 厘米，通高 6.5 厘米

Porcelain Medicine Bottle

Qing Dynasty

Porcelain

Mouth Diameter 1.4 cm/ Belly Diameter 3.3 cm/

Height 6.5 cm

圆瓶状，直口，平底，白釉上绘灰黑色人物脸谱图案，配木塞，小巧玲珑，工艺较好。盛药器具。保存基本完好。1957 年入藏。

中华医学会 / 上海中医药大学医史博物馆藏

On the white-glazed cylinder bottle are painted black opera facial masks. The bottle has a flat bottom and a straight mouth with a wooden cork. It is exquisitely designed and well processed. The basically well-preserved medicine container was collected in 1957. Preserved in Chinese Medical Association/ Museum of Chinese Medicine, Shanghai University of Traditional Chinese Medicine

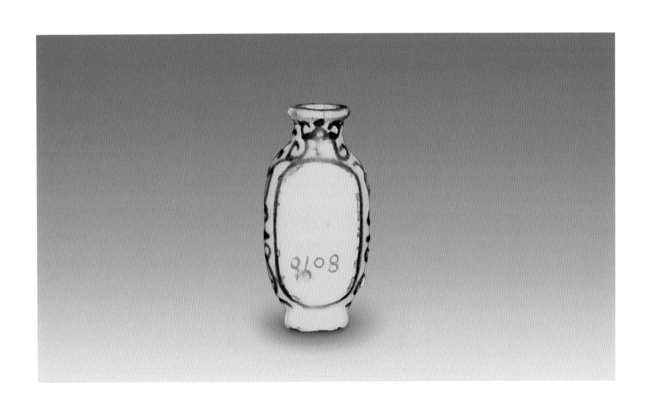

小兰花扁药瓶

清

瓷质

口径 1.5 厘米，底径 1.6 厘米，通高 5.5 厘米，
重 50 克

直口，扁腹，两肩饰小兰花。贮药器具。完整无损。

陕西医史博物馆藏

Oblate Medicine Bottle with Designs of Orchids

Qing Dynasty

Porcelain

Mouth Diameter 1.5 cm/ Bottom Diameter 1.6 cm/
Height 5.5 cm/ Weight 50 g

This bottle has a straight mouth and an oblate belly, with designs of little orchids on its shoulders. This medicine container remains intact.

Preserved in Shaanxi Museum of Medical History

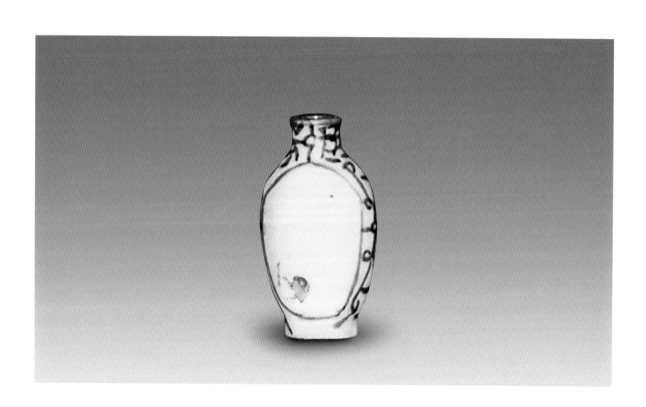

小兰花扁药瓶

清

瓷质

口径 0.8 厘米，底径 2.2 厘米，通高 7.5 厘米，
重 50 克

直口，扁腹，圈足，两侧为缠枝纹。贮药器具。
完整无损。

陕西医史博物馆藏

Oblate Medicine Bottle with Designs of Orchids

Qing Dynasty

Porcelain

Mouth Diameter 0.8 cm/ Bottom Diameter 2.2 cm/
Height 7.5 cm/ Weight 50 g

This bottle has a straight mouth, an oblate belly, and a ring
foot. Its body is decorated with designs of interlocking
branches. This medicine container remains intact.

Preserved in Shaanxi Museum of Medical History

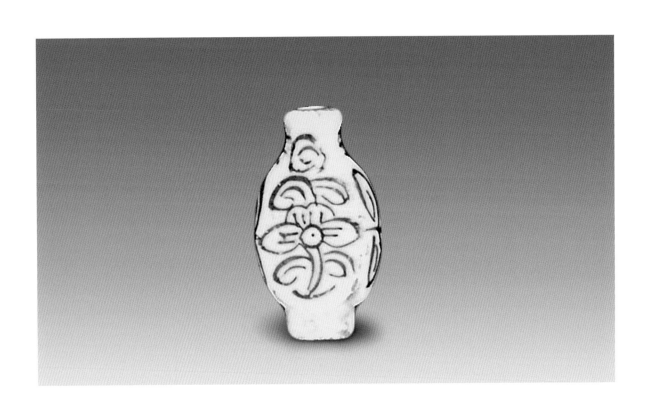

青花扁药瓶

清

瓷质

口径 1.7 厘米，底径 2 厘米，通高 6.3 厘米，重 50 克

直口，扁腹，圈足，表面饰青花图。贮药器具。完整无损。

陕西医史博物馆藏

Blue-and-white Oblate Medicine Bottle

Qing Dynasty

Porcelain

Mouth Diameter 1.7 cm/ Bottom Diameter 2 cm/ Height 6.3 cm/ Weight 50 g

This bottle has a straight mouth, an oblate belly, and a ring foot. Its body is decorated with designs of blue-and-white flowers. This medicine container remains intact.

Preserved in Shaanxi Museum of Medical History

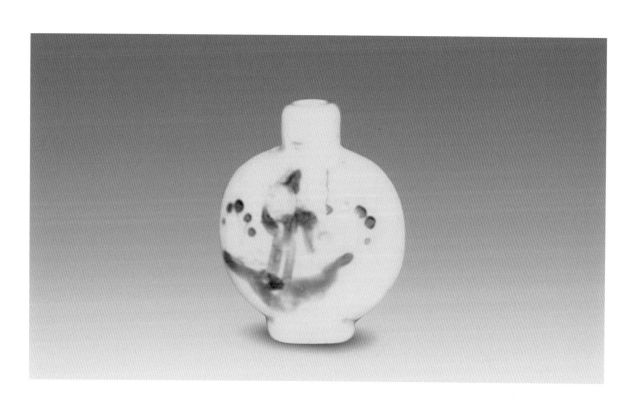

扁药瓶

清

瓷质

口径 1.3 厘米，底径 2 厘米，通高 5.5 厘米，重 50 克

直口，扁圆腹，圈足，表面饰人物图案。贮药器具。完整无损。

陕西医史博物馆藏

Oblate Medicine Bottle

Qing Dynasty

Porcelain

Mouth Diameter 1.3 cm/ Bottom Diameter 2 cm/ Height 5.5 cm/ Weight 50 g

This bottle has a straight mouth, an oblate belly, and a ring foot. Its body is decorated with a figure design. This medicine container remains intact.

Preserved in Shaanxi Museum of Medical History

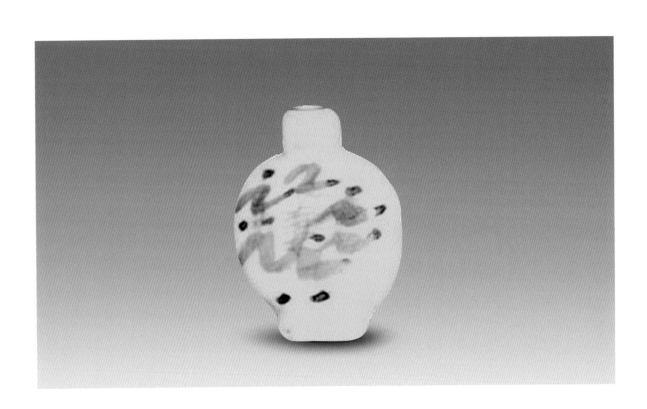

青花扁药瓶

清

瓷质

口径 1.5 厘米，底径 2.5 厘米，通高 5.9 厘米，
重 50 克

直口，扁圆腹，圈足，表面饰青花图。贮药器具。
完整无损。

陕西医史博物馆藏

Blue-and-white Oblate Medicine Bottle

Qing Dynasty

Porcelain

Mouth Diameter 1.5 cm/ Bottom Diameter 2.5 cm/
Height 5.9 cm/ Weight 50 g

This bottle has a straight mouth, an oblate belly, and a
ring foot. Its body is decorated with designs of blue-and-
white flowers. This medicine container remains intact.

Preserved in Shaanxi Museum of Medical History

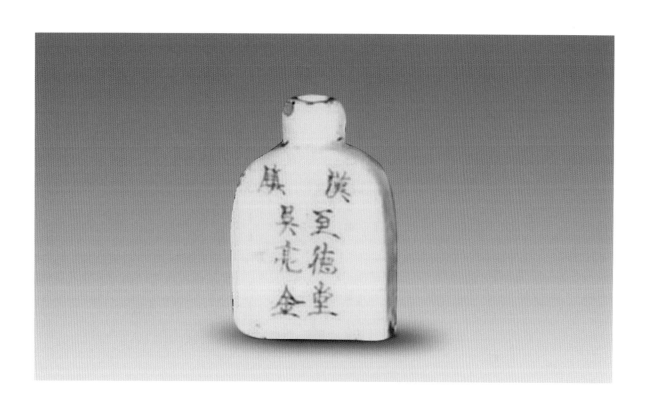

扁药瓶

清

瓷质

口径 1.2 厘米，底径 3.5 厘米，通高 5.2 厘米，
重 50 克

直口，直扁腹，圈足，上有字"汉镇至德堂吴亮
金"。贮药器具。完整无损。

陕西医史博物馆藏

Oblate Medicine Bottle

Qing Dynasty

Porcelain

Mouth Diameter 1.2 cm/ Bottom Diameter 3.5 cm/
Height 5.2 cm/ Weight 50 g

This bottle has a straight mouth, a straight and oblate
belly, and a ring foot, on which is found an inscription
of the name of the pharmacy together with the name of
the doctor "Han Zhen Zhi De Tang Wu Liang Jin". This
medicine container remains intact.

Preserved in Shaanxi Museum of Medical History

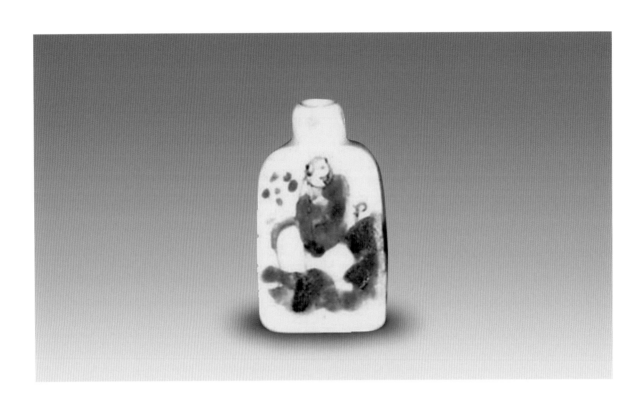

青花人物扁药瓶

Oblate Medicine Bottle with Blue-and-white Figure Design

清

瓷质

口径 0.7 厘米，底径 3.2 厘米，通高 5.7 厘米，重 50 克

直口，直扁腹，圈足，腹饰小兰花。贮药器具。完整无损。

陕西医史博物馆藏

Qing Dynasty

Porcelain

Mouth Diameter 0.7 cm/ Bottom Diameter 3.2 cm/ Height 5.7 cm/ Weight 50 g

This bottle has a straight mouth, a straight and oblate belly, and a ring foot. This medicine container remains intact.

Preserved in Shaanxi Museum of Medical History

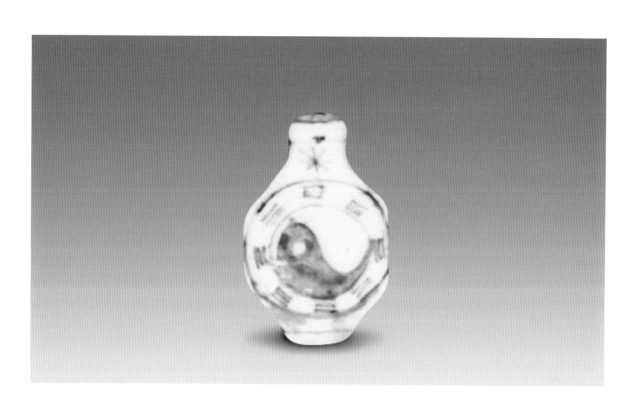

扁药瓶

清

瓷质

口径 1.5 厘米，底径 1.8 厘米，通高 5 厘米，重 10 克

小圆口，六边形扁腹，圈足，腹中间有"八卦太极图"。贮药器具。完整无损。

陕西医史博物馆藏

Oblate Medicine Bottle

Qing Dynasty

Porcelain

Mouth Diameter 1.5 cm/ Bottom Diameter 1.8 cm/ Height 5 cm/ Weight 10 g

This bottle has a small round mouth, an oblate flat hexagonal belly, and a ring foot. On the belly is a painting of "Circulating Tai Ji Diagram". This medicine container remains intact.

Preserved in Shaanxi Museum of Medical History

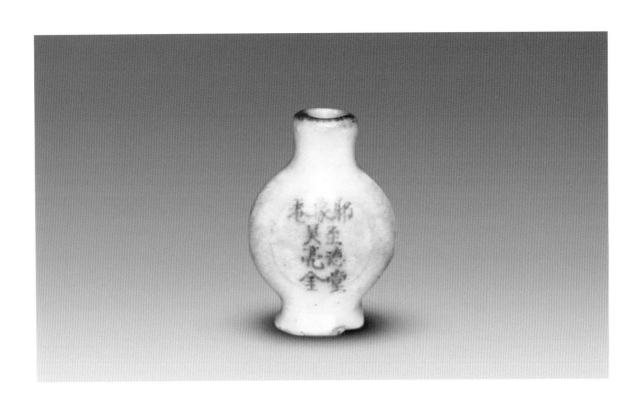

扁瓷药瓶

清

瓷质

口径 1.5 厘米，底径 2.5 厘米 ×2 厘米，高 6 厘米，重 38 克

Oblate Porcelain Medicine Bottle

Qing Dynasty

Porcelain

Mouth Diameter 1.5 cm/ Bottom Diameter 2.5 cm×2 cm/ Height 6 cm/ Weight 38 g

平口沿，扁腹，平底，青瓷，腹一面有"郭
家巷""至德堂吴亮金"字样。贮药器具。
完整无损。2001 年 9 月入藏，陕西省西安市
古玩市场征集。

陕西医史博物馆藏

This bottle has a flat mouth rim, an oblate belly, and
a flat bottom. On one side of the belly are inscribed
the name of the pharmacy together with the doctor's
name, "Zhi De Tang Wu Liang Jin", and the name
of the alley where the pharmacy is located, "Guo Jia
Xiang". This well-preserved medicine container was
collected from the Antique Market in Xi'an, Shaanxi
Province, in September 2001.

Preserved in Shaanxi Museum of Medical History

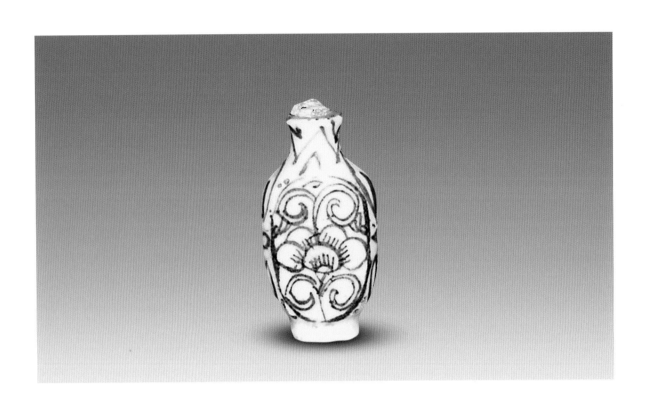

青花扁药瓶

清

瓷质

口径 1.2 厘米，底径 2 厘米，通高 6 厘米，重 30 克

小喇叭口，扁腹，圈足，颈和肩处有三角纹，腹上有小兰花图。贮药器具。完整无损。

陕西医史博物馆藏

Blue-and-white Oblate Medicine Bottle

Qing Dynasty

Porcelain

Mouth Diameter 1.2 cm/ Bottom Diameter 2 cm/ Height 6 cm/ Weight 30 g

This bottle has a slightly flared mouth, an oblate belly, and a ring foot. Its neck and shoulders are decorated with triangle patterns, while on the belly are painted designs of little orchids. This medicine container remains intact.

Preserved in Shaanxi Museum of Medical History

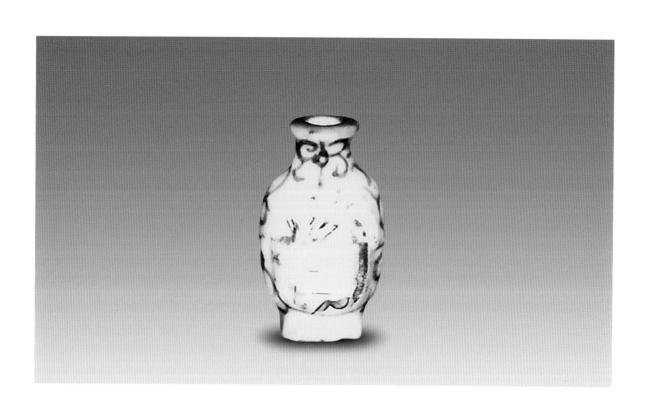

青花扁药瓶

清

瓷质

口径 1.5 厘米，底径 1.8 厘米，通高 4.8 厘米，
重 20 克

小喇叭口，扁腹，圈足，两侧为缠枝纹，中为一
动物图。贮药器具。完整无损。

陕西医史博物馆藏

Blue-and-white Oblate Medicine Bottle

Qing Dynasty

Porcelain

Mouth Diameter 1.5 cm/ Bottom Diameter 1.8 cm/
Height 4.8 cm/ Weight 20 g

This bottle has a slightly flared mouth, an oblate belly,
and a ring foot. The two sides are decorated with designs of
interlocking branches, while the front face has a painting of
an animal. This medicine container remains intact.

Preserved in Shaanxi Museum of Medical History

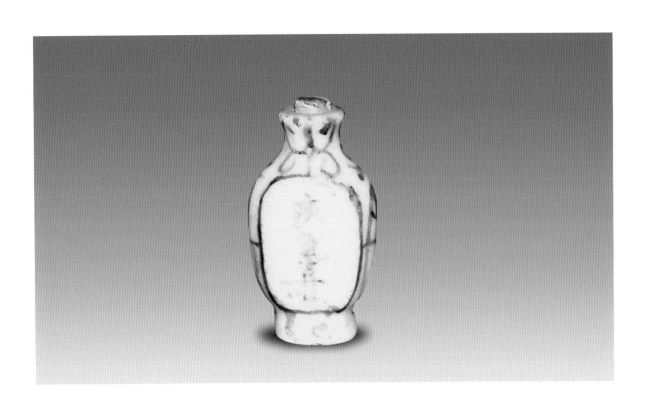

扁药瓶

清

瓷质

口径 1.2 厘米，底径 1.5 厘米，通高 5.1 厘米，
重 25 克

小喇叭口，扁腹，圈足，两侧为缠枝纹，腹上有
"痧气丹"。贮药器具。完整无损。

陕西医史博物馆藏

Oblate Medicine Bottle

Qing Dynasty

Porcelain

Mouth Diameter 1.2 cm/ Bottom Diameter 1.5 cm/
Height 5.1 cm/ Weight 25 g

This bottle has a slightly flared mouth, an oblate belly,
and a ring foot. The two sides are decorated with designs
of interlocking branches, while its belly is inscribed with
"Sha Qi Dan" (Pills for Eruptive Disease). This medicine
container remains intact.

Preserved in Shaanxi Museum of Medical History

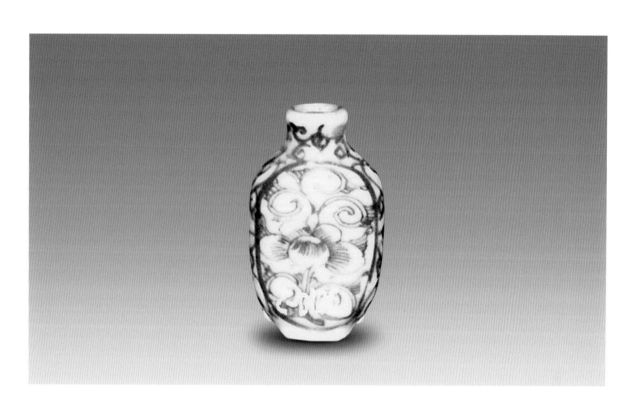

青花扁瓷药瓶

清

瓷质

口径 1.4 厘米，底径 5.4 厘米，通高 1.2 厘米，
重 23 克

小喇叭口，扁腹，平底，周身饰缠枝纹。贮药器
具。完整无损。

陕西医史博物馆藏

Blue-and-white Oblate Porcelain Medicine Bottle

Qing Dynasty

Porcelain

Mouth Diameter 1.4 cm/ Bottom Diameter 5.4 cm/
Height 1.2 cm/ Weight 23 g

This oblate bottle has a slightly flared mouth, an oblate
belly, and a flat bottom. Its body is decorated with
designs of interlocking branches. This medicine container
remains intact.

Preserved in Shaanxi Museum of Medical History

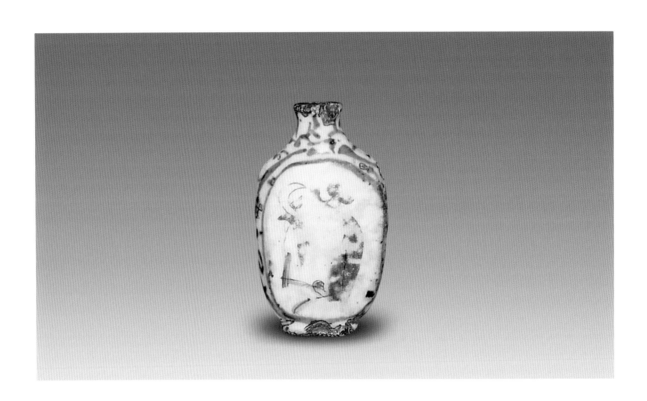

彩绘瓷药瓶

清

瓷质

口径 1.5 厘米，底径 2.4 厘米 ×1.4 厘米，高 7 厘米，重 43 克

平口沿，扁腹，浅圈足，腹部有人物图案，颈肩及两侧有蓝色条纹图案。贮药器具。口、底略残。2001 年 9 月入藏，陕西省西安市古玩市场征集。

陕西医史博物馆藏

Painted Porcelain Medicine Bottle

Qing Dynasty

Porcelain

Mouth Diameter 1.5 cm/ Bottom Diameter 2.4 cm×1.4 cm/ Height 7 cm/ Weight 43 g

This bottle has a flat mouth rim, an oblate belly, and a shallow ring foot. Its belly is decorated with designs of human figures, while its neck, shoulders and the two sides with blue string patterns. The mouth and bottom of this medicine container are slightly damaged. It was collected from the Antique Market in Xi'an, Shaanxi Province, in September 2001.

Preserved in Shaanxi Museum of Medical History

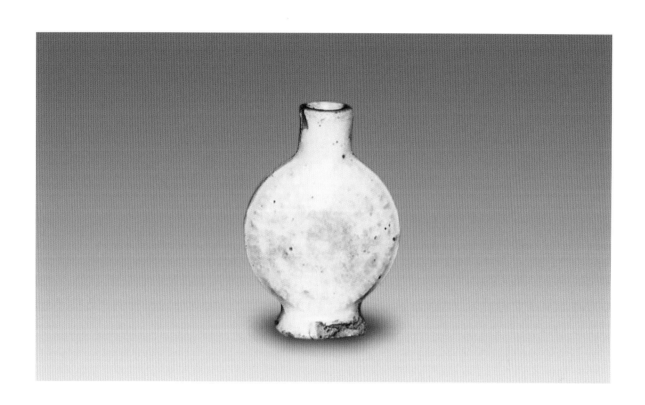

扁瓷药瓶

清

瓷质

口径 1.3 厘米，底径 2.5 厘米 ×1.8 厘米，高 6 厘米，重 31 克

直口，扁圆腹，平底，腹部两面有放射状浮雕图案。盛药器具。口沿残。2001 年 9 月入藏，陕西省西安市古玩市场征集。

陕西医史博物馆藏

Oblate Porcelain Medicine Bottle

Qing Dynasty

Porcelain

Mouth Diameter 1.3 cm/ Bottom Diameter 2.5 cm×1.8 cm/ Height 6 cm/ Weight 31 g

This bottle has a straight mouth, an oblate belly, and a flat bottom. The front and the back of its belly are decorated with radiative relief patterns. This medicine container is slightly damaged on the mouth rim. It was collected from the Antique Market in Xi'an, Shaanxi Province, in September 2001.

Preserved in Shaanxi Museum of Medical History

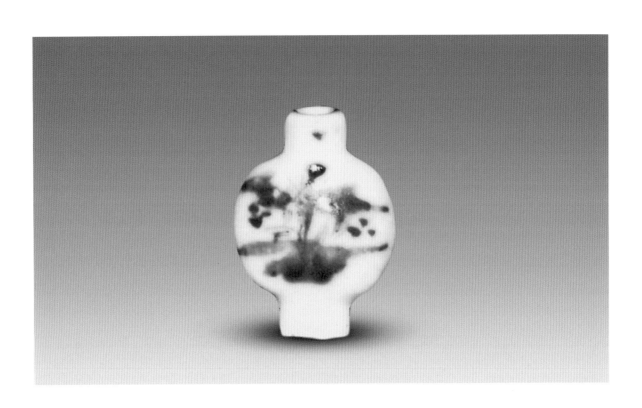

扁药瓶

清

瓷质

口径 1.5 厘米，底径 1.5 厘米 ×2 厘米，通高 5.6 厘米，重 17 克

直口，扁腹，圈足，腹一面饰有青花花卉。盛药器具。完整无损。2001 年 9 月入藏，陕西省西安市古玩市场征集。

陕西医史博物馆藏

Oblate Medicine Bottle

Qing Dynasty

Porcelain

Mouth Diameter 1.5 cm/ Bottom Diameter 1.5 cm×2 cm/ Height 5.6 cm/ Weight 17 g

This bottle has a straight mouth, an oblate belly, and a ring foot. One side of its belly is decorated with blue-and-white floral motifs. This medicine container is well preserved. It was collected from the Antique Market in Xi'an, Shaanxi Province, in September 2001.

Preserved in Shaanxi Museum of Medical History

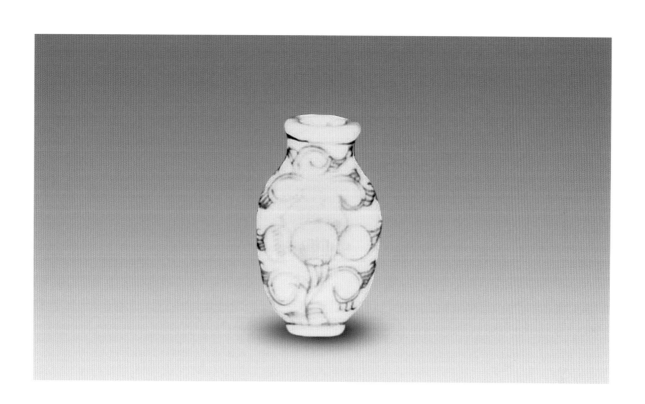

青花小药瓶

清

瓷质

口径 1.2 厘米，底径 1 厘米，高 3.6 厘米，重 8 克

平口沿，扁腹，浅圈足，周身饰青花缠枝花卉纹。

盛药器具。完整无损。2001 年 9 月入藏，陕西

省西安市古玩市场征集。

陕西医史博物馆藏

Small Blue-and-white Porcelain Medicine Bottle

Qing Dynasty

Porcelain

Mouth Diameter 1.2 cm/ Bottom Diameter 1 cm/ Height 3.6 cm/ Weight 8 g

The bottle has a flat mouth rim, an oblate belly, and a shallow ring foot. Its body is decorated with designs of blue-and-white interlocking floral patterns. This well-preserved medical utensil was collected from the Antique Market in Xi'an, Shaanxi Province, in September 2001.

Preserved in Shaanxi Museum of Medical History

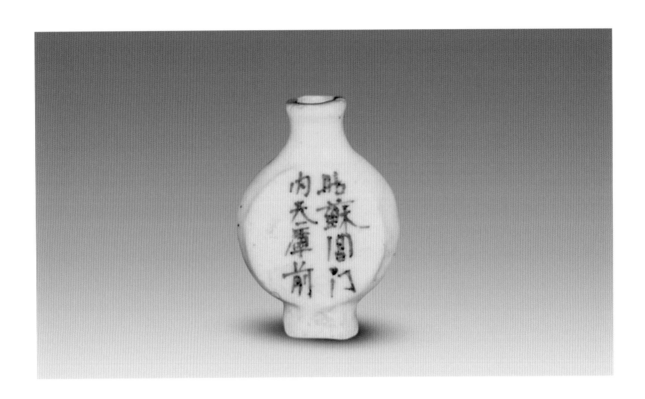

扁瓷药瓶

清

瓷质

口径 1.5 厘米，底径 2 厘米 ×1.6 厘米，高 6 厘米，重 35 克

Oblate Porcelain Medicine Bottle

Qing Dynasty

Porcelain

Mouth Diameter 1.5 cm/ Bottom Diameter 2 cm×1.6cm/ Height 6 cm/ Weight 35 g

平口沿，扁圆腹，平底，腹上有"姑苏阊门
内天库前"字样，另一面有"诵芬堂雷"字
样。盛药器具。完整无损。2001 年 9 月入藏，
陕西省西安市古玩市场征集。

陕西医史博物馆藏

This bottle has a flat mouth rim, an oblate belly, and
a flat bottom. One side of its belly is inscribed with
the address of the pharmacy"Gu Su Lü Men Nei Tian
Ku Qian" while the other side with the name of the
pharmacy "Song Fen Tang Lei". This well-preserved
medicine container was collected from the Antique
Market in Xi'an, Shaanxi Province, in September 2001.
Preserved in Shaanxi Museum of Medical History

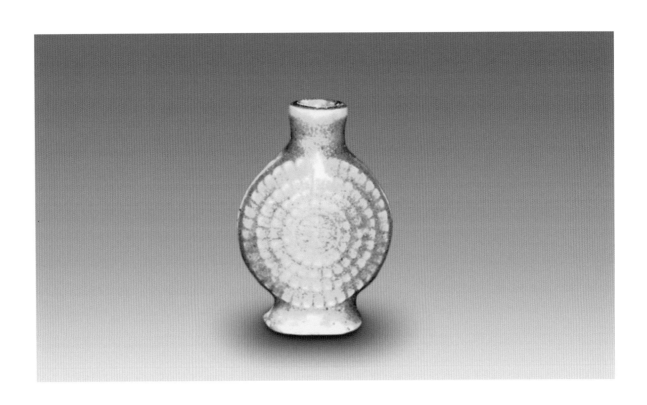

蓝瓷药瓶

清

瓷质

口径 1.6 厘米，底径 2.7 厘米 ×2 厘米，高 6.2 厘米，重 47 克

Blue Porcelain Medicine Bottle

Qing Dynasty

Porcelain

Mouth Diameter 1.6 cm/ Bottom Diameter 2.7 cm ×2 cm/ Height 6.2 cm/ Weight 47 g

平口沿，圆肩，扁腹，平底，施霁蓝釉，内装粉状药物，腹贴有药名档签，腹部有放射图案。盛药器具。完整无损。2002年4月入藏，陕西省咸阳市古玩市场征集。

陕西医史博物馆藏

The bottle has a flat mouth rim, a rounded shoulder, an oblate belly, and a flat bottom. In the bottle is found some powdered drug. Attached with a label of the medicine's name, the belly of the sacrificial-blue glazed bottle is decorated with radiative patterns. This well-preserved medical utensil was collected from the Antique Market in Xianyang, Shaanxi Province, in April 2002.

Preserved in Shaanxi Museum of Medical History

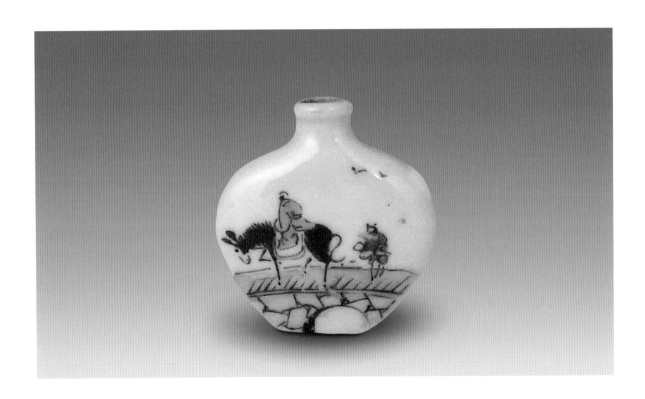

扁药瓶

清

瓷质

口径 1.6 厘米，宽 4.9 厘米，通高 5.1 厘米，厚 1.8 厘米

Oblate Medicine Bottle

Qing Dynasty

Porcelain

Mouth Diameter 1.6 cm/ Width 4.9 cm/ Height 5.1 cm/ Thickness 1.8 cm

扁瓶状，直口，平底，白釉，彩绘有骑者、小桥、
母鸡、草木等图案，画工简洁美观。盛药器具。
保存基本完好。1954 年入藏。

中华医学会 / 上海中医药大学医史博物馆藏

This oblate bottle has a straight mouth and a flat
bottom. Its white-glazed body is decorated with the
painting of a rider, a small bridge, a hen, some plants
and so on. The painting is of both simplicity and
prettiness. This basically well-preserved medicine
container was collected in 1954.

Preserved in Chinese Medical Association/ Museum
of Chinese Medicine, Shanghai University of
Traditional Chinese Medicine

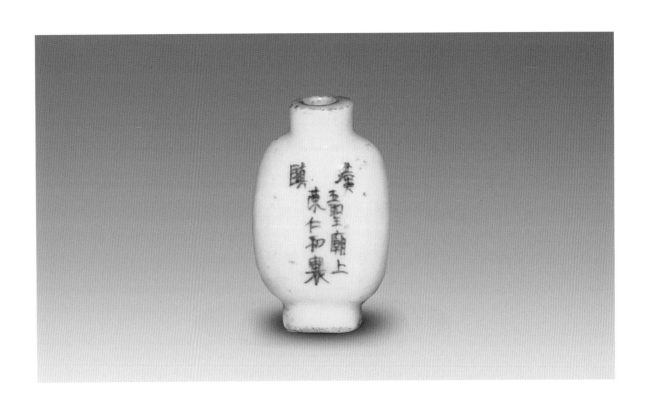

瓷药瓶

清

瓷质

口径 1.7 厘米，底径 2.2 厘米 ×1.8 厘米，高 6.4 厘米，重 40 克

平口沿，直口，椭圆形腹，平底，腹部有"汉镇五圣庙上陈仁和制"。盛药器具。完整无损。2001年 9 月入藏，陕西省西安市古玩市场征集。

陕西医史博物馆藏

Porcelain Medicine Bottle

Qing Dynasty

Porcelain

Mouth Diameter 1.7 cm/ Bottom Diameter 2.2 cm×1.8 cm/ Height 6.4 cm/ Weight 40 g

The bottle has a flat mouth rim, a straight mouth, an oval belly, and a flat bottom. Its belly is inscribed with the address of the pharmacy together with the doctor's name "Han Zhen Wu Sheng Miao Shang Chen Ren He Zhi". This well-preserved medical utensil was collected from the Antique Market in Xi'an, Shaanxi Province, in September 2001.

Preserved in Shaanxi Museum of Medical History

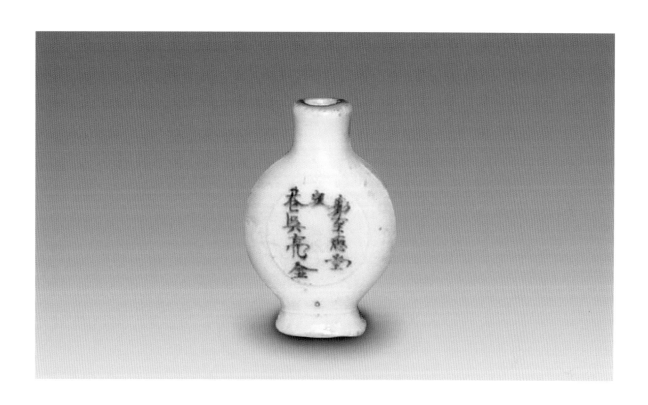

影青瓷药瓶

清

瓷质

口径 1.9 厘米，底径 3 厘米 ×2.3 厘米，高 7 厘米，
重 50 克

直口，扁腹，平底，腹一面有"穷家巷至德堂
吴亮金"字样，影青。医药器具。完整无损。

2001 年 9 月入藏，陕西省西安市古玩市场征集。

陕西医史博物馆藏

Misty Blue Porcelain Medicine Bottle

Qing Dynasty

Porcelain

Mouth Diameter 1.9 cm/ Bottom Diameter 3 cm ×2.3 cm/
Height 7 cm/ Weight 50 g

The misty blue glazed bottle has a straight mouth, an
oblate belly, and a flat bottom. One side of its belly is
inscribed with the address of the pharmacy together
with the doctor's name "Qiong Jia Xiang Zhi De Tang
Wu Liang Jin". This well-preserved medical utensil was
collected from the Antique Market in Xi'an, Shaanxi
Province, in September 2001.

Preserved in Shaanxi Museum of Medical History

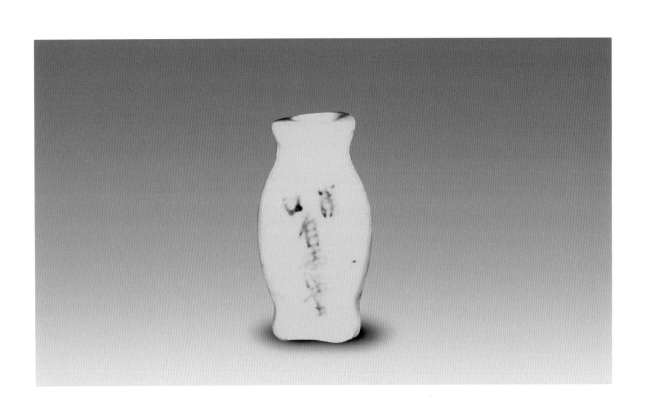

小瓷药瓶

清

瓷质

口径 1.4 厘米，底径 1.5 厘米 ×1.1 厘米，
高 3.6 厘米，重 9 克

平口沿，扁腹，平底，腹部有"汉口至德堂"字
样。盛药器具。完整无损。2001 年 9 月入藏，
陕西省西安市古玩市场征集。

陕西医史博物馆藏

Small Porcelain Medicine Bottle

Qing Dynasty

Porcelain

Mouth Diameter 1.4 cm/ Bottom Diameter 1.5 cm ×1.1 cm/
Height 3.6 cm/ Weight 9 g

The bottle has a flat mouth rim, an oblate belly, and a
flat bottom. Its belly is inscribed with the name of the
pharmacy "Han Kou Zhi De Tang". This well-preserved
medical utensil was collected from the Antique Market in
Xi'an, Shaanxi Province, in September 2001.

Preserved in Shaanxi Museum of Medical History

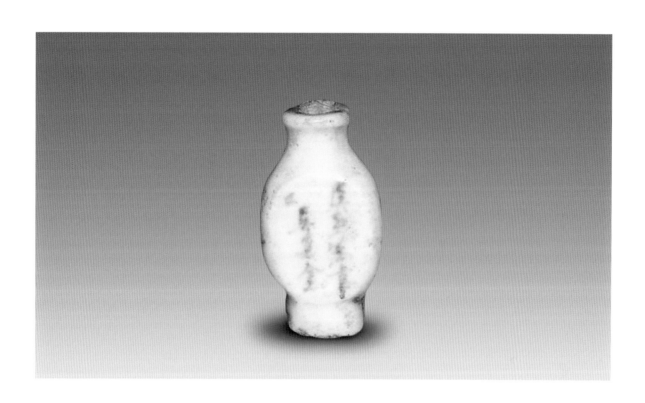

小瓷药瓶

清

瓷质

口径 1.5 厘米，底径 1.8 厘米 ×1.4 厘米，
高 5.5 厘米，重 25 克

平口沿，扁腹，浅圈足，腹部有"汉口至德堂吴
亮金"字样。盛药器具。完整无损。2001 年
9 月入藏，陕西省西安市古玩市场征集。

陕西医史博物馆藏

Small Porcelain Medicine Bottle

Qing Dynasty

Porcelain

Mouth Diameter 1.5 cm/ Bottom Diameter 1.8 cm ×1.4 cm/
Height 5.5 cm/ Weight 25 g

The bottle has a flat mouth rim, an oblate belly, and a
shallow ring foot. Its belly is inscribed with the name of
the pharmacy together with the doctor's name "Han Kou
Zhi De Tang Wu Liang Jin". This well-preserved medical
utensil was collected from the Antique Market in Xi'an,
Shaanxi Province, in September 2001.

Preserved in Shaanxi Museum of Medical History

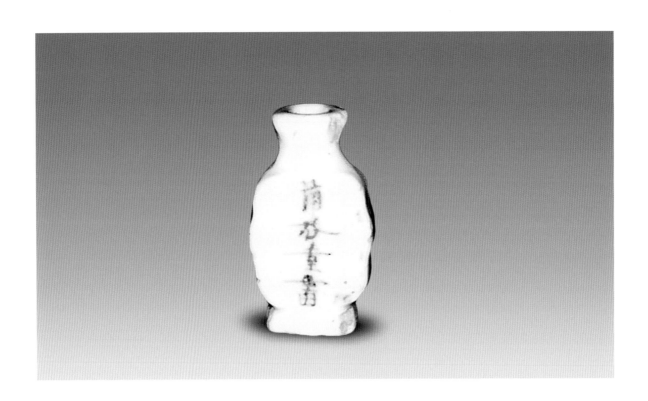

小瓷药瓶

清

瓷质

口径 0.9 厘米，底径 1.7 厘米 ×1.4 厘米，通高 4.3 厘米，重 18 克

Small Porcelain Medicine Bottle

Qing Dynasty

Porcelain

Mouth Diameter 0.9 cm/ Bottom Diameter 1.7 cm ×1.4 cm/ Height 4.3 cm/ Weight 18 g

平口沿，短颈，平肩，扁方形腹，平底，腹部有"姑苏阊门内天库前"，另一面为"诵芬堂雷"字样。药具。口沿、底略残。2001 年 9 月入藏，陕西省西安市古玩市场征集。

陕西医史博物馆藏

The bottle has a flat mouth rim, a short neck, a flat shoulder, an oblate square belly, and a flat bottom. On one side of its belly is inscribed the address of the pharmacy "Gu Su Lü Men Nei Tian Ku Qian", while on the other the name of the pharmacy "Song Fen Tang Lei". This medical utensil is slightly damaged on the mouth rim and the bottom. It was collected from the Antique Market in Xi'an, Shaanxi Province, in September 2001.

Preserved in Shaanxi Museum of Medical History

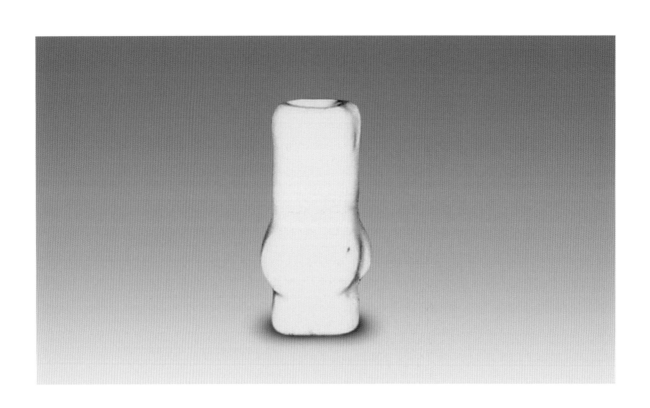

小瓷药瓶

清

瓷质

口径 1 厘米，底径 1.3 厘米，高 3.2 厘米，重 8 克
柱状，直口，小扁腹，平底，素面。盛药器具。
完整无损。2001 年 9 月入藏，陕西省西安市古
玩市场征集。

陕西医史博物馆藏

Small Porcelain Medicine Bottle

Qing Dynasty

Porcelain

Mouth Diameter 1 cm/ Bottom Diameter 1.3 cm/ Height
3.2 cm/ Weight 8 g

The bottle, with no decoration, has a straight mouth, a
tubular body, an oblate belly, and a flat bottom. This well-
preserved medical utensil was collected from the Antique
Market in Xi'an, Shaanxi Province, in September 2001.

Preserved in Shaanxi Museum of Medical History

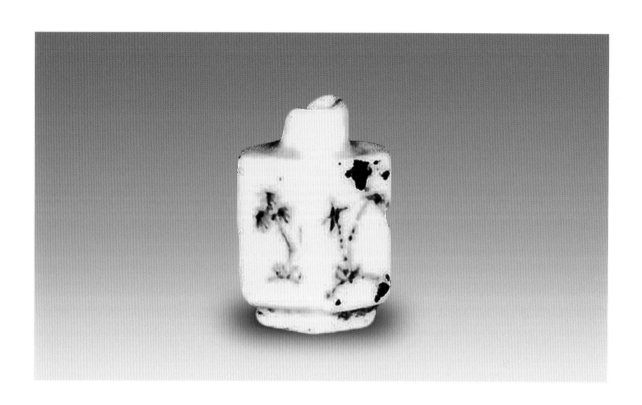

药瓶

清

瓷质

口径 1 厘米，底径 1.9 厘米，高 3.5 厘米，重 12 克

直口，平肩，菱形腹，菱形平底，腹四面各绘有不同花卉。医药器具。口沿残。2002 年入藏，陕西省咸阳市古玩市场征集。

陕西医史博物馆藏

Medicine Bottle

Qing Dynasty

Porcelain

Mouth Diameter 1 cm/ Bottom Diameter 1.9 cm/ Height 3.5 cm/ Weight 12 g

The bottle has a straight mouth, a flat shoulder, a prismatic belly and bottom. The four sides of the belly are decorated with designs of various floral patterns. This medical utensil has a damaged mouth rim. It was collected from the Antique Market in Xianyang, Shaanxi Province, in 2002.

Preserved in Shaanxi Museum of Medical History

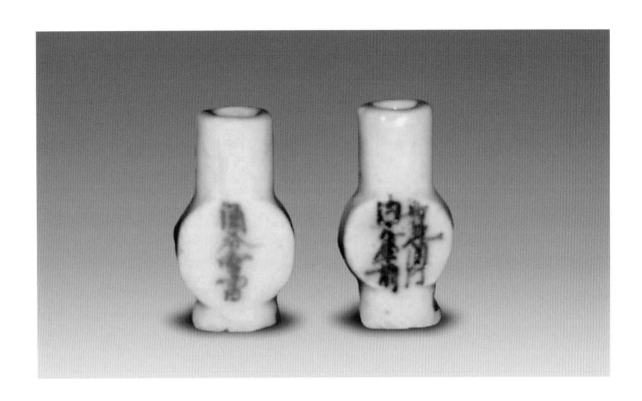

小瓷药瓶

清

瓷质

口径 1.2 厘米，底径 1.5 厘米，高 3.9 厘米，重 13 克

Small Porcelain Medicine Bottle

Qing Dynasty

Porcelain

Mouth Diameter 1.2 cm/ Bottom Diameter 1.5 cm/ Height 3.9 cm/ Weight 13 g

直口，扁腹，平底，腹部有"姑苏阊门内天库前"，另一面为"诵芬堂雷"字样。盛药器具。完整无损。2001 年 9 月入藏，陕西省西安市古玩市场征集。

陕西医史博物馆藏

The bottle has a straight mouth, an oblate belly, and a flat bottom. On one side of its belly is inscribed the address of the pharmacy, "Gu Su Lü Men Nei Tian Ku Qian", with the name of the pharmacy "Song Fen Tang Lei" on the other. This well-preserved medical utensil was collected from the Antique Market in Xi'an, Shaanxi Province, in September 2001.

Preserved in Shaanxi Museum of Medical History

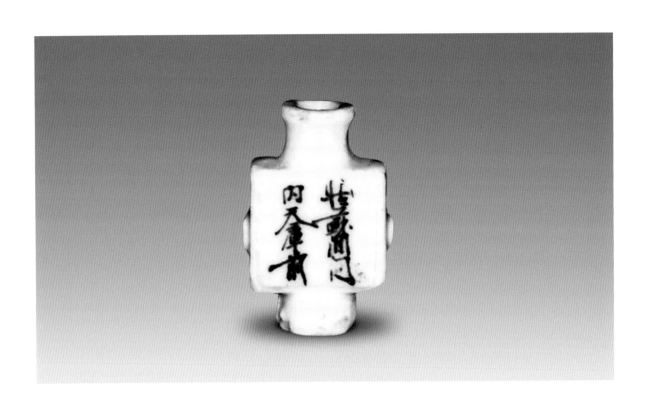

小瓷药瓶

清

瓷质

口径 1.4 厘米，底径 1.6 厘米 ×1.3 厘米，高 4.6 厘米，重 20 克

Small Porcelain Medicine Bottle

Qing Dynasty

Porcelain

Mouth Diameter 1.4 cm/ Bottom Diameter 1.6 cm ×1.3 cm/ Height 4.6 cm/ Weight 20 g

平口沿，短颈，平肩，扁方形腹，平底，高
圈足。腹部一面有"诵芬堂雷"，另一面有"姑
苏阊门内天库前"字样，腹两侧有一对凸耳。
盛药器具。完整无损 。2002 年入藏，陕西
省咸阳市征集。

陕西医史博物馆藏

The bottle has a flat mouth rim, a short neck, a flat
shoulder, an oblate square belly, a flat bottom, and
a ring foot. On one side of its belly is inscribed the
address of the pharmacy, "Gu Su Lü Men Nei Tian
Ku Qian", with the name of the pharmacy "Song Fen
Tang Lei" on the other. A pair of projecting lugs is
attached to the other two sides. This well-preserved
medical utensil was collected from Xianyang City,
Shaanxi Province, in 2002.

Preserved in Shaanxi Museum of Medical History

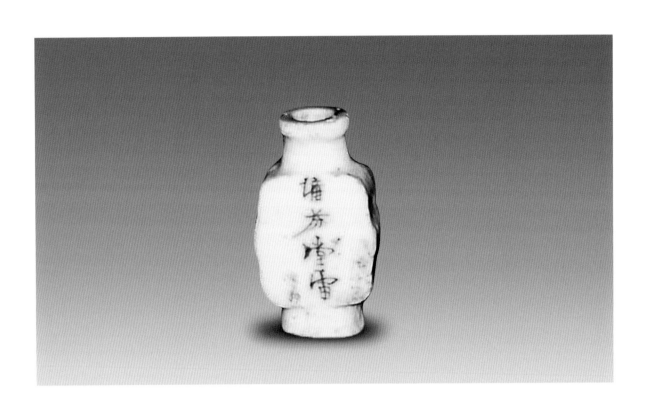

瓷药瓶

清

瓷质

口径 1.5 厘米，底径 1.9 厘米，高 5 厘米，重 27 克

Porcelain Medicine Bottle

Qing Dynasty

Porcelain

Mouth Diameter 1.5 cm/ Bottom Diameter 1.9 cm/ Height 5 cm/ Weight 27 g

平口沿，束颈，折肩，扁方形腹，平底，腹一面有"姑苏阊门内天库前"，另一面有"诵芬堂雷"字样。盛药器具。完整无损。2001 年 9 月入藏，陕西省西安市古玩市场征集。

　　　　　　　　　　　　陕西医史博物馆藏

The bottle has a flat mouth rim, a contracted neck, an angular shoulder, an oblate square belly, and a flat bottom. On one side of its belly is inscribed the address of the pharmacy, "Gu Su Lü Men Nei Tian Ku Qian", with the name of the pharmacy "Song Fen Tang Lei" on the other. This well-preserved medical utensil was collected from the Antique Market in Xi'an, Shaanxi Province, in September 2001.

Preserved in Shaanxi Museum of Medical History

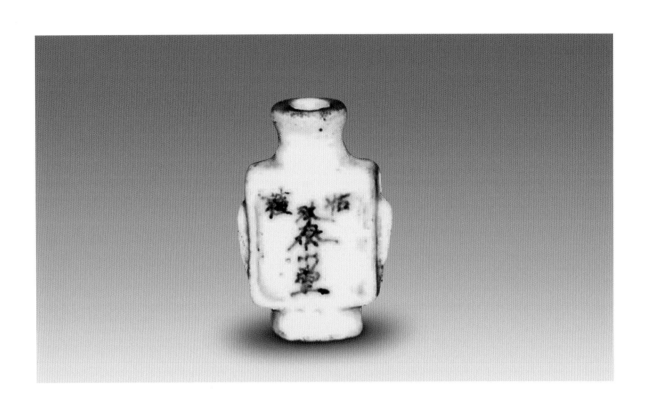

方瓷药瓶

清

瓷质

口径 1.3 厘米，底径 1.7 厘米，高 4.2 厘米，重 17 克

Square Porcelain Medicine Bottle

Qing Dynasty

Porcelain

Mouth Diameter 1.3 cm/ Bottom Diameter 1.7 cm/ Height 4.2 cm/ Weight 17 g

平口沿，平肩，扁方形腹，平底，腹两侧有
一对凸耳，腹有"阊门外渡，僧桥南□"，
另一面为"姑苏沐泰山堂"字样。药具。
完整无损。2001 年 9 月入藏，陕西省西安
市古玩市场征集。

陕西医史博物馆藏

The bottle has a flat mouth rim, a flat shoulder, an
oblate square belly, a flat bottom and two projecting
lugs attached to the two sides of the belly. One
side of its belly is inscribed with the address of the
pharmacy "Lü Men Wai Du, Seng Qiao Nan □ "
with the name of the pharmacy "Gu Su Mu Tai Shan
Tang" on the other. This well-preserved medical
utensil was collected from the Antique Market in
Xi'an, Shaanxi Province, in September 2001.

Preserved in Shaanxi Museum of Medical History

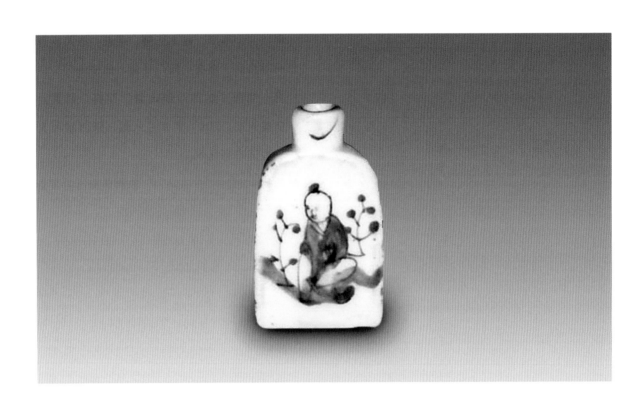

人物青花瓷药瓶

清

瓷质

口径 1.3 厘米，底径 3.4 厘米 ×1.3 厘米，高 5.6 厘米，重 35 克

Blue-and-white Porcelain Medicine Bottle with Figure Design

Qing Dynasty

Porcelain

Mouth Diameter 1.3 cm/ Bottom Diameter 3.4 cm ×1.3 cm / Height 5.6 cm/ Weight 35 g

直口，圆肩，扁方形腹，平底，腹一面有人物图案。完整无损。药具。2001 年 9 月入藏，陕西省西安市古玩市场征集。

陕西医史博物馆藏

The bottle has a straight mouth, a rounded shoulder, an oblate belly, and a flat bottom. On one side of its belly is painted a figure. This well-preserved medical utensil was collected from the Antique Market in Xi'an, Shaanxi Province, in September 2001.

Preserved in Shaanxi Museum of Medical History

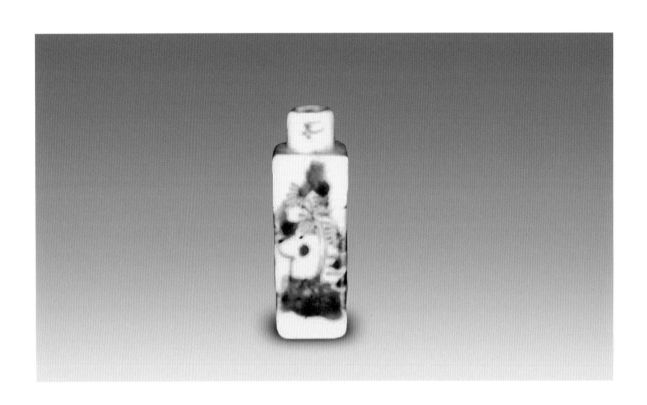

小方形瓷药瓶

清

瓷质

口径 1.1 厘米，底径 7 厘米，通高 6 厘米，重 30 克

直口，长方形腹，圈足，腹饰兰花图。贮药器具。完整无损。

陕西医史博物馆藏

Small Square Porcelain Medicine Bottle

Qing Dynasty

Porcelain

Mouth Diameter 1.1 cm/ Bottom Diameter 7 cm/ Height 6 cm/ Weight 30 g

The bottle has a straight mouth, a rectangular belly decorated with orchid patterns, and a ring foot. This medicine container remains intact.

Preserved in Shaanxi Museum of Medical History

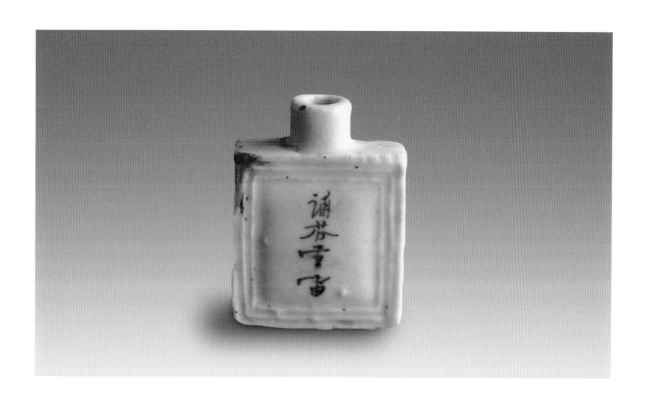

药瓶

清

瓷质

口径 5 厘米，高 6.5 厘米，厚 2 厘米

圆井形口，器身为方形，腹部有铭文 "诵芬堂雷"，应为药铺名称。由民间征集。

成都中医药大学中医药传统文化博物馆藏

Medicine Bottle

Qing Dynasty

Porcelain

Mouth Diameter 5 cm/ Height 6.5 cm/ Thickness 2 cm

The bottle has a square body and a well-shaped mouth. Its belly is inscribed with the name of the pharmacy "Song Fen Tang Lei". It was collected from a private owner. Preserved in Museum of Traditional Chinese Medicine Culture, Chengdu University of Traditional Chinese Medicine

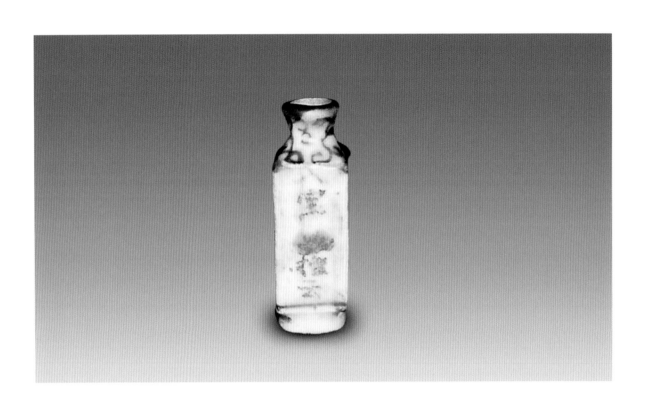

方瓷药瓶

清

瓷质

口径 1.9 厘米，底径 1.6 厘米，高 5.7 厘米，重 25 克

Square Porcelain Medicine Bottle

Qing Dynasty

Porcelain

Mouth Diameter 1.9 cm/ Bottom Diameter 1.6 cm/ Height 5.7 cm/ Weight 25 g

唇口，束颈，平肩，方腹，浅圈足，腹四面
有彩绘，颈肩处有蓝花纹。药具。底略残。
2002 年入藏，陕西省咸阳市古玩市场征集。

陕西医史博物馆藏

The bottle has a round mouth rim, a contracted
neck, a flat shoulder, a square belly, and a shallow
ring foot. The four sides of the belly are decorated
with colored painting, while its neck and shoulder
with blue decorative patterns. This medical utensil,
slightly damaged, was collected from the Antique
Market in Xianyang, Shaanxi Province, in 2002.

Preserved in Shaanxi Museum of Medical History

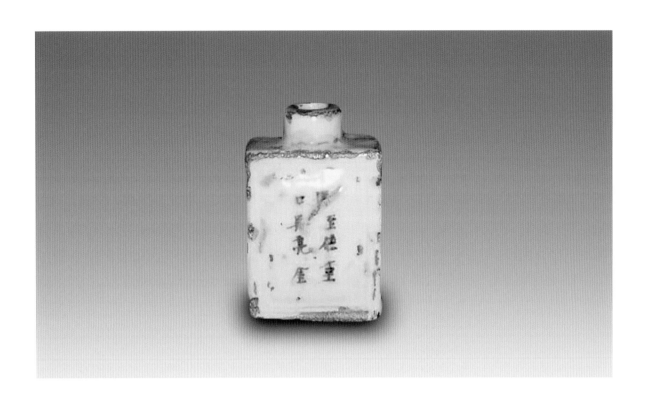

方形瓷药瓶

清

瓷质

口径 1.7 厘米，底径 3.8 厘米，高 6 厘米，重 50 克

Square Porcelain Medicine Bottle

Qing Dynasty

Porcelain

Mouth Diameter 1.7 cm/ Bottom Diameter 3.8 cm/ Height 6 cm/ Weight 50 g

直口，方平腹，平底，腹一面有"汉口至德堂吴亮金"字样。医药器具。完整无损。陕西省西安市古玩市场征集。

陕西医史博物馆藏

The bottle has a straight mouth, a flat square body, and a flat bottom. One side of its belly is inscribed with the name of the pharmacy together with the name of the doctor, "Han Kou Zhi De Tang Wu Liang Jin". This well-preserved medical utensil was collected from the Antique Market in Xi'an, Shaanxi Province.

Preserved in Shaanxi Museum of Medical History

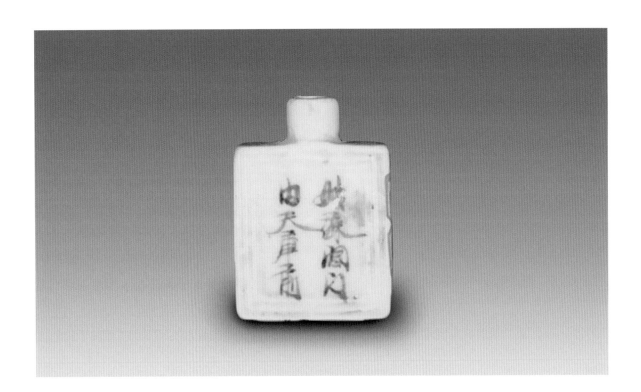

小瓷药瓶

清

瓷质

口径 1.5 厘米，底径 5 厘米，通高 5.2 厘米，重 50 克

Small Porcelain Medicine Bottle

Qing Dynasty

Porcelain

Mouth Diameter 1.5 cm/ Bottom Diameter 5 cm/ Height 5.2 cm/ Weight 50 g

直口，方平腹，平底，腹上有"雨谷堂雷""姑
苏阊门内天库前"字样。贮药器具。完整无损。
江苏省苏州市雷允上中药店专用贮药瓶。

陕西医史博物馆藏

The bottle has a straight mouth, a flat square
body, and a flat bottom. One side of its belly is
inscribed with the address of the pharmacy, "Gu Su
Lü Men Nei Tian Ku Qian" with the name of the
pharmacy "Yu Gu Tang Lei" on the other. This well-
preserved medicine container was exclusively used
in Leiyunshang Chinese Medicinal Herb Store in
Suzhou, Jiangsu Province.

Preserved in Shaanxi Museum of Medical History

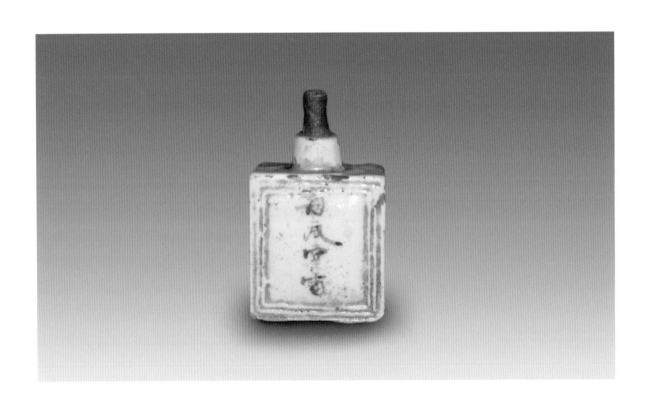

方形瓷药瓶

清

瓷质

口径 1.9 厘米，底径 5.6 厘米 ×2.3 厘米，高 7.5 厘米，重 100 克

Square Porcelain Medicine Bottle

Qing Dynasty

Porcelain

Mouth Diameter 1.9 cm/ Bottom Diameter 5.6 cm×2.3 cm/ Height 7.5 cm/ Weight 100 g

直口，平肩，方平腹，平底，腹一面有"诵
芬堂雷"字样，一面有红色药签。医药器具。
保存完整。陕西省西安市古玩市场征集。

　　　　　　　　　陕西医史博物馆藏

The bottle has a straight mouth, a flat shoulder, a flat
square belly, and a flat bottom. One side of its belly
is inscribed with the name of the pharmacy "Song
Fen Tang Lei" with a red medicine label on the other.
This well-preserved medical utensil was collected
from the Antique Market in Xi'an, Shaanxi Province.
Preserved in Shaanxi Museum of Medical History

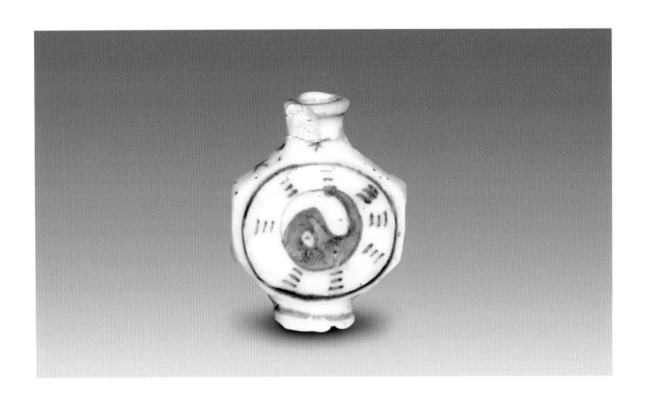

八卦瓷药瓶

清

瓷质

口径 1.4 厘米，底径 1.4 厘米 ×1.7 厘米，高 5 厘米，重 22 克

Porcelain Medicine Bottle with Design of Eight Diagrams

Qing Dynasty

Porcelain

Mouth Diameter 1.4 cm/ Bottom Diameter 1.4 cm ×1.7 cm/ Height 5 cm/ Weight 22 g

平口沿，短颈，溜肩，扁腹，圈足，肩及两

侧有不规则符号，两腹为太极图案。药具。

口残。2001 年 9 月入藏，陕西省西安市古玩

市场征集。

陕西医史博物馆藏

The bottle has a flat mouth rim, a short neck, a

sloping shoulder, an oblate belly, and a ring foot. The

shoulder and the two sides are decorated with irregular

symbols, and the front and back sides of the belly

with diagram of the Supreme Ultimate. This medical

utensil is slightly damaged on the mouth. It was

collected from the Antique Market in Xi'an, Shaanxi

Province, in September 2001.

Preserved in Shaanxi Museum of Medical History

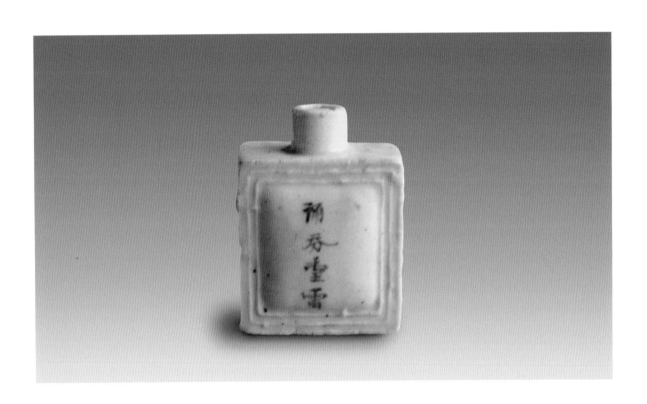

药瓶

清

瓷质

口径 3 厘米，高 8 厘米

Medicine Bottle

Qing Dynasty

Porcelain

Mouth Diameter 3 cm/ Height 8 cm

圆井形口，器身为方形，平底，腹部有铭文"诵芬堂雷"，应为药铺名称。由民间征集。

成都中医药大学中医药传统文化博物馆藏

The bottle has a well-shaped mouth, a square body, and a flat bottom. Its belly is inscribed with the name of the pharmacy "Song Fen Tang Lei". It was collected from a private owner.

Preserved in Museum of Traditional Chinese Medicine Culture, Chengdu University of Traditional Chinese Medicine

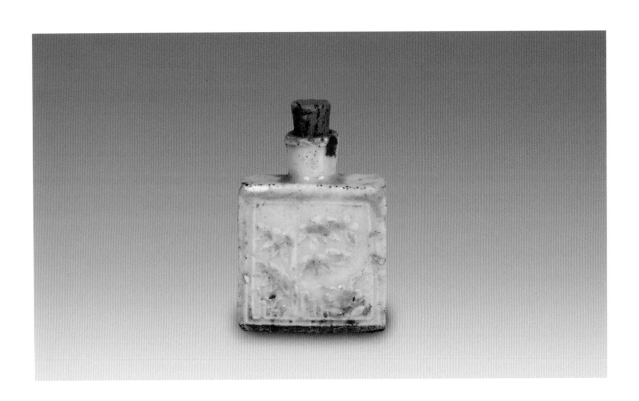

瓷药瓶

清

瓷质

口外径 1.8 厘米，口内径 1.05 厘米，宽 4.95 厘米，高 6.5 厘米，厚 2.2 厘米

Porcelain Medicine Bottle

Qing Dynasty

Porcelain

Mouth Outer Diameter 1.8 cm/ Mouth Inner Diameter 1.05 cm/ Width 4.95 cm/ Height 6.5 cm/ Thickness 2.2 cm

扁瓶状，直口，平底，底无釉、无款，通身施灰白釉，釉下浮雕植物图案。盛药器具。保存基本完好。1955 年入藏。

中华医学会 / 上海中医药大学医史博物馆藏

The oblate bottle has a straight mouth and an unglazed flat bottom with no inscription. This bottle is covered with grayish-white glaze, under which are incised relief floral motifs. This well-preserved medicine container was collected in 1955.

Preserved in Chinese Medical Association/ Museum of Chinese Medicine, Shanghai University of Traditional Chinese Medicine

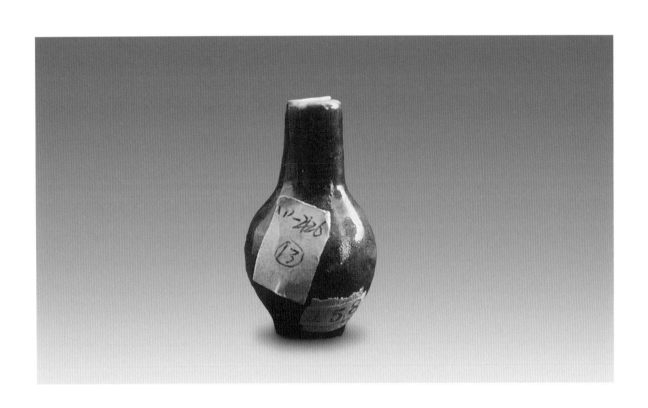

小药瓶

清

瓷质

口外径 1 厘米，腹径 2.55 厘米，底径 1.7 厘米，
通高 4.35 厘米，重 16 克

平口，长颈，溜肩，鼓腹，圈足，平底，外施雾
蓝釉。用于装药。

广东中医药博物馆藏

Small Medicine Bottle

Qing Dynasty

Porcelain

Mouth Outer Diameter 1 cm/ Belly Diameter 2.55 cm/
Bottom Diameter 1.7 cm/ Height 4.35 cm/ Weight 16 g

This bottle has a flat mouth, a long neck, a sloping
shoulder, a drum-like belly, a ring foot, and a flat bottom.
It is coated with blue glaze. The bottle served as a
medicine container.

Preserved in Guangdong Chinese Medicine Museum

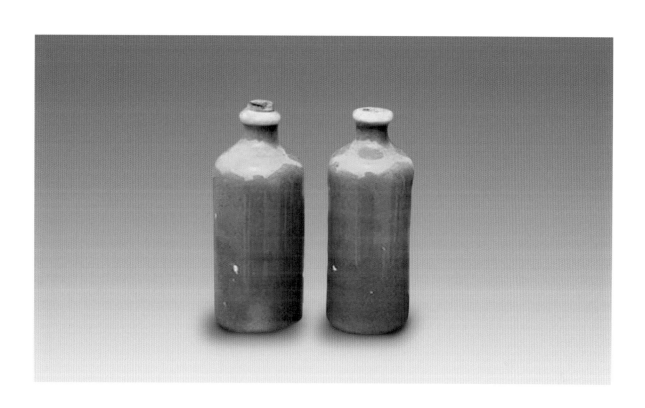

霁蓝圆形小药瓶

清

瓷质

口外径 1.57 厘米，底径 3.23 厘米，通高
7.68 厘米，共重 110 克

两件。圆柱形，平口，短颈，平底。用于装药。

广东中医药博物馆藏

Small Sacrificial-blue Round Medicine Bottles

Qing Dynasty

Porcelain

Mouth Outer Diameter 1.57 cm/ Bottom Diameter 3.23 cm/
Height 7.68 cm/ Gross Weight 110 g

These two bottles are cylindrical in shape with flat
mouths, short necks, and flat bottoms. They were used for
storing medicine.

Preserved in Guangdong Chinese Medicine Museum

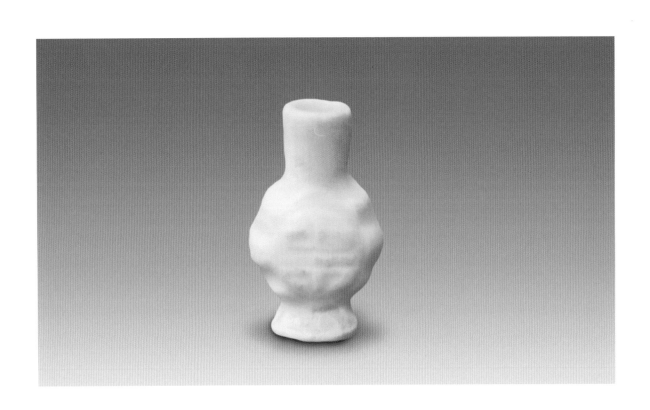

小药瓶

清

瓷质

口外径 1.3 厘米，腹径 2.5 厘米，底径 1.6 厘米，
通高 4.1 厘米，重 11 克

平口，长颈，溜肩，鼓腹，平底，圈足外撇，扁
药瓶。用于装药。

广东中医药博物馆藏

Small Medicine Bottle

Qing Dynasty

Porcelain

Mouth Outer Diameter 1.3 cm/ Belly Diameter 2.5 cm/
Bottom Diameter 1.6 cm/ Height 4.1 cm/ Weight 11 g

This bottle has a flat mouth, a long neck, a sloping
shoulder, a drum-like belly, a flat bottom, a flared ring
foot.It is oblate and served as a medicine container.

Preserved in Guangdong Chinese Medicine Museum

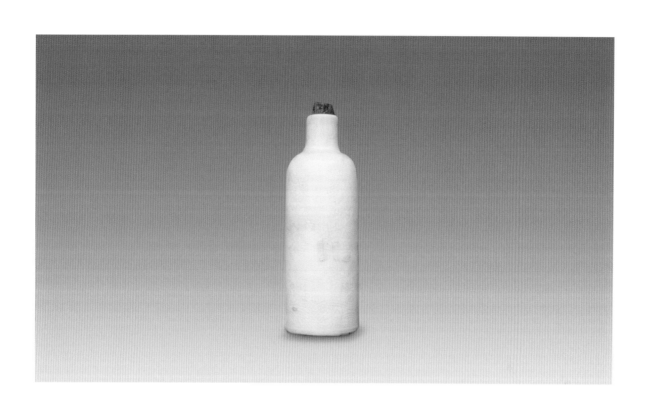

小药瓶

清

瓷质

口外径 1.05 厘米，腹径 2.4 厘米，通高 6.5 厘米，
重 27 克

直口，紧颈，溜肩，直腹，平底，圈足，配木质
盖，上绘龙纹图案。用于装药。

广东中医药博物馆藏

Small Medicine Bottle

Qing Dynasty

Porcelain

Mouth Outer Diameter 1.05 cm/ Belly Diameter 2.4 cm/
Height 6.5 cm/ Weight 27 g

This bottle has a straight mouth,with a wooden lid, a
straight neck, a sloping shoulder, a straight belly, a flat
bottom, and a ring foot. Dragon patterns are on its body.
It served as a medicine container.

Preserved in Guangdong Chinese Medicine Museum

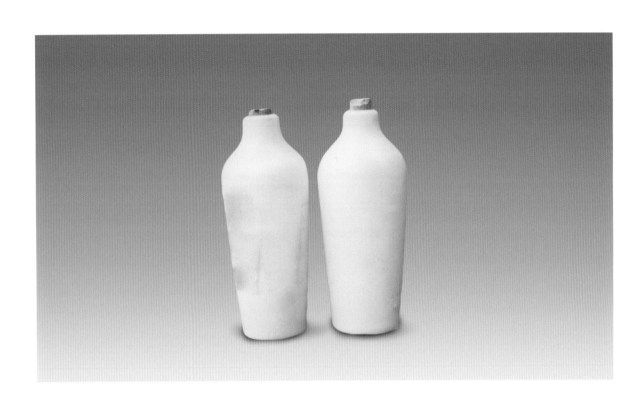

小药瓶

清

瓷质

左：口外径 1.15 厘米，腹径 2.7 厘米，底径 2 厘米，通高 6.8 厘米，重 30 克

右：口外径 1.1 厘米，腹径 2.7 厘米，底径 2.1 厘米，通高 6.7 厘米，重 31 克

Small Medicine Bottles

Qing Dynasty

Porcelain

Left: Mouth Outer Diameter 1.15 cm/ Belly Diameter 2.7 cm/ Bottom Diameter 2 cm/ Height 6.8 cm/ Weight 30 g

Right: Mouth Outer Diameter 1.1 cm/ Belly Diameter 2.7 cm/ Bottom Diameter 2.1 cm/ Height 6.7 cm/ Weight 31 g

直口，短颈，溜肩，直腹，平底，圈足，配
木质盖，施白釉。用于装药。

广东中医药博物馆藏

Each has a straight mouth, with a wooden lid, a
short neck, a sloping shoulder, a straight belly, a flat
bottom, and a ring foot. They are glazed in white and
served as medicine containers.

Preserved in Guangdong Chinese Medicine Museum

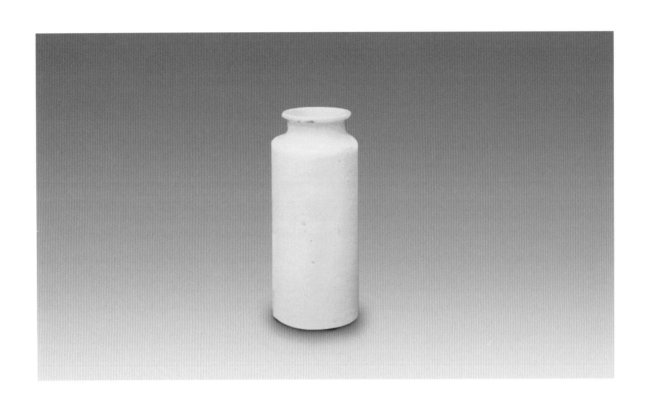

甜白釉圆柱形药瓶

清

瓷质

口外径 4.34 厘米，腹径 5.84 厘米，底径 5.84 厘米，
通高 13.2 厘米，瓶深 12.4 厘米，重 182.5 克

圆柱形，敞口外撇，束颈，直腹，平底，圈足，
上施甜白釉。用于装药。

广东中医药博物馆藏

Lovely-white-glazed Cylindrical Medicine Bottle

Qing Dynasty

Porcelain

Mouth Outer Diameter 4.34 cm/ Belly Diameter 5.84 cm/
Bottom Diameter 5.84 cm/ Height 13.2 cm/ Depth 12.4 cm/
Weight 182.5 g

This cylindrical bottle has a flared mouth, a contracted
neck, a straight belly, a flat bottom, and a ring foot. It is
glazed in white. It served as a medicine container.

Preserved in Guangdong Chinese Medicine Museum

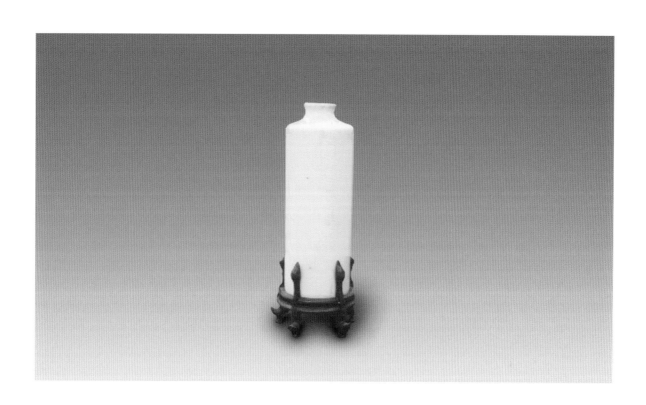

甜白暗花药瓶（带底座）

清

瓷质

口外径1.2厘米，底径3.55厘米，通高
9.29厘米，瓶深9.2厘米，重72克

圆柱形，口微敞，束颈，平底。用于装药。

广东中医药博物馆藏

Lovely-white-glazed Medicine Bottle Incised with Veiled Design (with Base)

Qing Dynasty

Porcelain

Mouth Outer Diameter 1.2 cm/ Bottom Diameter 3.55 cm/
Height 9.29 cm/ Depth 9.2 cm/ Weight 72 g

The cylindrical bottle has a slightly flared mouth, a
contracted neck, and a flat bottom. It was used as a
medicine container.

Preserved in Guangdong Chinese Medicine Museum

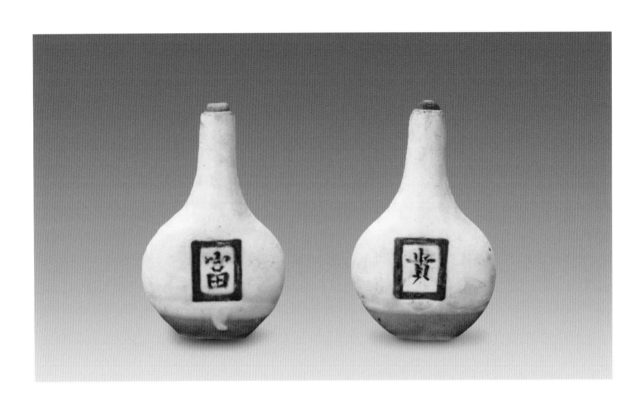

仿宋长颈小药瓶

清

瓷质

口外径 2.3 厘米，通高 11.2 厘米，瓶颈长 4.75 厘米，腹身长 7.35 厘米，腹身宽 3.3 厘米，腹身高 6.5 厘米，重 115 克

Imitative Song-dynasty-style Medicine Bottle with Long Neck

Qing Dynasty

Porcelain

Mouth Outer Diameter 2.3 cm/ Height 11.2 cm/ Bottleneck Length 4.75 cm/ Body Length 7.35 cm/ Body Width 3.3 cm/ Body Height 6.5 cm/ Weight 115 g

扁圆形，平口，细长颈，鼓腹，圈足，上书 "富贵" 二字。用于装药。

广东中医药博物馆藏

The oblate bottle has a flat mouth, a thin and long neck, a drum-like belly, and a ring foot. On its belly are written two Chinese characters "Fu" (wealth) and "Gui"(honour). The bottle was used as a medicine container.

Preserved in Guangdong Chinese Medicine Museum

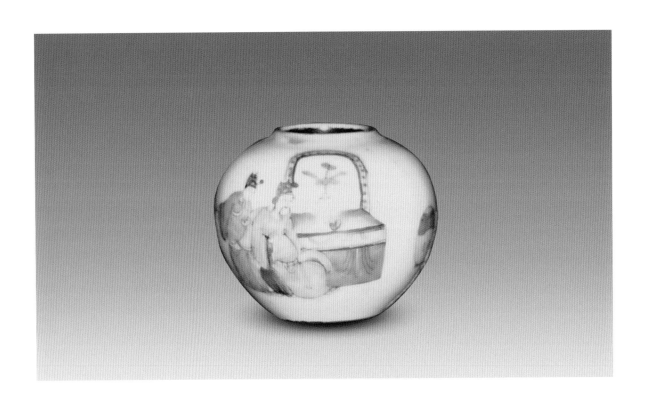

小药罐

清

瓷质

重 27 克

圆口，圆肩，鼓腹，圈足，腹饰白底粉彩人物图案。贮药器具。完整无损。

陕西医史博物馆藏

Small Medicine Pot

Qing Dynasty

Porcelain

Weight 27 g

The pot has a rounded mouth, a rounded shoulder, a drum-like belly, and a ring foot. Its belly is decorated with a figure design in famille rose on a white ground. This medical container remains intact.

Preserved in Shaanxi Museum of Medical History

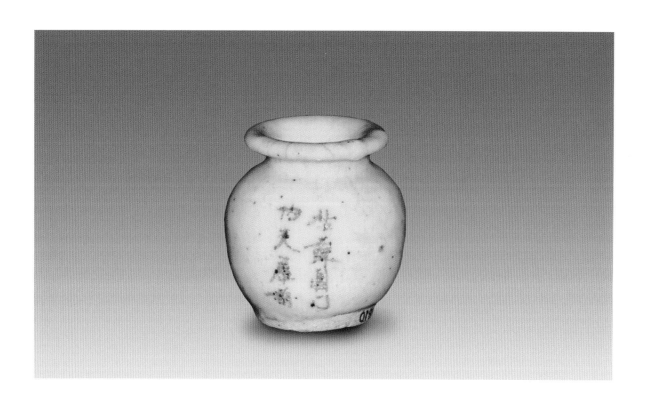

瓷药瓶

清

瓷质

口径 4.1 厘米，底径 3.5 厘米，通高 5.5 厘米，
重 50 克

小口，圆唇，圆腹，圈足，腹有"内夫犀前""姑
苏国门"字样。医药器具。口沿有裂印。

陕西医史博物馆藏

Porcelain Medicine Bottle

Qing Dynasty

Porcelain

Mouth Diameter 4.1 cm/ Bottom Diameter 3.5 cm/
Height 5.5 cm/ Weight 50 g

The bottle has a small mouth with rounded lip, a rounded
belly, and a ring foot. Its belly is inscribed with the
address of the pharmacy. This medical utensil has a crack
on the mouth rim.

Preserved in Shaanxi Museum of Medical History

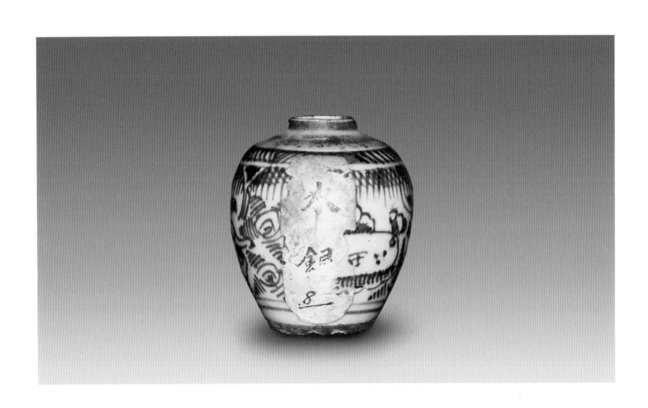

"水银"药瓶

清

瓷质

小直口，圆肩，鼓腹，圈足，腹部有兰花回纹饰，并贴一"水银"标签。贮药器具。完整无损。陕西省周至县广育堂遗物征集。

陕西医史博物馆藏

Medicine Bottle

Qing Dynasty

Porcelain

The bottle has a little straight mouth, a rounded shoulder, a drum-like belly, and a ring foot. Its belly is decorated with orchid fret patterns, with a label of "Shui Yin" attached to it. This medical utensil remains intact. It was collected from the relic of Guang Yu Tang in Zhouzhi County, Shaanxi Province.

Preserved in Shaanxi Museum of Medical History

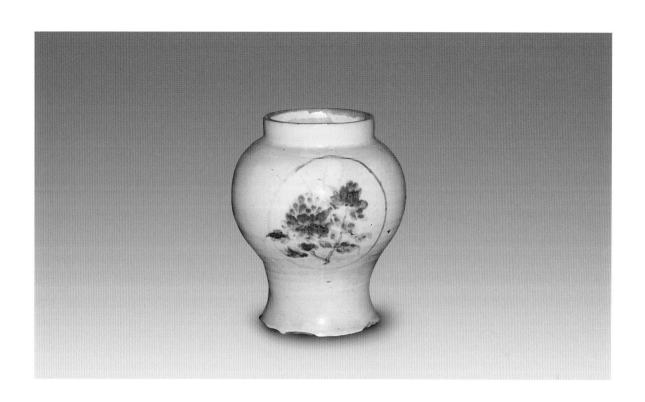

白瓷带盖药瓶

清

瓷质

口径 10 厘米，底径 11 厘米，通高 19 厘米，重 1500 克

子母口，直颈，鼓腹，圈足，腹饰月季花图，药标签为"六一散"。贮药器具。底有残。陕西省铜川市黄堡镇征集。

陕西医史博物馆藏

White Porcelain Medicine Bottle with Lid

Qing Dynasty

Porcelain

Mouth Diameter 10 cm/ Bottom Diameter 11 cm/ Height 19 cm/ Weight 1,500 g

The bottle has a snap lid, a straight neck, a drum-like belly, and a ring foot. On its belly is painted a China rose pattern with a label of the medicine "Liu Yi San" attached to it. This medicine container, with its bottom damaged, was collected from Huangbao Town of Tongchuan City, Shaanxi Province.

Preserved in Shaanxi Museum of Medical History

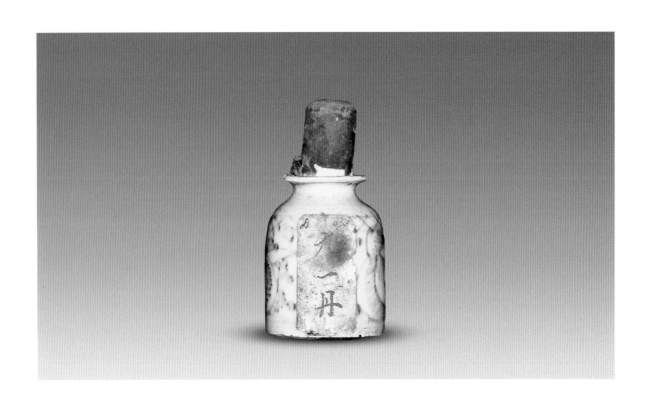

药瓶

清

瓷质

小喇叭口，短颈，直腹，平底，腹饰青花，上贴"九一丹"标签，带一木质瓶塞。贮药用具。口有残。

陕西医史博物馆藏

Medicine Bottle

Qing Dynasty

Porcelain

The blue-and-white bottle has a slightly flared mouth with a wooden cork, a short neck, a straight belly, and a flat bottom. To its belly is attached a label of the drug name "Jiu Yi Dan". This medicine container has a damaged mouth.

Preserved in Shaanxi Museum of Medical History

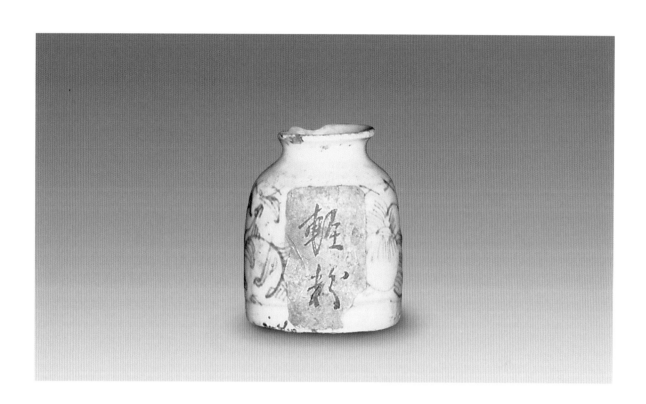

药瓶

清

瓷质

小喇叭口，短颈，斜腹，平底，腹部有青花纹饰，

上贴"轻粉"标签。贮药用具。口有残缺。

陕西医史博物馆藏

Medicine Bottle

Qing Dynasty

Porcelain

The bottle has a slightly flared mouth, a short neck, a flat

bottom and an oblique belly decorated with blue-and-

white flower patterns. A"Qing Fen"label is stuck on its

body. The mouth of this medicine container is damaged.

Preserved in Shaanxi Museum of Medical History

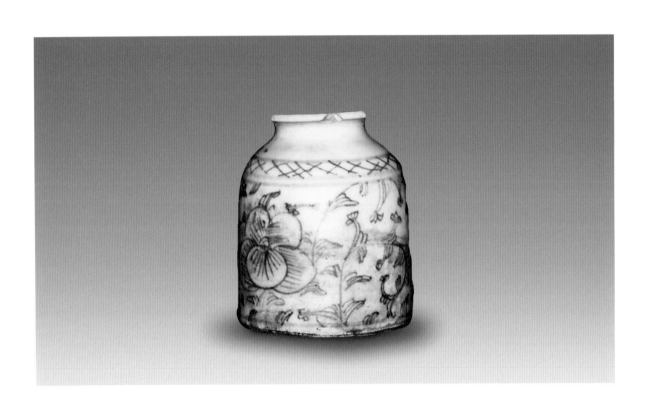

药瓶

清

瓷质

小喇叭口，短颈，圆肩，直腹，腹饰青花花草纹饰，平底。贮药用器。口有残。

陕西医史博物馆藏

Medicine Bottle

Qing Dynasty

Porcelain

The bottle has a slightly flared mouth, a short neck, a rounded shoulder, a flat bottom, and a straight belly decorated with blue-and-white floral patterns. The mouth of this medicine container is damaged.

Preserved in Shaanxi Museum of Medical History

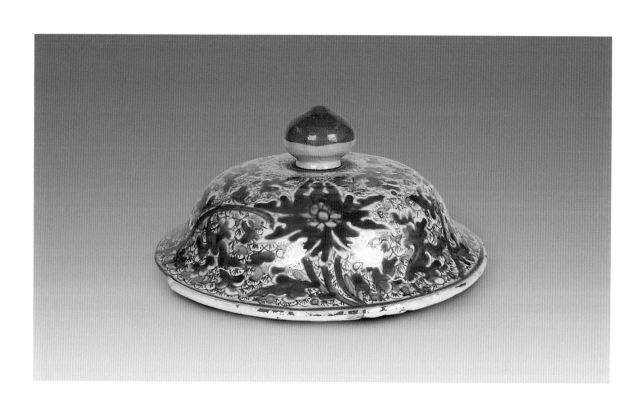

青花加彩药罐盖

清

瓷质

直径 26.5 厘米，通高 13 厘米

盖形，青花加彩瓷，原瓷盖钮破损后配以木钮。原配药缸缺失。1959 年入藏。

中华医学会 / 上海中医药大学医史博物馆藏

Blue-and-white Glazed Medicine Pot Lid with Color

Qing Dynasty

Porcelain

Diameter 26.5 cm/ Height 13 cm

The collection is a blue-and-white glazed lid with color. The wooden knob on the lid is a substitute for the original one since it was broken. The original jar was lost. It was collected in 1959.

Preserved in Chinese Medical Association/ Museum of Chinese Medicine, Shanghai University of Traditional Chinese Medicine

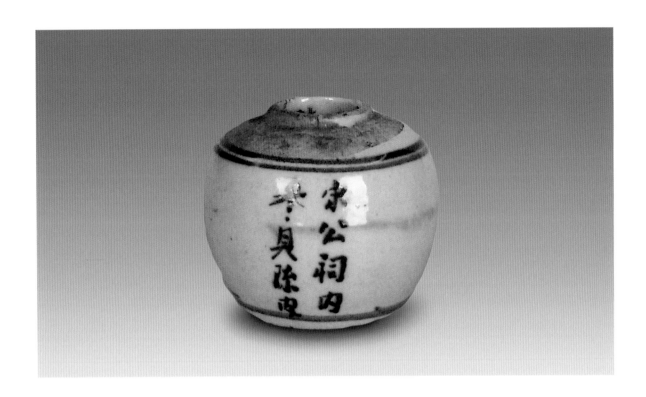

瓷药瓶

清

瓷质

口外径 2.5 厘米，口内径 1.9 厘米，腹径 5.6 厘米，通高 4.9 厘米

Porcelain Medicine Bottle

Qing Dynasty

Porcelain

Mouth Outer Diameter 2.5 cm/ Mouth Inner Diameter 1.9 cm/ Belly Diameter 5.6 mm/ Height 4.9 cm

圆形，施乳白釉，瓶颈与圈足皆无釉，瓶底无款识，瓶身有 "宋公祠内参贝陈皮" "益寿监制" 蓝字，制作工艺一般。盛药器具。保存基本完好。

中华医学会／上海中医药大学医史博物馆藏

The round bottle, covered with opalescent glaze except the neck and the ring foot, was made with common craftsmanship. On its belly are inscribed the drug ingredients "Song Gong Ci Nei Shen Bei Chen Pi""Yi Shou Jian Zhi" in blue, with no inscription on its bottom. This medicine container remains basically intact.

Preserved in Chinese Medical Association/ Museum of Chinese Medicine, Shanghai University of Traditional Chinese Medicine

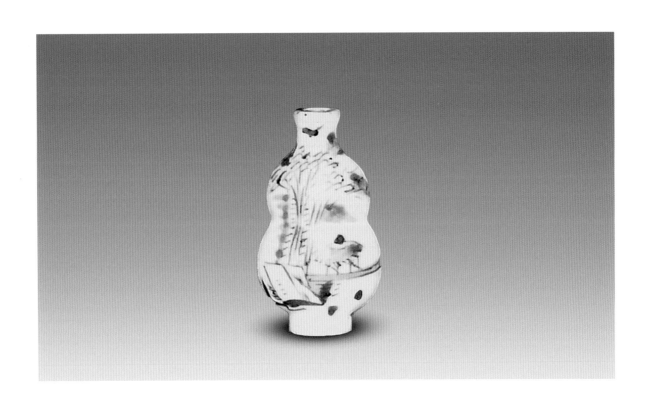

扁葫芦药瓶

清

瓷质

口径 1.2 厘米，底径 1.8 厘米，通高 6.5 厘米，
重 50 克

直口，葫芦状腹，圈足。贮药器具。完整无损。

陕西医史博物馆藏

Oblate Gourd-shaped Medicine Bottle

Qing Dynasty

Porcelain

Mouth Diameter 1.2 cm/ Bottom Diameter 1.8 cm/ Height 6.5 cm/ Weight 50 g

The bottle has a straight mouth, a gourd-shaped belly, and a ring foot. This medicine container remains intact.

Preserved in Shaanxi Museum of Medical History

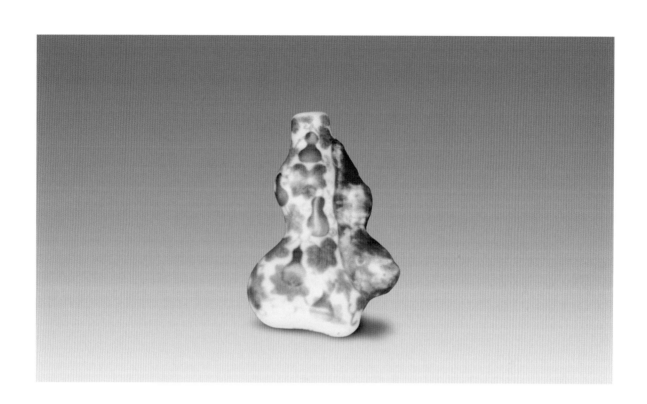

小药瓶

清

瓷质

口外径 1 厘米，腹径 4 厘米，通高 5.7 厘米，重
20 克

扁葫芦形，上绘葫芦图案。用于装药。

广东中医药博物馆藏

Small Medicine Bottle

Qing Dynasty

Porcelain

Mouth Outer Diameter 1 cm/ Belly Diameter 4 cm/
Height 5.7 cm/ Weight 20 g

The oblate gourd-shaped bottle is painted with gourd
patterns. It was used for storing medicine.

Preserved in Guangdong Chinese Medicine Museum

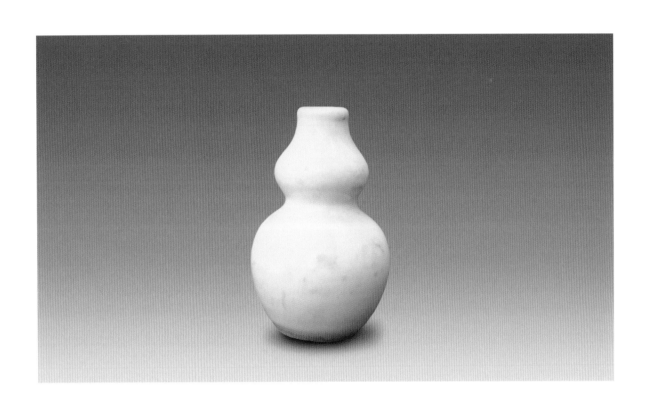

小药瓶

清

瓷质

口外径 2.2 厘米，腹径 4.65 厘米，底径 2.8 厘米，

通高 7.4 厘米，重 77 克

葫芦状，直口，短颈，束腰，鼓腹，平底，圈足。

用于装药。

广东中医药博物馆藏

Small Medicine Bottle

Qing Dynasty

Porcelain

Mouth Outer Diameter 2.2 cm/ Belly Diameter 4.65 cm/

Bottom Diameter 2.8 cm/ Height 7.4 cm/ Weight 77 g

This bottle is gourd-shaped, and has a straight mouth, a

short neck, a contracted waist, a drum-like belly, a flat

bottom, and a ring foot. It served as a medicine container.

Preserved in Guangdong Chinese Medicine Museum

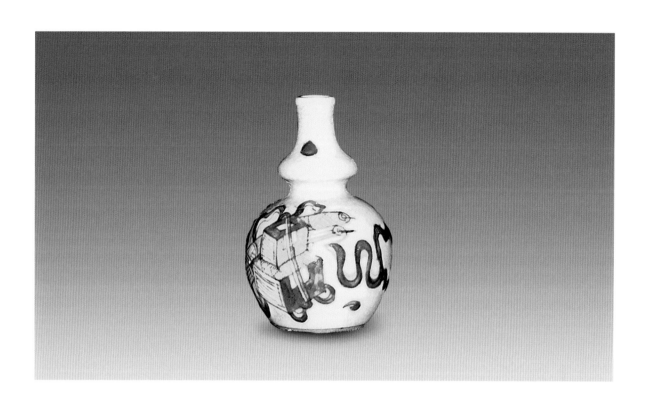

葫芦药瓶

清

瓷质

口径 1.8 厘米，底径 3.4 厘米，通高 8.2 厘米，
重 100 克

葫芦状，直口，圈足，瓶身饰蓝色图案，瓶底有
"成化年制"字样。贮药器具。完整无损。

陕西医史博物馆藏

Gourd-shaped Medicine Bottle

Qing Dynasty

Porcelain

Mouth Diameter 1.8 cm/ Bottom Diameter 3.4 cm/
Height 8.2 cm/ Weight 100 g

The bottle has a straight mouth, a gourd-shaped body,
and a ring foot. Its body is decorated with blue patterns.
Its bottom is inscribed with "Cheng Hua Nian Zhi", the
time when the medicine bottle was made. This medicine
container remains intact.

Preserved in Shaanxi Museum of Medical History

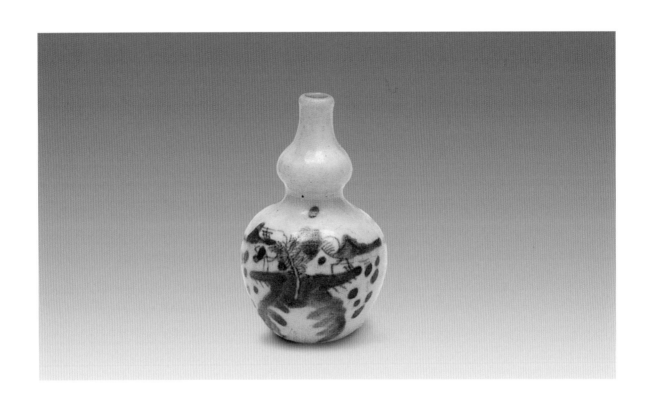

药瓶

清

瓷质

底径 4.5 厘米，高 9 厘米

葫芦状，直口，束腰，鼓腹，平底，瓶身饰青花图案。用于盛药。由民间征集。

成都中医药大学中医药传统文化博物馆藏

Medicine Bottle

Qing Dynasty

Porcelain

Bottom Diameter 4.5 cm/ Height 9 cm

This bottle is gourd-shaped, and has a straight mouth, a contracted waist, a drum-like belly, and a flat bottom.It is decorated with blue-and-white patterns. It served as a medicine container, It was collected from a private owner. Preserved in Museum of Traditional Chinese Medicine Culture, Chengdu University of Traditional Chinese Medicine

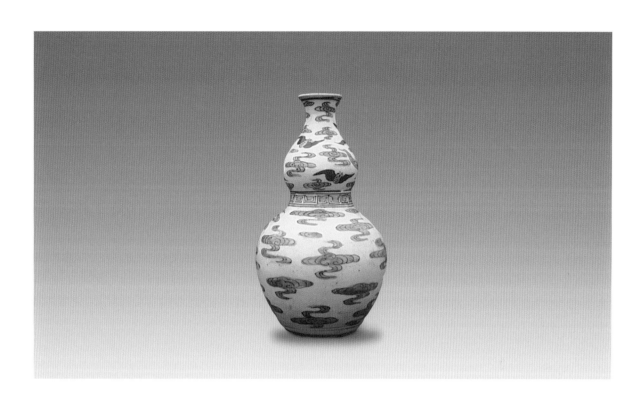

青花葫芦形大药瓶

清

瓷质

口外径4.3厘米，瓶颈径2.8厘米，腹径12.3厘米，

通高21.8厘米，重618克

葫芦形，敞口，器身绘祥云、蝙蝠，腰部绘回形

纹，平底。用于盛药。

广东中医药博物馆藏

Big Blue-and-white Glazed Gourd-shaped Medicine Bottle

Qing Dynasty

Porcelain

Mouth Outer Diameter 4.3 cm/ Bottleneck Diameter 2.8 cm/ Belly Diameter 12.3 cm/ Height 21.8 cm/ Weight 618 g

With a flared mouth and a flat bottom, this gourd-shaped bottle was used as a medicine container.On its body is painted clouds and bats, while on its waist is patterns of zigzag lines.

Preserved in Guangdong Chinese Medicine Museum

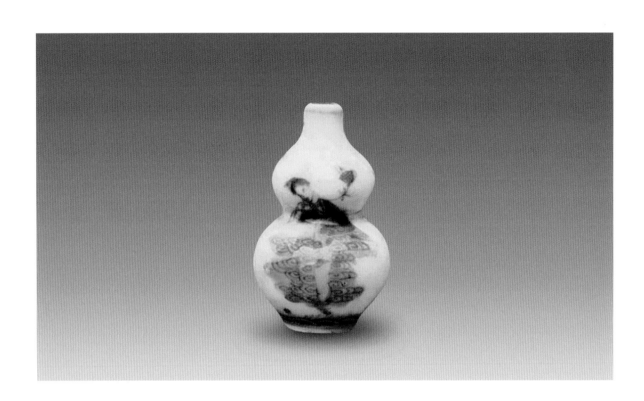

青花仕女葫芦小药瓶

清

瓷质

口外径 1.2 厘米，上葫芦直径 3.06 厘米，下葫芦直径 4.1 厘米，底径 2.3 厘米，通高 6.38 厘米，重 42 克

Small Blue-and-white Medicine Bottle

Qing Dynasty

Porcelain

Mouth Outer Diameter 1.2 cm/ Upper Diameter 3.06 cm/ Lower Diameter 4.1 cm/ Bottom Diameter 2.3 cm/ Height 6.38 cm/ Weight 42 g

葫芦形，底部有矮圈足，束腰，瓶身饰青花
人物像。用于装药。

广东中医药博物馆藏

The gourd-shaped bottle has a short ring foot and a
contracted waist with a blue-and-white portrait on the
body. It was used for storing medicine.
Preserved in Guangdong Chinese Medicine Museum

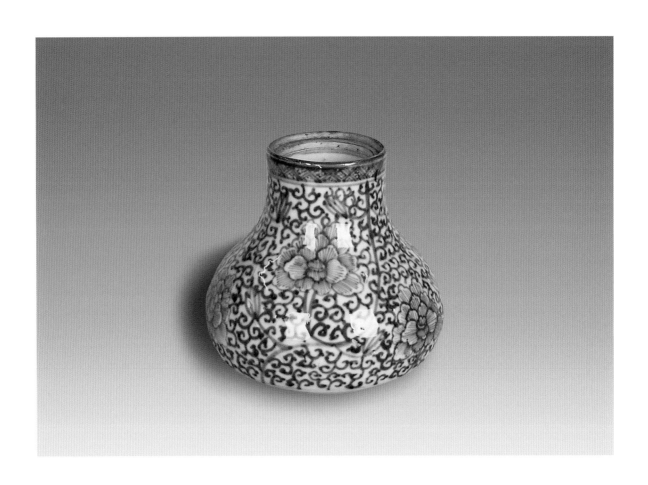

青花瓷瓶

清

瓷质

口外径 6.45 厘米，口内径 5.05 厘米，腹径 13.3 厘米，通高 12 厘米

Blue-and-white Porcelain Bottle

Qing Dynasty

Porcelain

Mouth Outer Diameter 6.45 cm/ Mouth Inner Diameter 5.05 cm/ Belly Diameter 13.3 cm/ Height 12 cm

圆瓶状，瓷胎细腻，器身绘青花团花缠枝图，

底面有旋纹无款识。煎药器具。

中华医学会／上海中医药大学医史博物馆藏

The round bottle has a delicate pottery body painted

with blue-and-white patterns of clustered flowers and

intertwining branches. There are spiral patterns but

no inscription on the bottom. The bottle was utilized

for decocting medicine.

Preserved in Chinese Medical Association/ Museum

of Chinese Medicine, Shanghai University of

Traditional Chinese Medicine

索　引
（馆藏地按拼音字母排序）

上海中医药博物馆

中华医学会 / 上海中医药大学医史博物馆

Index

Shaanxi Museum of Medical History

参考文献

[1] 李经纬.中国古代医史图录 [M].北京：人民卫生出版社，1992.

[2] 傅维康，李经纬，林昭庚.中国医学通史：文物图谱卷 [M].北京：人民卫生出版社，2000.

[3] 和中浚，吴鸿洲.中华医学文物图集 [M].成都：四川人民出版社，2001.

[4] 上海中医药博物馆.上海中医药博物馆馆藏珍品 [M].上海：上海科学技术出版社，2013.

[5] 西藏自治区博物馆.西藏博物馆 [M].北京：五洲传播出版社，2005.

[6] 崔乐泉.中国古代体育文物图录：中英文本 [M].北京：中华书局，2000.

[7] 张金明，陆雪春.中国古铜镜鉴赏图录 [M].北京：中国民族摄影艺术出版社，2002.

[8] 文物精华编辑委员会.文物精华 [M].北京：文物出版社，1964.

[9] 谭维四.湖北出土文物精华 [M].武汉：湖北教育出版社，2001.

[10] 常州市博物馆.常州文物精华 [M].北京：文物出版社，1998.

[11] 镇江博物馆.镇江文物精华 [M].合肥：黄山书社，1997.

[12] 贵州省文化厅，贵州省博物馆.贵州文物精华 [M].贵阳：贵州人民出版社，2005.

[13] 徐良玉.扬州馆藏文物精华 [M].南京：江苏古籍出版社，2001.

[14] 昭陵博物馆，陕西历史博物馆.昭陵文物精华 [M].西安：陕西人民美术出版社，1991.

[15] 南通博物苑.南通博物苑文物精华 [M].北京：文物出版社，2005.

[16] 邯郸市文物研究所.邯郸文物精华 [M].北京：文物出版社，2005.

[17] 张秀生，刘友恒，聂连顺，等.中国河北正定文物精华 [M].北京：文化艺术出版社，1998.

[18] 陕西省咸阳市文物局.咸阳文物精华 [M].北京：文物出版社，2002.

[19] 安阳市文物管理局.安阳文物精华 [M].北京：文物出版社，2004.

[20] 深圳市博物馆.深圳市博物馆文物精华 [M].北京：文物出版社，1998.

[21]《中国文物精华》编辑委员会.中国文物精华（1993）[M].北京：文物出版社，1993.

[22] 夏路，刘永生 . 山西省博物馆馆藏文物精华 [M]. 太原：山西人民出版社，1999.

[23] 文物精华编辑委员会 . 文物精华 [M]. 北京：文物出版社，1957.

[24] 山西博物院，湖北省博物馆 . 荆楚长歌：九连墩楚墓出土文物精华 [M]. 太原：山西人民出版社，2011.

[25] 刘广堂，石金鸣，宋建忠 . 晋国雄风：山西出土两周文物精华 [M]. 沈阳：万卷出版公司，2009.

[26] 沈君山，王国平，单迎红 . 滦平博物馆馆藏文物精华 [M]. 北京：中国文联出版社，2012.

[27] 张家口市博物馆 . 张家口市博物馆馆藏文物精华 [M]. 北京：科学出版社，2011.

[28] 浙江省文物考古研究所 . 浙江考古精华 [M]. 北京：文物出版社，1999.

[29] 故宫博物院 . 故宫雕刻珍萃 [M]. 北京：紫禁城出版社，2004.

[30] 故宫博物院紫禁城出版社 . 故宫博物院藏宝录 [M]. 上海：上海文艺出版社，1986.

[31] 首都博物馆 . 大元三都 [M]. 北京：科学出版社，2016.

[32] 新疆维吾尔自治区博物馆 . 新疆出土文物 [M]. 北京：文物出版社，1975.

[33] 王兴伊，段逸山 . 新疆出土涉医文书辑校 [M]. 上海：上海科学技术出版社，2016.

[34] 刘学春 . 刍议医药卫生文物的概念与分类标准 [J]. 中华中医药杂志，2016，31（11）:4406-4409.

[35] 上海古籍出版社 . 中国艺海 [M]. 上海：上海古籍出版社，1994.

[36] 紫都，岳鑫 . 一生必知的 200 件国宝 [M]. 呼和浩特：远方出版社，2005.

[37] 谭维四 . 湖北出土文物精华 [M]. 武汉：湖北教育出版社，2001.

[38] 张建青 . 青海彩陶收藏与鉴赏 [M]. 北京：中国文史出版社，2007.

[39] 银景琦 . 仡佬族文物 [M]. 南宁：广西人民出版社，2014.

[40] 廖果，梁峻，李经纬 . 东西方医学的反思与前瞻 [M]. 北京：中医古籍出版社，2002.

[41] 梁峻，张志斌，廖果，等 . 中华医药文明史集论 [M]. 北京：中医古籍出版社，2003.

[42] 郑蓉，庄乾竹，刘聪，等 . 中国医药文化遗产考论 [M]. 北京：中医古籍出版社，2005.